Advanced Nanohybrids for Biomedical Applications

This book is focused on the applications of various advanced nanohybrids in biomedical sectors to provide solutions for different pressing challenges. Through detailed discussions and case studies, it explores how these advanced nanomaterials can address critical issues and offer new perspectives with practical approaches. It provides a comprehensive exploration of the properties of advanced nanohybrids that are used for the diagnosis of inflammatory diseases, and in nano-drugs for several cancers and wound healing applications. It also addresses contemporary trends in biomedical electronics and biosensors, and the use of cutting-edge plasmonic nanomaterials in biomedicine.

Features:

- Provides comprehensive understanding of the current applications of nanohybrids in biomedical areas.
- Presents state-of-the-art technologies and research invested in nanohybrids.
- Discusses current hot topics such as semiconductor-based nanohybrids and plasmonic metal-based nanohybrids.
- Evaluates the role of nanozymes as anticancer drug agents and as novel antibiotics for antimicrobial resistant microorganisms.
- Includes case studies from across the world, especially from regions where high-level research is underway.

Advanced Nanohybrids for Biomedical Applications is an excellent reference for researchers, professionals, graduate, and senior undergraduate students in biomedical engineering, biotechnology, and biomaterials.

Advanced Nanohybrids for Biomedical Applications

Edited by Firdoz Shaik, Weiqing Zhang, and
Ranjit Pabbati

CRC Press
Taylor & Francis Group
Boca Raton London New York

CRC Press is an imprint of the
Taylor & Francis Group, an **informa** business

Designed cover image: iStock

First edition published 2026
by CRC Press
2385 NW Executive Center Drive, Suite 320, Boca Raton FL 33431

and by CRC Press
4 Park Square, Milton Park, Abingdon, Oxon, OX14 4RN

CRC Press is an imprint of Taylor & Francis Group, LLC

ISBN: 978-1-032-91526-5 (hbk)
ISBN: 978-1-032-91527-2 (pbk)
ISBN: 978-1-003-56372-3 (ebk)

DOI: 10.1201/9781003563723

Typeset in Times
by Apex CoVantage, LLC

Contents

Preface

The increased demand for advanced healthcare solutions, fueled by the enhancement in drug-resistant infections, chronic diseases, and the need for personalized medicine, has driven the investigation of innovative and effective biomedical technologies. Nanoscience, owing to its unique physicochemical characteristics and multifunctional potential, has evolved as an effective tool in the advancement of next-generation biomedical platforms. Among these innovations, **nanohybrids** – engineered nanostructures integrating multiple components at the nanoscale – have shown outstanding promise across various biomedical domains.

This volume, titled *Advanced Nanohybrids for Biomedical Applications*, is meticulously compiled to present recent advancements, current trends, and future prospects in the field of nanohybrids for healthcare and medical innovations. The book comprises ten chapters, each focused on a substantial area highlighting the role of nanohybrids in developing therapeutic, diagnostic, and regenerative biomedical technologies.

The introductory chapter provides a comprehensive overview of the evolving role of nanotechnology in reshaping biomedical science. Subsequent chapters explore into the synthesis strategies, structural tunability, and functionalization of nanohybrids, investigating their implementations in drug delivery, antimicrobial therapy, biosensing, photothermal therapy, tissue engineering, and more. Specific attention is paid to carbon-based, metallic, and magnetically responsive nanohybrids, demonstrating their abilities in overcoming traditional therapeutic limitations and enabling targeted, stimuli-responsive biomedical therapies.

Furthermore, the book explores emerging areas such as nanohybrid-based scaffolds for regenerative medicine, nanozyme-integrated platforms for smart biosensing, and the integration of artificial intelligence for designing nanohybrids with enhanced biomedical efficacy. These interdisciplinary discussions highlight the convergence of materials science, biotechnology, clinical research, and computational modeling in driving innovative nanomedical solutions.

This volume is organized to serve as an essential resource for graduate students, researchers, clinicians, and professionals working in nanomedicine, biomedical engineering, pharmaceutical sciences, and related fields. It offers an in-depth foundation and forward-looking insights into how nanohybrids can revolutionize healthcare by enabling safer, more efficient, and personalized biomedical interventions.

We hope that this book will motivate further research, promote cross-disciplinary collaborations, and expedite the development of nanohybrid-based technologies to improve human health and medical outcomes.

Firdoz Shaik
Vignan's Foundation for Science, Technology and Research, Vadlamudi, India

Weiqing Zhang
Guangxi Medical University, Nanning, Guangxi, China

Ranjit Pabbati
Jawaharlal Nehru Technological University Hyderabad, Telangana, India

About the Editors

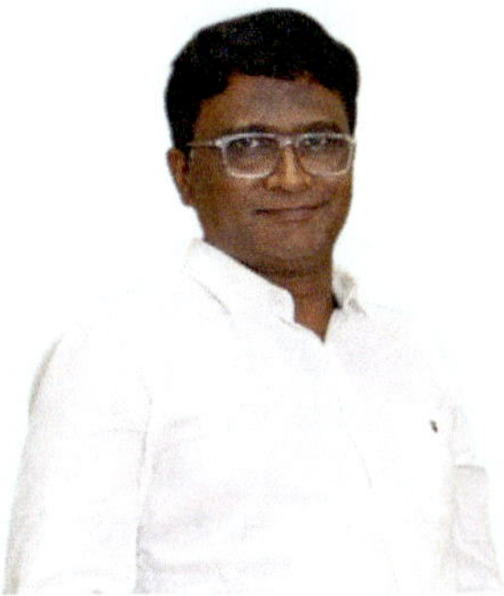

Dr. Firdoz Shaik earned his PhD in chemical and biomolecular engineering from the National University of Singapore in 2015. He completed his M.Tech in nanotechnology from the Indian Institute of Technology Roorkee in 2010, following a B.Tech in biotechnology from JNTU-Hyderabad in 2007. Over the course of more than seven years, he has held various academic and research positions – including postdoctoral fellow, academic staff (teaching), and scientist – at esteemed institutions such as the Technion–Israel Institute of Technology, Haifa, and its Guangdong Technion-Israel Institute of Technology (GTIIT) campus. Currently, he is serving as Associate Professor at the Department of Biotechnology, Vignan's Foundation for Science and Technology, India.

Dr. Firdoz possesses deep expertise in the rational design of advanced nanostructures, with a particular focus on bio-semiconductor hybrids and nanozymes tailored for environmental and biomedical applications. His interdisciplinary research, bridging materials science and biotechnology, has added significant value to this volume. He has authored and co-authored over 40 peer-reviewed publications in reputed international journals.

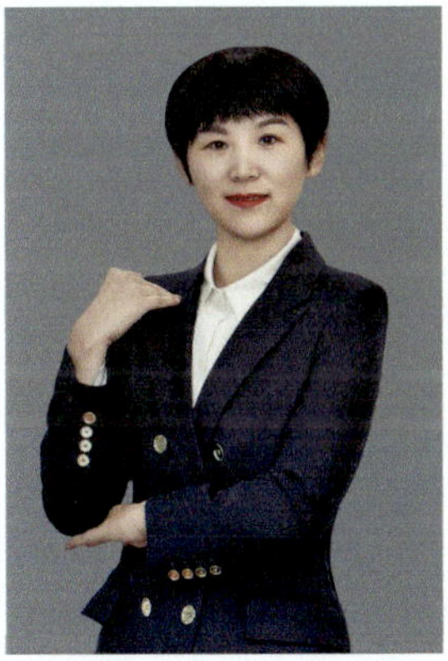

Dr. Weiqing Zhang received her PhD in chemical and biomolecular engineering from the National University of Singapore in 2014. She obtained her M.Sc in inorganic chemistry from the University of Science and Technology of China in 2008, and her B.Sc in chemistry from Hebei Normal University in 2005. She conducted postdoctoral research at both the National University of Singapore and Nanyang Technological University for four years and previously served as Associate Professor at Tianjin University of Technology. Currently, she is a professor at the Department of Experimental Research, Guangxi Medical University Cancer Hospital, China. Dr. Zhang's research focuses on the development of advanced noble metal-based nanohybrids for energy and biomedical applications, with particular emphasis on nanozyme catalysis, photothermal therapy, and tumor-targeted nanomedicine. She has authored or co-authored more than 40 peer-reviewed research articles in high-impact scientific journals.

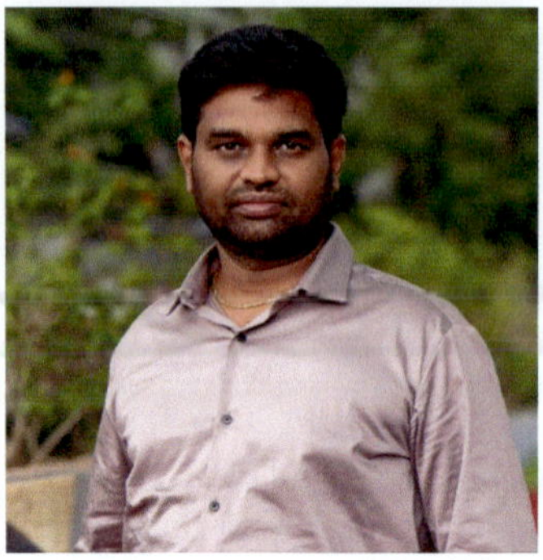

Dr. Ranjit Pabbati completed his B.Tech (2003–2007), M.Tech (2007–2009), and PhD in biotechnology at Jawaharlal Nehru Technological University, Hyderabad, India. His research work focused on the area of medicinal plant biotechnology for evaluation of its antimicrobial activity on various pathogenic bacteria and antioxidant activity. He also worked to understand the secondary metabolite biosynthesis pathways for mapping of genes involved in antimicrobial activity by transcriptome analysis using next generation sequencing techniques. He has 14 years of teaching experience, teaching undergraduate and postgraduate students. He has mentored undergraduate and postgraduate students for their projects. He has received an internal grant from the Technical Education Quality Improvement Programme of the Government of India (TEQIP) and worked in the area of plant biotechnology. Currently he is working as Assistant Professor at the Centre for Biotechnology, University College of Engineering Science and Technology Hyderabad, Jawaharlal Nehru Technological University, Hyderabad, Telangana, India. He has published 25 book chapters, three books, 25 research papers, and three review articles in reputed journals. He has one patent for design from the Indian Patent Agency in 2023.

Contributors

Sai Bhavani
Department of Environmental Sciences
Osmania University
Hyderabad, Telangana, India

Suchika Burra
Department of Biotechnology
Vignan's Foundation for Science, Technology and Research
Vadlamudi, Guntur, India

Kalyani Chepuri
Centre for Biotechnology
University College of Engineering Science and Technology
JNTU Hyderabad
Telangana, Hyderabad, India

Subhasri Das
Centre for Biotechnology
University College of Engineering Science and Technology
JNTU Hyderabad
Telangana, Hyderabad, India

Manikanta Dunna
Graduate School of Biomedical Sciences
Texas Tech University Health Sciences Center
Lubbock, Texas, USA

Thulasi Gandamalla
Centre for Biotechnology
University College of Engineering Science and Technology
JNTU Hyderabad
Telangana, Hyderabad, India

Vadakavila Geethikalal
Centre for Biotechnology
University College of Engineering Science and Technology
JNTU Hyderabad
Telangana, Hyderabad, India

Kathuroju Harikrishna
Centre for Biotechnology
University College of Engineering Science and Technology
JNTU Hyderabad
Telangana, Hyderabad, India

Akhila Karumuri
Department of Biotechnology
Vignan's Foundation for Science, Technology and Research
Vadlamudi, Guntur, India

B S R S Sai Kaustubh
Centre for Biotechnology
University College of Engineering Science and Technology
JNTU Hyderabad
Telangana, Hyderabad, India

Srinivas Kunta
Agricultural Research Organization
The Volcani Institute
Rishon LeZion, Israel

Himabindu Kurra
Department of Biotechnology
Vaagdevi Degree and P.G. College
Warangal, Telangana

Balla Sai Mrudula
Centre for Biotechnology
University College of Engineering Science and Technology
JNTU Hyderabad
Telangana, Hyderabad, India

Suchitra Nakka
Centre for Biotechnology
University College of Engineering Science and Technology
JNTU Hyderabad
Telangana, Hyderabad, India

Manaswini Narapusetty
Department of Biotechnology
Vignan's Foundation for Science, Technology and Research
Vadlamudi, Guntur, India

Anand Kumar Nelapati
Department of Biotechnology
Vignan's Foundation for Science, Technology and Research
Vadlamudi, Guntur, Andhra Pradesh, India

Madeeha Owais
Centre for Biotechnology
University College of Engineering Science and Technology
JNTU Hyderabad
Telangana, Hyderabad, India

Ranjit Pabbati
Jawaharlal Nehru Technological University
Hyderabad, Telangana, India

Siddhartha Palasala
Centre for Biotechnology
University College of Engineering Science and Technology
JNTU Hyderabad
Telangana, Hyderabad, India

Mahendar Porika
Department of Biotechnology
Kakatiya University
Warangal, Telangana, India

Surya Prakash DV
Department of Biotechnology
Meerut Institute of Engineering and Technology
Meerut, Uttar Pradesh, India

Chittepu Pranitha
Centre for Biotechnology
University College of Engineering Science and Technology
JNTU Hyderabad
Telangana, Hyderabad, India

Joshika Rerelly
Centre for Biotechnology
University College of Engineering Science and Technology
JNTU Hyderabad
Telangana, Hyderabad, India

Shreyas Sadineni
Centre for Biotechnology
University College of Engineering Science and Technology
JNTU Hyderabad
Telangana, Hyderabad, India

Firdoz Shaik
Department of Biotechnology
Vignan's Foundation for Science, Technology and Research
Vadlamudi, Guntur, India

Sandeep Sirohi
Department of Botany
Hariom Saraswati P.G College
Haridwar, Dhanauri Uttarakhand, India

Taniya Sribhashyam
Department of Biotechnology
University College of Science and Technology
Jawaharlal Nehru Technological University
Hyderabad, Telangana, India

Prathipati Supriya
Centre for Biotechnology
University College of Engineering Science and Technology
JNTU Hyderabad
Telangana, Hyderabad, India

Radhika Tippani
Department of Biotechnology
Kakatiya University
Warangal, Telangana, India

Parnika Vashist
Department of Biotechnology
Meerut Institute of Engineering and Technology
Meerut, Uttar Pradesh, India

P. Paul Vijay
Centre for Biotechnology
University College of Engineering Science and Technology
JNTU Hyderabad
Telangana, Hyderabad, India

Weiqing Zhang
Department of Research
Guangxi Medical University Cancer Hospital
Nanning, China

Acknowledgments

We extend our sincere appreciation to all the contributors of this book for their invaluable time, dedication, and dedicated support throughout the development of this project. Their commitment and collaboration played a crucial role in the timely completion of this volume. We are also deeply thankful to the anonymous reviewers for their thoughtful and constructive feedback, which greatly improved the quality of the book and facilitated the inclusion of additional expert chapters.

We extend our special appreciation to the editorial and production team at CRC Press, Taylor & Francis Group, whose guidance and persistent support were vital in successfully bringing this project to completion within a limited timeframe. It has been a true honor to collaborate with such a professional and supportive team.

Last but certainly not least, Dr. Firdoz Shaik extends heartfelt thanks to the Indian Council of Medical Research (ICMR) for their generous financial support (EM/Dev/IG/17/1129/2023), which was crucial in the successful completion of this book. We are deeply grateful to Vignan's Foundation for Science, Technology & Research and Guangxi Medical University for their consistent encouragement and strong institutional support. Our sincere appreciation also goes to all the editors whose insightful suggestions during the proposal and finalization stages significantly enhanced the quality and impact of this volume.

Firdoz Shaik
Department of Biotechnology, Vignan's Foundation for Science, Technology & Research, Vadlamudi, Andhra Pradesh, India

Weiqing Zhang
Department of Research, Guangxi Medical University Cancer Hospital, Guangxi Medical University, Nanning, Guangxi, China

Ranjit Pabbati
Jawaharlal Nehru Technological University Hyderabad, Telangana, India

1 Editorial Overview of Nanotechnology in Biomedical Applications

Firdoz Shaik, Weiqing Zhang, and Ranjit Pabbati

1.1 INTRODUCTION

1.1.1 An Outline of Nanotechnology

Designing, creating, characterizing, and using materials and technologies in the nanoscale regime, usually between 1 and 100 nm (Xia et al., 2023), are collectively referred to as nanotechnology. At this scale, materials exhibit unique optical, electrical, magnetic, and biological properties that distinguish them from their bulk counterparts (Huang et al., 2021). Because of their quantum effects and high surface-area-to-volume ratio, nanoparticles are extremely adaptable and can be used for different applications. Significant improvements in medical distribution, therapies, diagnostics, and regenerative medicine are made possible by the exquisite control these nanoscale materials offer over interactions at the molecular and cellular levels (Kiparissides & Kammona, 2015).

1.1.2 Evolution of Nanotechnology in the Biomedical Field

The last several decades have seen a notable advancement in the use of nanotechnology in biomedicine (Coccia & Finardi, 2012). The goal of early research in the 1990s was to comprehend the interactions between biological systems and nanoparticles. This has developed into the creation of therapeutic nanostructures for the treatment of infections, cancer, and genetic abnormalities (Chaturvedi et al., 2019), nano diagnostics for the early detection of disease, and nanocarriers for the transport of drugs (Alrushaid et al., 2023). Novelties such as the use of lipid nanoparticles (LNPs) in COVID-19 mRNA vaccines, imaging agents that are enabled by nanotechnology for tumor localization, and biosensing nanozymes show how nanotechnology is being integrated into routine biological processes (Yang, Z. et al., 2024). The field is still developing thanks to interdisciplinary contributions from computer modeling, materials science, molecular biology, and bioengineering (Tadmor & Tidor, 2005).

DOI: 10.1201/9781003563723-1

1.1.3 Importance and Scope of the Editorial Overview

A comprehensive understanding of this ever-evolving topic is necessary given the quick speed of research and the increasing therapeutic significance of nanotechnology in healthcare. Highlighting important ideas, new developments, and persistent difficulties in nano biomedicine is the goal of this editorial chapter. It provides a basis for comprehending how traditional medical methods are being transformed by nanotechnology, allowing for more individualized and focused therapies (Chattopadhyay et al., 2025). Offering insights into drug transport, diagnostics, therapy, regulatory considerations, and future directions, the coverage spans from basic concepts to translational applications. The goal of this overview is to help scientists, medical professionals, and legislators fully utilize nanotechnology to enhance global health outcomes (Riehemann et al., 2009).

1.2 FUNDAMENTALS OF NANOTECHNOLOGY IN BIOMEDICINE

1.2.1 Definition and Scale of Nanomaterials

Nanomaterials are substances that have a minimum of one dimension within the nanoscale range. New and improved physical, chemical, and biological capabilities that are not seen in their bulk forms are displayed by materials at this scale (1 to 100nm) (Huang et al., 2021). In biomedicine, these nanoscale structures are made to interact with biological systems at the molecular and cellular levels, providing accurate imaging therapy and diagnostic capabilities. Their size is similar to that of biomolecules, which enables highly effective cellular uptake and interaction with certain biological targets (Mosquera et al., 2018).

1.2.2 Key Physicochemical Properties Relevant to Biomedical Use

Their physicochemical properties have a significant impact on whether nanomaterials are biologically suitable. One of these is a high surface-area-to-volume ratio, which improves reactivity and facilitates the surface's functionalization with medications, imaging agents, or targeting ligands (Comanescu, 2023).

- Size and shape have an impact on clearance, biodistribution, and cellular uptake (Wei et al., 2018).
- Surface charge, which influences how well it interacts with cell membranes and blood circulation time (Fröhlich, 2012).
- For stability in vivo, solubility and dispersibility in biological fluids are crucial.
- Electrical, magnetic, and optical characteristics that make sophisticated imaging and sensing applications possible.
- Minimizing toxicity and guaranteeing safe clinical translation depend on biocompatibility.
- Certain biomedical needs can be satisfied by carefully adjusting these characteristics during synthesis.

1.2.3 Types of Nanomaterials Used

Numerous nanomaterials have been investigated and refined for use in biomedicine, each with unique benefits.

- **Metal-based nanomaterials:** Gold, silver, iron oxide, and other metallic nanoparticles are examples of metal-based nanomaterials. These are utilized in antibacterial, photothermal, drug delivery, and imaging applications. For example, gold nanoparticles have exceptional optical characteristics for therapy and diagnostics and are very biocompatible (Singh, A. et al., 2023).
- **Carbon-based nanomaterials**: Materials such as carbon nanotubes, fullerenes, and graphene are well known due to their enormous surface area, mechanical strength, and exceptional electrical conductivity. They have discovered applications in medication delivery, brain interface, and biosensing (Joshi et al., 2021).
- **Nanomaterials made of polymers:** These are often made up of biodegradable polymers such as chitosan, PEG, and PLGA. They make it possible for targeted distribution, controlled medication release, and low toxicity. In therapeutic drug delivery systems, polymeric micelles and nanoparticles are frequently utilized (Lu & Park, 2013).
- **Lipid-based nanomaterials:** Lipid-based materials, including liposomes and solid lipid nanoparticles, are the most medically advanced nanocarriers. As demonstrated by lipid-based COVID-19 mRNA vaccines, they offer controlled and targeted release, shield hydrophilic or hydrophobic medications from degradation, and encapsulate them (Lu et al., 2017).

These nanomaterials provide platforms for combined therapeutic, regenerative, and diagnostic applications, making them the foundation of nano biomedicine.

1.3 NANOTECHNOLOGY-ENABLED DRUG DELIVERY SYSTEMS

1.3.1 Targeted Medication Administration and Regulated Release

Creating targeted drug administration systems is one of nanotechnology's most revolutionary medical achievements (Hu et al., 2018). These nanoscale carriers are designed to minimize side effects and increase therapeutic efficacy by delivering therapeutic compounds directly to sick tissues, such as tumors or inflammatory areas, while preserving healthy cells. These nanocarriers are able to identify and attach to particular cell receptors through functionalization with targeting ligands. To ensure the best possible drug concentration at the target location throughout time, nanocarriers also provide controlled release profiles, in which the drug is released in a sustained or stimuli-responsive way (Bose & Wong, 2015).

1.3.2 Liposomes, Dendrimers, and Polymeric Nanoparticles

Various nanocarrier platforms have been developed, each with unique structures and functionalities:

- **Liposomes**: These circular vesicles, which may transport both hydrophilic and hydrophobic medications, are made up of an aqueous core encased in a phospholipid bilayer. Numerous FDA-approved formulations, including Doxil ® for cancer therapy, are the result of their biocompatibility and capacity to encapsulate medications.
- **Dendrimers**: These are artificial polymers with several surface functional groups that resemble trees and have many branches. High drug-loading capacity, surface modification, and multiple agent co-delivery are all made possible by their exact architecture. Additionally, dendrimers can be designed to improve cellular absorption and release drugs in response to stimuli.
- **Polymeric nanoparticles**: Constructed from biodegradable polymers like PLGA and PEG, these nanoparticles offer regulated and prolonged release of medications. Their surfaces can be customized to increase target specificity, prevent immune clearance, and lengthen circulation duration (Wakaskar, 2018).

Each of these systems offers flexibility in drug loading, release kinetics, and targeting capabilities, making them essential tools in modern therapeutics (Asl et al., 2023).

1.3.3 Overcoming Biological Barriers Using Nanocarriers

The existence of biological barriers that prevent drug absorption and accumulation at target areas presents a serious problem for drug delivery. Particularly well suited to get beyond these physiological barriers are nanocarriers, including:

- **Blood–brain barrier (BBB)**: Drug administration for neurological conditions is made possible by specific nanocarriers that are designed to pass through the BBB via receptor-mediated transcytosis (Xie et al., 2019).
- **Tumor microenvironment**: Nanocarriers can benefit from the enhanced permeability and retention (EPR) effect in tumors because of leaky vasculature, which permits passive accumulation (Ji et al., 2013).
- **Immune clearance**: Polyethylene glycol (PEGylation) surface modification can lengthen circulation time by decreasing identification by the mononuclear phagocyte system (MPS).
- **Gastrointestinal degradation**: By shielding medications from acidic conditions and enzymatic breakdown, oral nanocarriers can increase oral bioavailability.

By addressing these barriers, nanotechnology enhances the precision, effectiveness, and safety of therapeutic interventions, paving the way for personalized and disease-specific treatment strategies.

1.4 NANOTECHNOLOGY IN DIAGNOSTICS

1.4.1 Laboratory-on-a-Chip Devices and Nano Sensors

Nano sensors, as well as lab-on-a-chip technology analytical instruments known as nano sensors, employ nanoscale materials for very sensitive and specific identification and measurement of chemical or biological components (Li et al., 2012). Nano sensors can identify minuscule amounts of pathogens, environmental pollutants, or biomarkers by utilizing the distinct electrical, optical, and catalytic characteristics of nanomaterials. A lot of the time, these sensors are incorporated into lab-on-a-chip (LOC) platforms, which are tiny devices that integrate several laboratory operations onto one chip. LOC systems allow biological materials to be analyzed quickly and multiplexed, in small quantities with little user skill. In clinical situations where prompt choices are necessary, this combination of nanotechnology and microfluidics speeds up diagnostic operations (Luka et al., 2015).

1.4.2 Imaging Using Nanoparticles and Quantum Dots

By improving the resolution, contrast, and targeting of conventional imaging techniques, nanotechnology has completely transformed bioimaging (Smith et al., 2006). Fluorescence imaging commonly uses semiconductor nanocrystals called quantum dots (QDs) because of their brightness, photostability, and tunable emission wavelengths. In order to enable early and accurate localization, QDs can be coupled with targeting molecules to specifically label infections, cancer cells, or tissue markers.

Apart from QDs, metallic and magnetic nanoparticles are also important for imaging.

- In computed tomography (CT) imaging, gold nanoparticles improve contrast.
- In magnetic resonance imaging (MRI), iron oxide nanoparticles are employed as contrast agents, specifically for tumor detection and cell migration tracking (Bulte & Kraitchman, 2004).
- Research is being done on multimodal imaging platforms that integrate optical, magnetic, and radioactive detection using nanoparticles doped with silica and lanthanides.

These nanomaterials enable **real-time, non-invasive visualization** of molecular and cellular processes, facilitating earlier diagnosis and personalized treatment planning (Xi et al., 2012).

1.4.3 Point-of-Care Screening and Prompt Disease Identification

Rapid, inexpensive, and portable detection methods made possible by nanotechnology have greatly enhanced point-of-care (POC) diagnostics. Nanomaterial-based biosensors have been added to wearable technology to check health in real time, electrochemical chips, and paper-based lateral flow assays (LFAs). In LFAs, for instance, gold nanoparticles are widely employed to detect infectious illnesses such as HIV, COVID-19, and malaria. Nanotechnology enables early illness detection even in environments with limited resources by lowering reliance on centralized laboratory infrastructure (Noah & Ndangili, 2019).

Prompt clinical intervention, improved illness care, and successful epidemic control are made possible by these advancements (Laxminarayan et al., 2006). Additionally, new opportunities for pre-symptomatic diagnosis and monitoring of chronic ailments, including cancer, cardiovascular disorders, and neurodegenerative disease, are made possible by the ability to identify biomarkers unique to a disease at incredibly low concentrations.

1.5 THERAPEUTIC APPLICATIONS

1.5.1 Cancer Therapy (Photothermal, Photodynamic, Chemotherapy Enhancement)

Nanotechnology provides more accurate and creative ways to fight cancer than conventional chemotherapy and radiation (Nirmala et al., 2023). In photothermal therapy (PTT), tumor cells are destroyed by using nanomaterials such as graphene oxide or gold nanoshells, which transform near-infrared (NIR) light into localized heat (Yang, L. et al., 2015; Zhang et al., 2025). Similar to this, photodynamic therapy (PDT) uses light-activated nanoparticles that are loaded with photosensitizers. These nanoparticles produce reactive oxygen species (ROS), which eliminate particular cancer cells with the least amount of damage to the tissues around them (Brenneisen & Reichert, 2018).

Additionally, to increase the specificity and effectiveness of chemotherapeutic agents, nanocarriers are necessary. Systemic toxicity is reduced by precisely delivering cytotoxic drugs to tumor cells while protecting healthy tissues. Through the co-delivery of gene-silencing compounds to downregulate efflux pumps or the facilitation of intracellular drug accumulation, nanoparticles can also overcome multidrug resistance (MDR) (Yuan et al., 2016).

1.5.2 Antimicrobial and Antiviral Nanomaterials

New approaches to treating viral infections and microbial resistance have been made possible by nanotechnology. Because they may break down microbial membranes, create reactive oxygen species (ROS), hinder DNA replication, and have broad-spectrum antibacterial properties. Examples of metallic nanoparticles include copper oxide, zinc oxide, and silver. These nanoparticles are being used in oral formulations, medical device coatings, and wound dressings (Oyarzun-Ampuero et al., 2015).

Nanoparticles can prevent viral entrance, replication, or assembly in the context of viral illnesses. Gold and silica nanoparticles, for instance, have demonstrated potential in combating viruses such as influenza and HIV (Draz & Shafiee, 2018). Furthermore, surface coatings enabled by nanotechnology are being created to offer antiviral defense in medical settings.

1.5.3 Gene Therapy and mRNA Delivery (e.g., LNPs for COVID-19 Vaccines)

In recent years, nucleic acid delivery systems – particularly for gene therapy and mRNA-based vaccines – have been one of the most significant uses of nanotechnology. As demonstrated by their application in COVID-19 vaccines, for mRNA distribution, lipid nanoparticles have emerged as the most widely used technique.

To guarantee effective protein expression, these nanoparticles shield the delicate mRNA from deterioration, stimulate endosomal escape, and facilitate cellular absorption. Transporting siRNA, plasmid DNA, and CRISPR components to treat genetic abnormalities, malignancies, and chronic diseases is also being studied using other nanocarriers, such as polymeric or inorganic nanoparticles (Parhiz et al., 2024).

1.6 NANO-BIO INTERACTIONS AND MECHANISTIC INSIGHTS

1.6.1 Cellular Uptake and Biodistribution

The interaction of nanomaterials with biological systems must be understood to maximize their safety and therapeutic effectiveness. Endocytosis, which includes routes mediated by clathrin, caveolae, or micropinocytosis, is one way that nanoparticles might enter cells (Sahay et al., 2010). Their surface, charge, chemistry, size, and shape all have a major impact on the absorption pathway, intracellular trafficking, and final fate. After internalization, nanoparticles may locate in the cytoplasm, lysosomes, or even the nucleus, which could affect how they function.

Organ-specific clearance processes, protein corona formation, and systemic delivery routes all affect biodistribution. The liver and spleen, for example, are frequently accumulated because of their function in the mononuclear phagocyte system (MPS) (Singh, G. et al., 2024).

1.6.2 Nano-Bio Interface: Toxicity, Immunogenicity, and Targeting

Functionality and safety may be affected by inadvertent interactions at the nano-bio interface. Proteins in biological fluids can be adsorbed by nanoparticles, creating a protein corona that changes the protein's biological identity and cellular adsorption. This can be used to target, but it can also cause toxicity or immunogenicity (Singh, D. 2024).

By lowering non-specific contacts and immune clearance, surface modification (such as PEGylation or ligand attachment) enhances biocompatibility. However, in order to evaluate ROS generation, DNA damage, inflammation, and long-term accumulation, toxicological evaluation is necessary (Altankov et al., 2000).

1.6.3 Mechanistic Understanding of Therapeutic Action

Nanomedicines often have complex therapeutic effects (Fan et al., 2023). For example, when used to treat cancer, nanoparticles can carry a chemotherapeutic drug and either produce immune modulation or disrupt the tumor vasculature. Mechanistic investigations such as molecular profiling, in vivo imaging, and in vitro experiments are essential to comprehending how nanoparticles bring about their effects at the cellular and systemic levels. Based on these insights, next-generation nanotherapeutics with improved efficacy, safety, and specificity are logically created (Pajuelo, 2023).

1.7 RECENT ADVANCES AND EMERGING TRENDS

1.7.1 Biosensing and Therapy Using Single-Atom Nanozymes (SAzymes)

One recent advancement is the use of single-atom nanozymes in nanotechnology, offering atomic-level catalytic activity comparable to that of enzymes. High catalytic efficiency, adjustable activity, and exceptional stability are exhibited by SAzymes, which are made up of separated metal atoms scattered on a supporting substrate. They exhibit oxidase-like or peroxidase-like activity, which enables the colorimetric, electrochemical, or chemiluminescent detection of disease biomarkers with ultra-high sensitivity in biosensing. Therapeutic applications for SAzymes include ROS-mediated oxidative stress regulation, antimicrobial activity, and catalytic tumor treatment (Song et al., 2022). They are excellent prospects for next-generation theranostics due to their accuracy, low dosage requirement, and multifunctionality potential.

1.7.2 Stimuli-Responsive (Smart) Nanomaterials

An intelligent nanomaterial is made to respond to certain internal or external stimuli, such as temperature, pH, light, magnetic fields, or redox potential. With site-specific, on-demand drug release provided by these materials, treatment effectiveness is increased while side effects are reduced. To illustrate, in acidic tumor environments, pH-sensitive nanoparticles can release drugs preferentially, and in response to local heating, thermo-responsive hydrogels can deliver payloads. Multi-stimuli-responsive systems for improved control and programmable behavior are two other recent advancements that make highly adaptive therapeutic and diagnostic platforms possible (Zhang, J. et al., 2023).

1.7.3 Integration with AI and Wearable Biomedical Devices

Artificial intelligence (AI), nanotechnology, and wearable technology are combining to bring in a new era of personalized and predictive healthcare. Artificial intelligence algorithms are capable of predicting toxicity, optimizing nanoparticle design, and analyzing intricate diagnostic outputs from nano sensors. Concurrently, continuous, non-invasive health monitoring is made possible by wearable technology that incorporates nanomaterials, such as stretchy nanoelectronics patches or graphene-based sensors. These technologies represent a revolutionary shift toward responsive and remote healthcare systems by tracking physiological parameters, identifying early disease indicators, and sending real-time data to healthcare providers (Ma et al., 2023).

1.8 REGULATORY AND ETHICAL CONSIDERATIONS

1.8.1 Regulatory Frameworks (FDA, EMA) and Clinical Translation

Clinical application of nanotechnology necessitates navigating intricate regulatory systems, despite encouraging laboratory outcomes. The Food and Drug Administration (FDA) in the United States and the European Medicines Agency (EMA) have established criteria for evaluating nanomedicines. which include pharmacokinetics, toxicity, efficacy, and quality control requirements. The distinct properties of nanomaterials, however, make standardization difficult and regulatory approaches constantly changing. The industry, regulatory agencies, and researchers must work closely together to expedite the approval and uptake of products enabled by nanotechnology (Vilela et al., 2024).

1.8.2 Safety, Toxicity Testing, and Standardization

Because of their small size, strong surface reactivity, and potential for bioaccumulation, nanomaterials present special safety challenges. It is essential to conduct toxicity testing, which includes genotoxicity, immunogenicity, in vivo biodistribution, and in vitro cytotoxicity. Standardized procedures are desperately needed to guarantee repeatability and accurate risk assessment. The development of standardized frameworks for assessing the safety of nanomaterials in various applications and geographical areas is an ongoing effort by regulatory bodies and scientific consortia (Ganguly et al., 2018).

1.8.3 Ethical Challenges and Public Perception

Like any new technology, there are a number of social and ethical issues with nanomedicine. Concerns include long-term health effects, equitable access to cutting-edge nanotechnologies, and informed consent in clinical trials employing nanomedicine. Furthermore, the adoption and incorporation of nanotechnology into healthcare systems may be influenced by how the general public views (Gupta et al., 2012). It is essential to engage stakeholders, communicate openly, and create inclusive policies to foster trust and proactively resolve moral quandaries.

1.9 CHALLENGES AND LIMITATIONS

1.9.1 Scalability and Reproducibility

A significant obstacle still stands in the way of the large-scale manufacture of nanomedicines, despite impressive laboratory-scale successes. The process of consistently creating nanoparticles with consistent surface properties, size, and shape is difficult and frequently prohibitively expensive. Clinical acceptance and regulatory approval may be hampered by the diversity introduced by the complexity of nanomaterial design, including functionalization and encapsulation. It will take advancements in manufacturing technologies, process standardization, and quality control to overcome this barrier.

1.9.2 Extended Biocompatibility and Approval

Ensuring the safe removal, biodistribution, and long-term biocompatibility of nanomaterials is essential for clinical success. Immune reactions or chronic toxicity may result from certain nanoparticles' ability to linger in the body or build up in organs like the brain, liver, or spleen. A thorough understanding of the safety profiles of various nanoplatforms requires extensive in vivo research evaluation, elimination mechanisms, immunological interactions, and degradation kinetics. For regulatory bodies to assess health hazards and guarantee patient safety, they need to have solid long-term data.

1.9.3 Cost-Effectiveness and Global Accessibility

In low- and middle-income nations, nanomedicines are frequently unavailable due to high development and manufacturing costs. This limits their applicability globally, particularly for common diseases like cancer, malaria, and tuberculosis. Decentralized distribution plans, scalable manufacturing techniques, and economical formulations must be given top priority in order to guarantee fair access. Bridging this gap and advancing inclusive healthcare solutions can be greatly aided by global funding initiatives and public-private collaborations.

1.10 CONCLUSION

There is no denying nanomedicine's revolutionary promise in the diagnosis, treatment, and management of complicated illnesses. But its full influence won't be possible until these developments are available to everyone, regardless of location or economic standing. There is a significant gap in the way healthcare is delivered globally, as evidenced by the current situation, where high development and manufacturing costs restrict the availability of nanomedicines in low-and middle-income nations. Each year, millions of people die from diseases including cancer, malaria, and tuberculosis, which are common in many underdeveloped areas. Because of infrastructure and financial limitations, the benefits of nanomedicine are still concentrated in wealthier countries, despite the potential for more accurate and efficient treatment of many health issues.

Developing cost-effective formulations, scalable production technologies, and decentralized distribution frameworks that are suited to the particular requirements of resource-constrained environments must be given top priority in order to rectify this imbalance. Innovations that can drastically lower production costs include the use of locally accessible biomaterials, green synthesis techniques, and streamlined manufacturing procedures. Enhancing knowledge transfer method, bolstering public-private collaborations, and participating in international financing and policy initiatives – like those led by the Gates Foundation, WHO, or GAVI – can also hasten the equitable distribution of nanomedicines.

Importantly, long-term sustainability depends on capacity-building initiatives including integrating nanomedicine into the current healthcare system, creating regional manufacturing facilities, and training local scientists. Fair access to nanomedicine requires not just financial resources but also public awareness, legislative backing, and international cooperation.

In conclusion, the ability of nanomedicine to lower health inequities and enhance quality of life globally should be used to gauge its success rather than just market size or scientific achievements. Only by embracing inclusive, cooperative, and morally sound methods can we make sure that nanotechnology lives up to its potential as driver of universal and revolutionary healthcare.

REFERENCES

Alrushaid, N., Khan, F. A., Al-Suhaimi, E. A., & Elaissari, A. (2023). Nanotechnology in cancer diagnosis and treatment. *Pharmaceutics*, *15*(3), 1025.

Altankov, G., Thom, V., Groth, T., Jankova, K., Jonsson, G., & Ulbricht, M. (2000). Modulating the biocompatibility of polymer surfaces with poly (ethylene glycol): Effect of fibronectin. *Journal of Biomedical Materials Research*, *52*(1), 219–230.

Asl, F. D., Mousazadeh, M., Taji, S., Bahmani, A., Khashayar, P., Azimzadeh, M., & Mostafavi, E. (2023). Nano drug-delivery systems for management of AIDS: Liposomes, dendrimers, gold and silver nanoparticles. *Nanomedicine*, *18*(3), 279–302.

Bose, A., & Wong, T. W. (2015). Nanotechnology-enabled drug delivery for cancer therapy. In *Nanotechnology applications for tissue engineering* (pp. 173–193). William Andrew Publishing.

Brenneisen, P., & Reichert, A. S. (2018). Nanotherapy and reactive oxygen species (ROS) in cancer: A novel perspective. *Antioxidants*, *7*(2), 31.

Bulte, J. W., & Kraitchman, D. L. (2004). Iron oxide MR contrast agents for molecular and cellular imaging. *NMR in Biomedicine: An International Journal Devoted to the Development and Application of Magnetic Resonance In Vivo*, *17*(7), 484–499.

Chattopadhyay, S., Goswami, A., & Sil, M. (2025). Nanobiotechnology: Traditional re-interpreting personalized medicine through targeted therapies and regenerative solutions. *Naunyn-Schmiedeberg's Archives of Pharmacology*, 1–24.

Chaturvedi, V. K., Singh, A., Singh, V. K., & Singh, M. P. (2019). Cancer nanotechnology: A new revolution for cancer diagnosis and therapy. *Current Drug Metabolism*, *20*(6), 416–429.

Coccia, M., & Finardi, U. (2012). Emerging nanotechnological research for future pathways of biomedicine. *International Journal of Biomedical Nanoscience and Nanotechnology*, *2*(3–4), 299–317.

Comanescu, C. (2023). Recent advances in surface functionalization of magnetic nanoparticles. *Coatings*, *13*(10), 1772.

Draz, M. S., & Shafiee, H. (2018). Applications of gold nanoparticles in virus detection. *Theranostics*, *8*(7), 1985.

Fan, D., Cao, Y., Cao, M., Wang, Y., Cao, Y., & Gong, T. (2023). Nanomedicine in cancer therapy. *Signal Transduction and Targeted Therapy*, *8*(1), 293.

Fröhlich, E. (2012). The role of surface charge in cellular uptake and cytotoxicity of medical nanoparticles. *International Journal of Nanomedicine*, 5577–5591.

Ganguly, P., Breen, A., & Pillai, S. C. (2018). Toxicity of nanomaterials: Exposure, pathways, assessment, and recent advances. *ACS Biomaterials Science & Engineering*, *4*(7), 2237–2275.

Gupta, N., Fischer, A. R., van der Lans, I. A., & Frewer, L. J. (2012). Factors influencing societal response of nanotechnology: An expert stakeholder analysis. *Journal of Nanoparticle Research*, *14*(5), 857.

Hu, Q., Li, H., Wang, L., Gu, H., & Fan, C. (2018). DNA nanotechnology-enabled drug delivery systems. *Chemical Reviews*, *119*(10), 6459–6506.

Huang, H., Feng, W., & Chen, Y. (2021). Two-dimensional biomaterials: Material science, biological effect and biomedical engineering applications. *Chemical Society Reviews*, *50*(20), 11381–11485.

Ji, T., Zhao, Y., Ding, Y., & Nie, G. (2013). Using functional nanomaterials to target and regulate the tumor microenvironment: Diagnostic and therapeutic applications. *Advanced Materials*, *25*(26), 3508–3525.

Joshi, P., Mishra, R., & Narayan, R. J. (2021). Biosensing applications of carbon-based materials. *Current Opinion in Biomedical Engineering*, *18*, 100274.

Laxminarayan, R., Chow, J., & Shahid-Salles, S. A. (2006). Intervention cost-effectiveness: overview of main messages. In *Disease control priorities in developing countries.* 2nd edition. The International Bank for Reconstruction and Development / The World Bank (Washington, DC) and Oxford University Press (New York).

Li, P., Lei, N., Sheadel, D. A., Xu, J., & Xue, W. (2012). Integration of nanosensors into a sealed microchannel in a hybrid lab-on-a-chip device. *Sensors and Actuators B: Chemical*, *166*, 870–877.

Lu, S., Yu, T., Wang, Y., Liang, L., Chen, Y., Xu, F., & Wang, S. (2017). Nanomaterial-based biosensors for measurement of lipids and lipoproteins towards point-of-care of cardiovascular disease. *Analyst*, *142*(18), 3309–3321.

Lu, Y., & Park, K. (2013). Polymeric micelles and alternative nanonized delivery vehicles for poorly soluble drugs. *International Journal of Pharmaceutics*, *453*(1), 198–214.

Luka, G., Ahmadi, A., Najjaran, H., Alocilja, E., DeRosa, M., Wolthers, K.,. . . Hoorfar, M. (2015). Microfluidics integrated biosensors: A leading technology towards lab-on-a-chip and sensing applications. *Sensors*, *15*(12), 30011–30031.

Ma, X., Guo, G., Wu, X., Wu, Q., Liu, F., Zhang, H.,. . . Guan, Y. (2023). Advances in integration, wearable applications, and artificial intelligence of biomedical microfluidics systems. *Micromachines*, *14*(5), 972.

Mosquera, J., García, I., & Liz-Marzán, L. M. (2018). Cellular uptake of nanoparticles versus small molecules: A matter of size. *Accounts of Chemical Research*, *51*(9), 2305–2313.

Nirmala, M. J., Kizhuveetil, U., Johnson, A., Nagarajan, R., & Muthuvijayan, V. (2023). Cancer nanomedicine: A review of nano-therapeutics and challenges ahead. *RSC Advances*, *13*(13), 8606–8629.

Noah, N. M., & Ndangili, P. M. (2019). Current trends of nanobiosensors for point-of-care diagnostics. *Journal of Analytical Methods in Chemistry*, *2019*(1), 2179718.

Oyarzun-Ampuero, F., Vidal, A., Concha, M., Morales, J., Orellana, S., & Moreno-Villoslada, I. (2015). Nanoparticles for the treatment of wounds. *Current Pharmaceutical Design*, *21*(29), 4329–4341.

Pajuelo, A. (2023). A perspective review of cancer therapy (part I): Immunotherapy, gene therapy, and nanotechnology. *Science Insights*, *43*(6), 1155–1165.

Parhiz, H., Atochina-Vasserman, E. N., & Weissman, D. (2024). mRNA-based therapeutics: Looking beyond COVID-19 vaccines. *The Lancet*, *403*(10432), 1192–1204.

Riehemann, K., Schneider, S. W., Luger, T. A., Godin, B., Ferrari, M., & Fuchs, H. (2009). Nanomedicine – challenge and perspectives. *Angewandte Chemie International Edition*, *48*(5), 872–897.

Sahay, G., Alakhova, D. Y., & Kabanov, A. V. (2010). Endocytosis of nanomedicines. *Journal of Controlled Release*, *145*(3), 182–195.

Singh, A., Banerjee, S. L., Gantait, A., Kumari, K., & Kundu, P. P. (2023). Metal-based nanoparticles: Synthesis and biomedical applications. In *Nanoparticles reinforced metal nanocomposites: Mechanical performance and durability* (pp. 365–408). Singapore: Springer Nature Singapore.

Singh, D. (2024). Nano-bio interfaces: Pioneering targeted approaches for disease treatment and prevention. *Journal of Macromolecular Science, Part B*, 1–18.

Singh, G., Preethi, L., & Thakur, N. (2024). Nano–bio dynamics: Mechanisms and challenges in shaping nanomaterials for biomedical use. In *Nanoparticles in cancer theranostics* (pp. 53–68). CRC Press.

Smith, A. M., Ruan, G., Rhyner, M. N., & Nie, S. (2006). Engineering luminescent quantum dots for in vivo molecular and cellular imaging. *Annals of Biomedical Engineering*, *34*(1), 3–14.

Song, H., Zhang, M., & Tong, W. (2022). Single-atom nanozymes: Fabrication, characterization, surface modification and applications of ROS scavenging and antibacterial. *Molecules*, *27*(17), 5426.

Tadmor, B., & Tidor, B. (2005). Interdisciplinary research and education at the biology-engineering-computer science interface: A perspective (reprinted article). *Drug Discovery Today*, *10*(23–24), 1706–1712.

Vilela, C., Lucas, J., Cunha, P., Cerqueira, R., Costa, J., Costa, J.,. . . Marquet, I. (2024). Regulatory and clinical translation. In *Multiscale cell-biomaterials interplay in musculoskeletal tissue engineering and regenerative medicine* (pp. 441–462). Academic Press.

Wakaskar, R. R. (2018). General overview of lipid–polymer hybrid nanoparticles, dendrimers, micelles, liposomes, spongosomes and cubosomes. *Journal of Drug Targeting*, *26*(4), 311–318.

Wei, Y., Quan, L., Zhou, C., & Zhan, Q. (2018). Factors relating to the biodistribution & clearance of nanoparticles & their effects on in vivo application. *Nanomedicine*, *13*(12), 1495–1512.

Xi, D., Dong, S., Meng, X., Lu, Q., Meng, L., & Ye, J. (2012). Gold nanoparticles as computerized tomography (CT) contrast agents. *Rsc Advances*, *2*(33), 12515–12524.

Xia, Y., Yang, P., Sun, Y., Wu, Y., Mayers, B., Gates, B.,. . . Yan, H. (2003). One-dimensional nanostructures: Synthesis, characterization, and applications. *Advanced Materials*, *15*(5), 353–389.

Xie, J., Shen, Z., Anraku, Y., Kataoka, K., & Chen, X. (2019). Nanomaterial-based blood-brain-barrier (BBB) crossing strategies. *Biomaterials*, *224*, 119491.

Yang, L., Tseng, Y. T., Suo, G., Chen, L., Yu, J., Chiu, W. J.,. . . Lin, C. H. (2015). Photothermal therapeutic response of cancer cells to aptamer–gold nanoparticle-hybridized graphene oxide under NIR illumination. *ACS Applied Materials & Interfaces*, *7*(9), 5097–5106.

Yang, Z., Guo, J., Wang, L., Zhang, J., Ding, L., Liu, H., & Yu, X. (2024). Nanozyme-enhanced electrochemical biosensors: Mechanisms and applications. *Small*, *20*(14), 2307815.

Yuan, Y., Cai, T., Xia, X., Zhang, R., Chiba, P., & Cai, Y. (2016). Nanoparticle delivery of anticancer drugs overcomes multidrug resistance in breast cancer. *Drug Delivery*, *23*(9), 3350–3357.

Zhang, H., Tang, X., & Jiang, Z. (2025). Next-generation Nanomaterial-based phototherapeutic strategies for tumor: From NIR responsiveness to smart activation. *Nanomedicine*, 1–25.

Zhang, J., Tang, W., Zhang, X., Song, Z., & Tong, T. (2023). An overview of stimuli-responsive intelligent antibacterial nanomaterials. *Pharmaceutics*, *15*(8), 2113.

2 Nanohybrids for Biosensors and Bioelectronics Applications

Kalyani Chepuri, Himabindu Kurra, Siddhartha Palasala, Balla Sai Mrudula, Subhasri Das, B S R S Sai Kaustubh, Prathipati Supriya, and Manikanta Dunna

2.1 INTRODUCTION

Diseases can be diagnosed in early stages by detecting certain organic or inorganic molecules that are present in living organisms, which enhances the survival rate and can aid in successful treatment strategies. This can be achieved by the medical device called a "Biosensor."

It was first developed by an American biochemist L.L Clark where he used the Clark electrode or oxygen electrode to determine the percentage of oxygen in the blood. Later on, the term biosensor was first used by Cammann in the year 1977. A biosensor can be defined as the analytical device that has the components like bioreceptor (enzyme, antibody, etc.), transducer (translates the observed signal into a useful output), and amplifier as shown in Figure 2.1 (Malik et al., 2023). The biosensor mainly relies on the principle of immobilization of biomolecules on the surface of a transducer. Numerous studies have been performed that mainly aim to develop new biosensor assemblies and immobilization approaches with the integration of various innovative materials (Batool et al., 2019).

An ideal biosensor is named for its certain unique characteristics which mostly include high sensitivity, selectivity, resolution, reproducibility, repeatability, and response time with good flow. Various advancements in the field of nanotechnology and the cumulative approach of interdisciplinarity made possible biosensors made up of nanoparticles, especially nanohybrids. These biosensors, which are made up of nanohybrids, have an excellent approach in various fields like chemistry, material science, physics, biomedicine, biology. These have gained huge popularity for their unique physio and chemical properties (Malik et al., 2023).

The progression in the field of biosensors can be classified into five generations. In the first generation the biosensor typically measures the composition of an analyte

 DOI: 10.1201/9781003563723-2

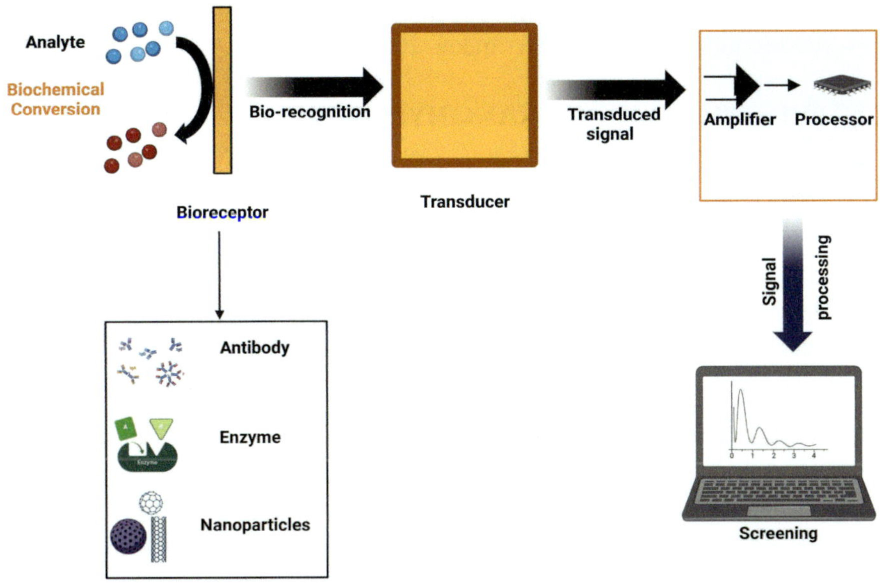

FIGURE 2.1 Working Principle of a biosensor: Biorecognition to signal processing.

and product of the bioreceptor reactions, which eventually produces a signal. In the second generation by the addition of co-reactants and the auxiliary enzymes the analytical efficiency of the biosensor was enhanced further. These sensors were called mediator amperometric biosensors. From the third to fifth generations of biosensors the bioreceptors were the key part in sensing the element where these became cost effective and highly sensitive with higher repeatability (Malik et al., 2023).

Bioelectronics, also known as biomolecular electronics, is a field of research with the conjunction of biology and electronics. The main aim of the bioelectronics was to process the systems and devices by utilizing biological materials and seeing assistance with the biological architectures. Electronics technology has been integrated into biology and medicine since the invention of the pacemaker and the development of the medical imaging industry (Wikipedia Contributors, 2025). At the end of the 18th century Luigi Galvani, an Italian physiologist, began to work on animals to understand the human physiology where he placed a detached leg of a frog on a brass hook and then he inserted a steal scalpel that touched the exposed sciatic nerve, which led to the twitching of frog leg. Then he described there is an electrical fluid in muscle that is responsible for the muscle movement. He named the electrical fluid "animal electricity," which is intrinsic to animals. Galvani is considered the father of bioelectronics. The application of bioelectronics in the field of medicine and other fields of science and research is one of the most groundbreaking and an innovative approach in the healthcare today. These are used to diagnose and cure several adverse health challenges like arrhythmias (heart problems), and chronic pain disorders. These innovations have shaped millions of patient lives. The medical bioelectronics market worldwide has already surpassed $22 billion and is expected to exceed $60 billion by 2030 (Stavrinidou, 2022).

2.2 FUNDAMENTALS OF NANOHYBRIDS

2.2.1 Classification of Nanohybrids

Nanohybrids are classified according to composition, structural arrangement, type of bonding, and dimensionality and can thus be designed as materials with customized and optimized properties. This characterization advances their usability across various fields of applications ranging from drug delivery, to biosensors and sustainable energy applications, since it facilitates absolute control over functional properties (Aich et al., 2014).

2.2.1.1 Based on the Composition

2.2.1.1.1 Organic-Inorganic Nanohybrids

Organic-inorganic nanohybrids are composite materials consisting of both organic and inorganic material at the nanoscale. These hybrids take the advantageous properties of the two materials to produce multifunctional systems with enhanced mechanical, electrical, optical, or biological properties (Sanchez et al., 2011). The synergism between the inorganic strength and stability with organic flexibility and function makes them valuable for utilization (Ananikov et al., 2019).

Example: Chitosan-LDH hybrids are used for gene therapy and drug delivery due to their controlled release properties (Chi et al., 2017).

2.2.1.1.2 Inorganic-Inorganic Nanohybrids

Nanoscale composites that combine two or more different inorganic materials are known as inorganic-inorganic nanohybrids. Thes hybrids exhibit exceptional mechanical strength, electrical conductivity, catalytic behavior, and thermal stability by integrating the unique properties of various inorganic materials (Choi et al., 2021).

Component **interactions** enhance overall functionality, resulting in **high efficiency** for energy storage, catalysis, electronics, and environmental remediation (Godja & Munteanu, 2024).

Example: Titanium dioxide-silica (TiO_2-SiO_2) nanohybrids – Utilized in photocatalytic processes, self-cleaning surfaces, and the purification of air and water (Khannyra et al., 2022).

2.2.1.1.3 Organic-Organic Nanohybrids

Organic-organic nanohybrids are nanomaterials that are composed of two or more distinct organic components. At the nano level the interaction between these materials results in enhanced properties that lead to increased mechanical strength, electrical conductivity, and thermal stability. These hybrids play an important role in different applications, such as drug delivery, organic electronics, and biodegradable materials (Lin et al., 2024).

Example: Polypyrrole-polyethylene glycol (PPy-PEG) nanohybrids – they are used in drug delivery systems because of their enhanced controlled release properties and biocompatibility (Zare et al., 2021).

2.2.1.2 Based on Bonding Type

2.2.1.2.1 Class I

Organic and inorganic components are bonded by weak intermolecular forces including van der Waals forces, hydrogen bonds, or electrostatic interactions. These hybrids maintain the unique individual properties of the components while forming a stable yet reversible structure (Rando et al., 2022).

Example: Polymer-silica nanocomposites – the silica nanoparticles are dispersed in a polymer matrix enhancing mechanical strength and thermal stability through hydrogen bonding and van der Waals forces (Mobin et al., 2019).

2.2.1.2.2 Class II

The inorganic and organic components have strong ionic or covalent bonds between them, which enhances nanoscale property integration and structural stability. These hybrids exhibit improved thermal stability, chemical resistance, and mechanical strength, which makes them ideal for a range of applications (Gomez-Romero et al., 2023).

Example: PMMA–SiO_2 Nanocomposites – These hybrids have covalent bonding between PMMA chains and silica, which increases mechanical strength and thermal stability (Mackenzie & Bescher, 2018).

2.2.1.3 Based on Structural Arrangement

2.2.1.3.1 Core-Shell Nanohybrids

Core-shell nanohybrids are crafted in such a way that a core material is surrounded by a well-designed shell layer, which is fashioned as a hierarchical structure. These structures support a high level of command over the surface properties, reactivity, and stability and simultaneously preserve the original functionalities of the core material (Singh & Bhateria, 2020).

Example: Prussian Blue@Porphyrinic Metal-Organic Framework (PB@PCN) core-shell nanohybrid is used in photothermal therapy due to its enhanced light absorption and efficiency in thermal conversion (Cheng et al., 2019).

2.2.1.3.2 Layered Nanohybrids

Layered nanohybrids are materials constituted of layers often with a thickness of a few nanometers that that were prepared from an assembly of substances with different properties and that together form a hybrid of many properties. With the presence of the layered architecture, such structures can easily be made through the intervening of the layers, where necessary functional sequences can be traversed, e.g., by the ion exchange, by the selective permeability, or by an increase in the mechanical strength due to a sequence of the layer stacked (Jin & Park, 2019).

Example: Gold nanoparticle-decorated layered double hydroxide (LDH–Au) nanohybrids – They are employed in fluorescence imaging and photothermal therapy of cancer cells (Komarala et al., 2017).

2.2.1.3.3 Intercalated Nanohybrids

Intercalated nanohybrids are composite materials formed by inserting guest molecules or ions between the layers of a host material, resulting in an increased interlayer spacing (Ivashchyshyn et al., 2012). Intercalation creates a well organized, layered structure that enhances properties such as ion exchange capacity and thermal stability.

Example: Phenolic antioxidant-intercalated Mg-Al LDH nanohybrid – Used in polymer stabilization owing to its improved thermal stability and controlled release of antioxidants (Lonkar et al., 2012).

2.2.1.3.4 Embedded Nanohybrids

Embedded nanohybrids are nanostructures in which nanoparticles are uniformly distributed within a matrix material, forming a composite that retains the properties of both the components. The embedding increases the material's mechanical strength and thermal stability, making it applicable for a range of various applications (Sanchez et al., 2001).

Example: Silver nanoparticle-embedded hybrid nanopaper – utilized in thermal management applications due to improved thermal conductivity (Li, Y. et al., 2021).

2.2.1.4 Based on Dimensionality

2.2.1.4.1 0D Nanohybrids

0D nanohybrids are composites with 0D nanostructures (nanoparticles, quantum dots, etc.) intercalated with a host matrix for modified physical and chemical properties (Wang et al., 2020).

Example: Graphitic carbon nitride (g-C_3N_4) with embedded nanoparticles – Utilized for water splitting in photocatalysis (Sinha et al., 2021).

2.2.1.4.2 1D Nanohybrids

1D nanohybrids are a type of composite that include one-dimensional (1D) nanostructures such as nanowires, nanotubes, and nanorods, which are incorporated into other materials in order to improve their mechanical, electrical, as well as optical properties. Their high aspect ratio and directional conductivity make them particularly efficient for different technological applications (Zhu et al., 2020).

Example: Peptide-gold nanoparticle 1D nanohybrids – utilized in targeted cancer therapy, these hybrids increase the near-infrared photothermal absorption and enhance the efficacy of the processes involved (Jeon et al., 2025).

2.2.1.4.3 2D Nanohybrids

2D nanohybrids are materials a combination of 2D structures like graphite, boron nitride, or transition metal dichalcogenides (TMDs) with other nanoscale materials. They display high surface-to-volume ratio while ultrathin, 2D materials possess layered structure and show unique electronic, optical, and mechanical properties dependent on the number of layers (Radhakrishnan et al., 2024).

Example: Graphene-MoS_2 nanohybrid – The hybrids are a combination of graphene and the nanomaterial MoS_2. Graphene-S Mo nanohybrid possesses the characteristics of high conductivity and the strong catalytic properties of MoS_2, enabling easy energy storage and supercapacitor charge/discharge cycles (Venkadajapathy & Sivaperumal, 2024).

2.2.1.4.4 3D Nanohybrids

3D nanohybrids are a kind of nanomaterials that include 3D structures such as interconnected porous networks, hierarchical structures, or scaffolded nanostructures. The hybrids leverage the high surface area, porosity, and multidirectional conductivity, which make them appropriate for several applications (Sefadi & Mochane, 2021).

Example: Graphene aerogel-metal oxide 3D nanohybrid – applied in supercapacitors and water purification due to its high porosity, extensive surface area, and exceptional electrical conductivity (Zhang et al., 2017).

2.3 SYNTHESIS AND FABRICATION TECHNIQUES OF NANOHYBRIDS

Nanohybrids are synthesized using different physical, chemical, and hybrid procedures. Each of these procedures has unique advantages that depend on the desired properties of biosensors and bioelectronics. The main fabrication methods include:

2.3.1 Sol-Gel Method

It is a wet chemical process to produce nanohybrids. The metal alkoxides hydrolyze and undergo polycondensation giving rise to nanohybrids. The formed gel is then dried and heated to increase the structural stability. It provides great composition and porosity control, making it suitable for use in biosensors (Thakur et al., 2022).

2.3.2 Hydrothermal/Solvothermal Processes

It is a technique where the precursors are dissolved in a solvent and then heated in a high-pressure vessel to induce crystallization. It is very effective in yielding nanohybrids of well-defined structure, controlled morphology, and phase purity. It is used extensively for metal oxide and carbon-based hybrids (Purohit et al., 2020).

2.3.3 Electrochemical Deposition

In this method a voltage is applied on an electrolyte solution of metal ions, causing the nanoparticles to deposit onto a conductive surface. The process allows for very accurate control over nanoparticle size and placement. This method is commonly used for fabrication of biosensor electrodes (Tripathy & Kim, 2018).

2.3.4 Chemical Vapor Deposition (CVD)

It is a technique in which the gaseous precursors decompose at high temperatures and deposit nanohybrids such as CNTs or graphene onto a substrate. The method can be used for precise control over thickness, purity, and structure. It is an extensive application in bioelectronics due to its scalability (Sreejith et al., 2015).

2.3.5 Physical Vapor Deposition (PVD)

In this method the nanohybrid thin films are deposited on substrates in a vacuum using either sputtering or thermal evaporation. By using this technique, we can produce uniform coating and have controlled thickness and composition. It is widely used in medical coatings and biosensors (Malik et al., 2023).

2.3.6 Langmuir-Blodgett and Self-Assembly

In this technique, nanohybrids are spread at a liquid-air interface and transferred to a solid substrate, resulting in formation of uniform thin films. Through this process we can achieve molecular-level precision for film organization. It is best for biosensors requiring well-ordered structures (Yoon et al., 2021).

2.3.7 Biogenic and Green Synthesis

Nanohybrids are synthesized using biological agents such as plant extracts or microbes as reducing agents. We can avoid toxic chemicals using this green process and while providing biocompatibility. It is becoming increasingly popular in medical and environmental applications (Mogha, 2023).

2.4 PHYSICOCHEMICAL PROPERTIES AND CHARACTERIZATION OF NANOHYBRIDS

The physicochemical properties of nanohybrids have an influence on their performance in biosensors and bioelectronics. These properties include surface chemistry, thermal stability, optical properties, electrochemical properties, and structural integrity.

Different analytical methods are employed to characterize these properties to establish their use in specific applications (Soto & Orozco, 2022).

2.4.1 Structural and Morphological Properties

The properties such as porosity, surface area, and interaction with biological molecules is greatly influenced by nanohybrids' morphology and structure. A well-defined structure improves sensitivity and signal transduction in biosensors. The morphology also determines the mechanical strength and stability of the material.

2.4.1.1 Transmission Electron Microscopy (TEM)

This shows the size, shape, lattice defects of the nanoparticles and atomic-resolution imaging, which are essential for optimizing nanohybrids for biosensors (Purohit et al., 2020).

2.4.1.2 Scanning Electron Microscopy (SEM)

Here we examine morphology of the surface, such as particle distribution, roughness, and porosity, which influence biosensor efficacy (Purohit et al., 2020).

2.4.1.3 Atomic Force Microscopy (AFM)

This enables us to quantify roughness of the surface and nanomechanics and offers one way to comprehend adhesion and biomolecule interactions with the nanohybrid surface (Sreejith et al., 2015)

2.4.2 Crystallinity and Phase Composition

The electronic, optical, and mechanical properties of nanohybrids are influenced by crystallinity. It has been observed that the conductivity and stability is improved in highly crystalline materials and for amorphous materials catalytic activity through defects.

2.4.3 X-ray Diffraction (XRD)

It helps in identifying the crystal structure, lattice parameters, and phase purity to ensure nanohybrids have necessary stability and electrical characteristics (Tripathy & Kim, 2018).

2.4.4 Optical and Electronic Properties

For nanohybrids that are used for biosensing and optoelectronic devices, optical properties like light absorption and photoluminescence play a pivotal role. The performance of electrochemical biosensors is influenced by electronic properties, i.e., charge transfer and conductivity.

UV-Visible spectroscopy (UV-Vis): It helps in quantifying the optical absorption and bandgap, which is very important for photoactive nanohybrids in biosensors (Malik et al., 2023).

Photoluminescence spectroscopy (PL): It enables to assess charge carrier dynamics and defect states, which facilitates enhancing electronic behavior in biosensing applications (Yoon et al., 2021).

2.4.5 Surface Chemistry and Functionalization

For nanohybrid stability, biocompatibility, and functionalization surface chemistry is very crucial. The biosensor's specificity is improved through the facilitation of selective biomolecule binding through accurate surface modifications.

2.4.5.1 Fourier Transform Infrared Spectroscopy (FTIR)

It detects molecular interactions and functional groups, which help in validating surface modifications in nanohybrids (Mogha, 2023).

2.4.5.2 X-ray Photoelectron Spectroscopy (XPS)

Here we examine oxidation states and elemental composition, which aid in the refinement of surface properties for enhanced biosensor performance (Thakur et al., 2022).

2.4.6 Thermal Stability

The ability of nanohybrids to resist temperature fluctuations without degradation is determined by thermal stability, which is a prerequisite for long-term use as biosensors.

2.4.6.1 Thermogravimetric Analysis (TGA)

It determines the weight loss caused by thermal degradation and also identifying the operation temperature range of nanohybrids (Purohit et al., 2020).

2.4.6.2 Differential Scanning Calorimetry (DSC)

The phase transformations like melting and crystallization can be monitored to refine the stability of polymer-based nanohybrids (Purohit et al., 2020)

2.4.7 Electrochemical Properties

The efficiency of nanohybrids in biosensors is affected by electrochemical characteristics like conductivity, capacitance, and charge transfer. High conductivity and low resistance improve sensitivity and signal transduction.

2.4.7.1 Cyclic Voltammetry (CV)

It evaluates redox behavior and efficiency of electron transfer in fine-tuning nanohybrids for electrochemical biosensors (Tripathy & Kim, 2018).

2.4.7.2 Electrochemical Impedance Spectroscopy (EIS)

It helps in quantifying capacitance and charge transfer resistance, ensuring nanohybrids are highly conductive with low detection limits (Tripathy & Kim, 2018).

2.5 NANOHYBRIDS IN BIOSENSORS

A sensor can be considered ideal or excellent if it has the following characteristics: high sensitivity, selectivity, resolution, reproducibility, repeatability, good flow, reaction speed, and outstanding detection range. Recently, nanoparticle (NP)-based biosensors have gained popularity due to their wide range of applications in practically every scientific and technical field. In biosensors, NPs are commonly employed to fill the nanoscale gap between the bioreceptor and the converter (Malik et al., 2023).

2.5.1 Role of Nanohybrids in Biosensing

The concurrent use of NPs and electrochemical techniques has produced biosensors with excellent sensitivity and decomposition power. This study outlines the development of NP-based biosensors, including dendrimers, carbon nanotubes (CNTs), noble metal and metal oxide nanoparticles (NPs), nanowires (NWs), nanorods (NRs), and quantum dots (QDs), as well as the current developments in biosensing technology brought about by the growth of nanotechnology (Naresh & Lee, 2021).

Since diseases that are identified early have a higher chance of successful therapies and survival, there is an urgent need to develop a device that can detect or feel the trouble-causing organic or inorganic biomolecule in a live creature. The biosensor was initially created in 1956 by American scientist L.L. Clark. The Clark electrode, also known as the oxygen electrode, was the electrode he utilized in this biosensor to measure the blood's oxygen content.

A biosensor is a type of analytical tool that consists of an amplifier (which amplifies and analyzes the final signal), a transducer (which transforms the observed signal into a useful output), and a bioreceptor (cell, enzyme, antibody, DNA, etc.). The term biosensor was first used by Cammann in 1977. Additionally, an analyte is a substance of interest that must be found (Naresh & Lee, 2021).

2.5.2 Types of Biosensors Using Nanohybrids

In order to improve sensitivity, selectivity, and stability in the detection of biological analytes, nanohybrid biosensors combine nanomaterials. These biosensors come in a variety of forms, each utilizing special qualities of hybrid nanomaterials. An outline of various kinds is provided Section 2.5.2.

2.5.2.1 Electrochemical Biosensors

The development of electrochemical biosensors relies on material science and technology advances. Analyzing the evolution of biosensors across generations, this is how the electrochemical biosensors have improved with different measuring techniques. First-generation biosensors used trapped glucose oxidase, leading to limitations such as deep enzyme sites hindering reagents' access and difficulties with electron transport due to enzyme core placement. Second-generation biosensors introduced oxidation mediators to enhance electron transfer, addressing many issues from the first generation. Third-generation biosensors wire enzymes to electrodes, boosting electron transport efficiency. Fourth-generation biosensors utilize nanomaterials for enhanced fabrication and detection of biomarkers like NH3. Fifth-generation biosensors leverage IoT and AI for real-time monitoring and precise diagnostics, offering potential for continuous healthcare tracking. The integration of AI with biosensors allows remote health monitoring and emergency alerts, promising a smart healthcare system with advanced monitoring capabilities (Sumitha & Xavier, 2023).

Electrochemical biosensors have been built using nanostructures of a variety of materials, including metal, oxide, semiconductor, composite, and nanohybrid nanoparticles. Despite the fact that nanomaterials exhibit a variety of roles in electrochemical biosensing schemes based on their unique characteristics, they have fundamental roles such as support for enzyme immobilization, nanomaterials as mediators, and nanomaterials as signal amplifiers (Batool et al., 2019).

2.5.2.2 Optical Biosensors

Optical biosensors are useful for environmental monitoring, drug development, food control, clinical diagnostics, and biological system detection. They can be combined onto a single chip and provide excellent sensitivity, durability, and dependability. This review presents state-of-the-art optical biosensor technologies, their principles, strengths, weaknesses, and future developments (Chen & Wang, 2020).

The most prevalent kind of biosensor is an optical biosensor. The most popular optical biosensors, surface plasmon resonance (SPR)-based biosensors, such as localized SPR and SPR imaging, are the primary emphasis. Other optical biosensor systems are also detailed, including surface-enhanced Raman scattering biosensors; ellipsometric, reflectometric, and interferometric interference spectroscopy; as well as bioluminescent optical fiber biosensors and evanescent wave fluorescence. The sensitive and specific detection of a variety of analytes, including as viruses, poisons, medications, antibodies, tumor biomarkers, and tumor cells, is made possible by the optical biosensors (Damborský et al., 2016).

2.5.2.3 Piezoelectric Biosensors

Globally, the new coronavirus (COVID-19) pandemic has resulted in significant mortality since late 2019. This pandemic sparked worries and investigation into the identification and management of viral illnesses. High specificity and sensitivity are necessary for a virus to be diagnosed accurately. Piezoelectric sensors are analytical tools that operate on micromechanical transducers with mass sensitivity. Alternate current and voltage are measured to reflect the change in mass caused by the interaction of biological elements and frequency. To mitigate a variety of viral illnesses, antiviral intervention techniques are necessary in addition to diagnosis. Antiviral therapy based on nanomaterials is effective, especially when using carbon, metal, and metal oxide (organic/inorganic) nanoparticles (Bhaskar et al., 2022)

Nowadays, there are three main categories of piezoelectric biomaterials used in dentistry: organic piezoelectric materials, piezoelectric composites, and inorganic piezoelectric materials (such as piezoelectric crystals and ceramics). Piezoelectric polymers are the primary classification for organic piezoelectric materials. Composite materials that combine piezoelectric and non-piezoelectric phases to produce a piezoelectric effect are known as piezoelectric composites. These materials can be prepared using a variety of methods, such as the sol-gel process, electrospinning, hydrothermal method, hot pressing method, and 3D bioprinting (Zeng et al., 2024).

2.5.2.4 Field-Effect Transistor(FET)-Based Biosensors

The field-effect transistor (FET) is regarded as the most promising option for the upcoming generation of biosensors because it is label-free, has straightforward operation, is low cost, has effortless integration, and provides direct detection of biomarkers in liquid environments. Researchers are working to increase the sensitivity of FET biosensors and expand their application scenarios from a variety of approaches in light of the rapidly developing fields of nanotechnology and biotechnology. The iteration and evolution of FET biosensors are reviewed from investigating the sensing mechanism in detecting biomolecules, the response signal type, the sensing performance optimization, and the integration strategy in order to allow researchers to fully comprehend and apply FET biosensors, concentrating on the multidisciplinary technical details (S. Chen et al., 2023).

2.6 NANOHYBRIDS IN BIOELECTRONICS

Bioelectronics is a domain of research where biology meets electronics. It utilizes various types of organic as well as inorganic materials to access the information from the biological systems and for designing new devices. Merging the science of bioelectronics with forms of nanotechnology could become a boon to mankind by offering unique opportunities in biology (Wikipedia Contributors, 2025).

2.6.1 Role of Nanohybrids in Bioelectronics

Nanohybrids consist of organic and inorganic components that are linked by non-covalent interactions at the nanometer level (Jachak et al., 2022). In bioelectronics, these materials have a remarkable ability to improve device performance because of their unique electrical, mechanical, and chemical properties, which are essential for efficient integration with biological environments. Nanobioelectronics is an interdisciplinary field that combines concepts from nanoscience, materials science, biology, and electronics to overcome existing limitations and open up new technological opportunities.

For instance, molecular recognition-based biosensors like those for proteins or DNA use surface-immobilized probes to selectively bind to target biomolecules dissolved in solution. This binding generates an electrical response proportional to the analyte concentration. In addition, bioelectronic interfaces can interface with electrogenic cells, like neurons or cardiac cells, to detect or generate electrical activity by facilitating the transduction between ionic and electronic signals within the interface of the device and biological tissue.

In the center of such devices are nanostructures, which are tasked with detecting, monitoring, and modulating biological processes. Their nanoscale sizes and high surface-to-volume ratios are essential for their operation in biological systems. Since their size is very close to that of biomolecules such as proteins and nucleic acids, nanostructures can interact with biological entities from the subcellular level up to tissues. This compatibility between scales facilitates easy interfacing of nanoelectronic devices and living tissues, which allows development in fields like synthetic tissue engineering and biomedical implants as represented in Figure 2.2. Additionally, the high surface area to volume increases sensitivity, which allows the sensing of trace amounts of analyte and the fabrication of miniature, highly sensitive biosensors (Zhang & Lieber, 2015).

2.6.2 Types of Bioelectronic Devices

2.6.2.1 Biofuel Cells

Biofuel cells are devices that function to convert chemical energy to electrical energy. The energy conversion is facilitated by metabolic reactions and processes that occur in a cell/living thing. They typically use enzymes or microorganisms to break down organic substances, such as glucose or other biomolecules. Although these biofuel cells have many potential applications, the major issues faced with them is the short life span and low power density. Integrating the nanomaterials with the biofuel cells has proven to be the strategy to increase its efficiency. Most biofuel cells (BFCs) developed so far are intended to supply energy for biomedical devices implanted for short-term use. Due to the non-specific orientation of the biocatalyst at the interface, the electron transfer to the planar electrode is quite challenging. Nanomaterials have the ability to facilitate efficient electron transfer between the biocatalyst and the

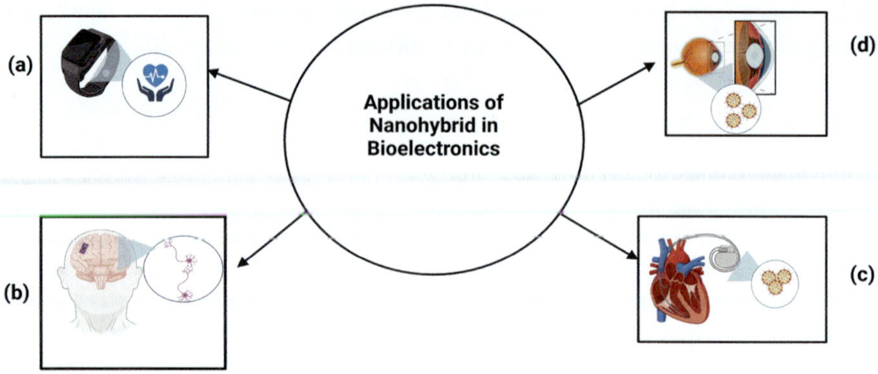

FIGURE 2.2 Applications of Nanohybrids in Bioelectronics: (a) Wearable biosensors: Smartwatch-based health monitoring using nanohybrid sensors. (b) Neural interfaces: Brain implants utilizing nanohybrids for neural signal transmission. (c) Cardiac pacemakers: Nanohybrid-enhanced bioelectronic pacemakers for heart regulation. (d) Artificial retina: Nanohybrid-based retinal implants for vision restoration.

planar electrode by decreasing the gap between the active site (the electron generating region in the biocatalyst) and the electrode. Various carbon nanostructures, conducting polymers, metals, and metal oxides are promising materials for enhancing the current output of BFCs (Mishra et al., 2021).

2.6.2.2 Neural Interfaces

This mismatch makes it difficult for rigid devices to fit properly with the tissue, causing signal instability and physical damage during both insertion and long-term use. When these devices are implanted, the body recognizes them as foreign objects and triggers an inflammatory response. Rigid materials make this response worse, forming a scar around the device that gradually reduces signal quality, hampers the device's ability to record or stimulate, and increases resistance in the electrodes. Constant tissue movement, pulsation, and friction against the rigid electrodes worsen the inflammation. Moreover, these rigid electrodes can't adjust to changes in tissue position, or the changes in tissue volume and density that happen over time due to development, aging, or disease (Boufidis et al., 2025).

2.6.2.3 Implantable Bioelectronics

To analyze various electrophysiological signals for providing treatment for various disorders, certain devices known as implantable bioelectronics evenly adhere to biological tissues and organs such as the heart, nerve, and brain (Xu et al., 2024). Until now, implantable bioelectronics serves three main purposes. They are – alleviating symptoms of chronic diseases, such as with cardiac pacemakers, deep brain stimulators for Parkinson's disease and tremors, and phrenic nerve stimulation for breathing problems; restoring lost or damaged body functions, like with retina prostheses, cochlear implants, and brain-machine interfaces for controlling prosthetic limbs; and monitoring health and tissue conditions, such as with implantable blood pressure sensors and sensors for tracking metabolic changes (Li, Y. et al., 2021). In addition to their diagnostic capabilities, implantable bioelectronic devices can also integrate therapeutic functions for continuous and on-demand treatments. So far, common strategies like electrical stimulation, drug delivery, thermal therapy, and photodynamic therapy have been developed for managing diabetes, promoting wound healing, stimulating neural activity, and treating heart conditions (Xu et al., 2024).

2.6.2.4 Wearable Bioelectronics

Wearable electronic devices are electronic gadgets designed to be integrated into the body, aiming to improve decision-making, sensory perception, and communication. Wearable bioelectronics are made up of fiber, 2D, piezoelectric, and conductive polymers. Wearable electronic devices are crucial in measuring and quantifying human physiological information and daily health assessment (Gürbüz & Ciftci, 2024). Wearable bioelectronics are highly adaptable and compatible with human skin, offering customizable designs. They enable early diagnosis and precise treatment for various conditions, including cardiovascular diseases and diabetes (Y. Zhang et al., 2025). They are also used for monitoring health, tracking fitness, and other biomedical applications. For example, wearable strain sensors can precisely detect body movements and facial expressions due to their ability to conform to the human body. Similarly, wearable pressure sensors provide non-intrusive monitoring of blood pressure and respiration rates. Today, wearable sensors and systems have become more advanced and multifunctional. Innovations in material design, synthesis, and the development of electronic nanomaterials are driving significant progress in wearable electronics and biosensing technologies (Ren et al., 2025).

2.6.3 Electrical and Mechanical Properties of Nanohybrids

2.6.3.1 Mechanical Properties

The properties that define the behavior of a material when they are subjected to the external forces or the environmental stress are called mechanical properties. They include brittleness, plasticity, hardness, ductility, fatigue strength elasticity toughness, rigidity, and yield stress. As we know, nanohybrids are made of organic as well as inorganic components; the inorganic, nonmetallic materials are generally brittle, meaning they tend to break or fracture easily under stress and lack significant flexibility while the organic components are typically more flexible and less prone to brittleness or rigidity, offering a contrast in mechanical behavior compared to inorganic materials (Joudeh & Linke, 2022). The addition of nanoparticles to a composite material can significantly enhance its strength and stiffness. Nanoparticles like carbon nanotubes (CNTs), graphene, and metal oxides possess exceptional mechanical properties that help strengthen the overall material.

Specifically, CNTs are known for their outstanding tensile strength and high modulus, making them particularly effective at improving the mechanical performance of polymer composites. For example, incorporating CNTs into polymer matrices such as epoxy resins has been shown to greatly increase both the tensile strength and Young's modulus of the composite (Rathinavel et al., 2021).

2.6.3.2 Electrical Properties

Organic and inorganic materials can be fused together into nanohybrids that boast multifunctional electrical properties suitable for multiple applications. Amongst the many electrical properties of nanohybrids, enhanced conductivity is a focal point. Conductive nanoparticles such as carbon nanotubes (CNTs), graphene, and metal nanoparticles are responsible for this property. These nanoparticles create conductive pathways in the insulating matrix, thereby enhancing the conductivity of the composite material (Deshmukh et al., 2020). A good example is MXene-PANI, where the combination of MXenes with polyaniline leads to unparalleled performance in electrochemical applications, especially with regard to energy storage systems (Kumar et al., 2024).

2.7 FABRICATION AND STRATEGIES

2.7.1 Self-Assembly and Functionalization

2.7.1.1 Self-Assembly

Self-assembly is the organization of molecules into an ordered structure without external direction. Furthermore, self-assembly is critical to maximize analyte binding and signal amplification. This approach provides a potent option for improving the sensitivity of the sensors, bioelectronic devices, etc. The methods of fabrication of nanomaterials can be classified based on the method used to determine the final material structure. Top-down approaches are those in which the sample is essentially a blank canvas, and an external stimulus is used to write patterns. The top-down method starts with a bulk material and shapes it to form nanostructures. It allows for fine control over positioning and size. On the other hand, bottom-up methods are where the final structure is coded in the material and the precursors self-organize into the required configuration.

In a bottom-up approach we try to build nanostructures from individual atoms and molecules. It relies heavily on self-assembly and helps us create very small and complex structures. Lately, there's been a lot of progress in combining these approaches, where high-level control helps steer and shape lower-level processes (Isaacoff & Brown, 2017).

2.7.1.2 Self-Assembled Quantum Dots

Quantum dots (QDs) are highly fluorescent nanoscale materials used in biosensing for ultra-sensitive detection of biomolecules, enabling advanced medical diagnostics and imaging. QDs often need to be modified to interact with biological molecules or electronic devices. Self-assembled monolayers (SAMs) assist by providing a stable organized layer of molecules that can be attached to QDs, which enhances stability and biocompatibility. Additionally, SAMs easily prevent oxidation of the QD, unwanted interactions, and surface defects, therefore allowing the QDs to have consistent fluorescence and electronic properties. QDs have been linked to nano sensors because they can act as a sensitive and tunable fluorescent probes that facilitate the detection of biomolecules, toxins, and environmental changes. QDs have size-dependent emission and therefore controlled emission and high brightness and stability

TABLE 2.1
Self-Assembly Methods Used in the Making of Quantum Dots

Method	Description	Reference
1. Molecular beam epitaxy (MBE method)	• Most advanced method for semiconductor QD synthesis. • Involves depositing atoms onto solid substances under ultra-high vacuum.	Hao et al., 2023
2. Gravity sedimentation method	• Uses gravity to settle colloidal QDs onto a substrate. • Settling process is influenced by particle size and solvent viscosity.	Hao et al., 2023
3. Colloidal solution method	• Uses the self-assembly properties of colloids to organize QDs in solution. • Self-assembled superstructures SODs exhibit tunable properties.	Hao et al., 2023
4. Electrochemical self-assembly method	• Uses an electric field to induce QD aggregation and self-organization. • Exhibits tunable control over QD assembly.	Hao et al., 2023

make them effective as signal reporters in fluorescence-based sensing systems for optical nano sensors. It had been noted during development that a range of characteristics of QDs makes them desirable to researchers for use in biosensing, medical imaging, drug delivery, and nano photonics. The recent developments made by researchers have focused on self-assembled QDs for their many benefits for optical biosensing applications, nanotechnology (NT), and material science. Although, the process is simply reorganizing QDs into well-organized nanostructures of varying shapes and sizes, researchers use various approaches such as DNA hybridization, surface modifications, and self-assembly to arrange QDs. Scaffolds present in DNA, peptides, and other biologically based biomolecular templates lend themselves to arranging QDs in ordered patterns for use in biosensors and bioelectronics. In biosensing, SAMs help immobilize QDs on sensor surfaces for specific and stable biomolecule detection. In solar cells and LEDs, SAMs help in the ordered assembly of QDs, improving light emission and energy transfer efficiency (Hao et al., 2023). The self-assembly of quantum dots can be achieved through four main techniques, as outlined in Table 2.1. These are: molecular beam epitaxy (MBE), gravity sedimentation, the colloidal solution approach, and electrochemical self-assembly.

Applications of quantum dots

1. **Biomedical imaging and biosensing**
   Quantum dots are in biological systems for fluorescent imaging. Gold nanoparticle-QD hybrids enhance biosensing by combining plasmonic and fluorescent properties. Example: QD-decorated gold nanoparticles improve cancer detection through multiplexed optical signals (Tian et al., 2012).

2. **Energy applications (Solar cells and LEDs)**
   A comprehensive study highlighted that QD-based μ-LEDs provide superior color rendering and are more suitable for ultrahigh-definition displays compared to conventional LCDs and OLEDs (Liu et al., 2020).

QDs combined with plasmonic nanoparticles increase charge separation efficiency in solar cells. Example: Incorporating gold nanoparticles (AuNPs) into organic solar cells (OSCs) enhances light-matter interactions by improving light absorption, scattering, and trapping through plasmonic and fluorescence effect (Phengdaam et al., 2024).

2.7.2 Functionalization

Functionalization is the process of modifying the surface of a biosensor to improve its performance. Addition of different materials or molecules to a biosensor interface relates to modification. The addition of materials is called functionalization of the biosensor interface. Functionalization of biosensor interfaces is an important component of biosensing systems. It is readily apparent that functionalization impacts many important aspects such as sensitivity, selectivity, accuracy, and rapidity (Wang et al., 2023).

2.7.2.1 Precise Detection

Functionalization helps to ensure that sensors only engage with their intended target molecules. When antibodies are utilized, enzyme-based biosensors become more specific – they can clearly detect the target analyte with less interference from false signals. In other words, these functionalization techniques impart the ability to recognize their targets to biosensors with both speed and specificity (Wang et al., 2023).

2.7.2.2 Heightened Sensitivity

Functionalization strengthens the interaction between the nanohybrid and the target. This results in an intense signal, which makes it easier for us to amplify the signal further. Specific chemical groups can facilitate efficient signal transfer – this ensures that the sensor produces a clear and reliable output when it detects its target. Modified interfaces can amplify sensing signals, making it easier to detect target analytes (Wang et al., 2023).

2.7.3 Surface Modification Techniques

Modification of surface includes the alteration of surfaces of sensor materials to achieve desired interactions with their surroundings. Biomolecule immobilization is achieved via adding specific chemical groups onto the surface – this is also called functionalizing. The main goal of surface modifications is to help biosensors detect their target analyte even at a lower concentration. For the effective functioning of these biosensors the surfaces where interactions take place with biomolecules need to be selective. These modifications help reduce non-specific interactions while enhancing the specific interactions. Surface modification techniques serve to functionalize nanomaterial surfaces through attachment of biological entities. Antibodies and aptamers are biological entities. These surface modification techniques fall into four classes. Thiol interacts with noble metal surfaces in 41% of cases. Streptavidin interacts with biotin in 33.7% of cases. Pi stacking interaction accounts for 23.8% of cases. NHS reacts with EDC carbodiimide in 1.4% of cases. These percentages come from a Google Scholar publication database search conducted in July 2017. The period reviewed was 1990 to 2017. Affinity is present between thiol compounds and noble metal surfaces. This affinity assisted in the creation of a self-assembled monolayer. Due to gold's inert nature, alkane chains with different terminal groups can be utilized, enabling the formation of a wide variety of functional groups on gold surfaces (Yüce & Kurt, 2017).

2.8 TYPES OF SURFACE MODIFICATION TECHNIQUES

2.8.1 Plasma Treatment

Plasma treatment uses ionized gas, called plasma, to change material properties. The properties affected are physical, chemical, as well as electrical. Plasma forms when an electric field with much energy is applied to a gas. This application causes the gas molecules to ionize. A combination of ions and free electrons next to reactive elements is the result.

These energetic particles bombard the surface, breaking chemical bonds and introducing specific functional groups. Oxygen plasma treatment improves the sensitivity of electrochemical biosensors by modifying the surface properties of screen-printed carbon electrodes-SPCEs. Oxygen plasma treatment introduces carboxyl groups on SPCE surfaces, improving electrochemical performance and biorecognition capabilities (Osaki et al., 2024).

2.8.2 Electrode Surface Modification

SPCEs were treated with oxygen plasma(O -plasma) at 75 W for 5 seconds. Carboxyl groups were introduced, enhancing hydrophilicity and charge transfer. O -plasma treatment is an effective, simple, and rapid technique to modify SPCE surfaces for biosensing. The method improves antibody attachment, electrochemical performance, and biosensor sensitivity.

2.8.3 Silane Coupling Agents

These are organosilicon compounds used to enhance adhesion between inorganic and organic materials. Silane coupling agents are bifunctional molecules with alkoxy groups that hydrolyze to form silanol groups. These silanols can form covalent bonds with inorganic surfaces (like silica, alumina, or metal oxides) while their organic functional groups interact with polymers. This dual reactivity enables them to effectively bridge inorganic fillers and organic matrices, improving interfacial adhesion (Aziz et al., 2021). The agents also facilitate the development of eco-friendly coatings and additives that enhance durability, reduce defects, and impart desirable properties such as hydrophobicity or controlled wettability (Aziz et al., 2021).

2.8.4 Polymer Coating PEGylation, Polydopamine

Polymer coatings are thin layers of polymeric materials applied to surfaces to enhance protection, functionality, and durability. These coatings are widely used in industries such as biomedicine, electronics, automotive, and aerospace due to their ability to provide corrosion resistance, waterproofing, anti-fouling properties, and controlled surface interactions.

Mussel-inspired surface chemistry (Kang et al., 2010): Drawing inspiration from mytilus edulis foot protein-5 (Mefp-5), which is rich in 3,4-dihydroxy-L-phenylalanine (DOPA), researchers have utilized dopamine's ability to undergo self-polymerization to create a polydopamine coating.

This coating efficiently modifies a variety of materials by improving their adhesion characteristics, making it a flexible method for surface alteration in many applications like microfluidics and lab-on-a-chip devices – It allows for accurate regulation of liquid flow by utilizing patterned wetting properties (Kang et al., 2010).

2.8.5 Self-Assembled Monolayers SAMs

SAMs are particularly stable, meaning they have greater chemical resistance than thiol-based SAMS and are therefore well suited for harsh environments where they can last for many years. Functionalization of SAMs can be done in two primary ways, using pre-functionalized silanes that are crafted before being applied to the substrate or through post deposition surface reactions which enable greater freedom in changing the monolayers after assembly. A number of alteration strategies are used to enhance the effectiveness of these compounds, including: amino acid ($-NH_2$) substitution where halides ($-Br$, $-Cl$) are replaced by some organic group; click chemistry whereby various functional groups are incorporated using highly efficient azide-alkyne cycloaddition; and supramolecular functionalization, which involves interactions of metal complexes with host chemicals.

These surface modifications significantly impact key properties such as wettability and adhesion, where tailored terminal groups enable switching between hydrophobic and hydrophilic states, and conductivity and reactivity, where the introduction of metal complexes enhances electronic properties for potential applications in biosensors and nanodevices (Haensch et al., 2010).

These have various applications such as chemical and biosensors – Functionalized SAMs enable highly sensitive biosensors for medical diagnostics, DNA/protein detection, and environmental monitoring, Nano-engineering and nanotechnology: Surface modifications allow for nanopatterning, smart coatings, and bioactive interfaces, advancing fields like molecular electronics; biomedical and biocompatible surfaces: SAMs can be designed for cell adhesion, protein immobilization, and implant coatings, improving interactions with biological systems (Kulkarni et al., 2022).

2.9 SCALABILITY AND MANUFACTURING CHALLENGES

Moving from prototype to mass-production of these biosensors is complicated to say the least. When discussing the scalability of nanohybrid biosensors, we're essentially addressing the ability to produce these sensors in large quantities, consistently, and cost-effectively, while maintaining their performance. This is a critical factor for their widespread adoption in real-world applications. One major challenge is the change in material properties during scale up. The precise control achievable at the nanometer level often diminishes when transitioning to larger scales (Darwish et al., 2024).

2.9.1 Synthesis Issues

Many nanohybrid synthesis methods are complex, involving multiple steps and specialized equipment. This can make it challenging to scale up production. Precise control over nanoparticle size, shape, and composition is crucial for consistent sensor performance, but achieving these at large scales can be difficult (Rahman et al., 2023).

2.9.2 Surface Functionalization

Ensuring uniform and reproducible surface functionalization across large batches of nanohybrids is a significant challenge. The stability of surface modifications over time and under various conditions is also a concern.

2.9.3 Cost-Effectiveness

The cost of nanomaterials and fabrication processes can be high, which can limit the scalability of nanohybrid biosensors. Developing cost-effective synthesis and fabrication methods is essential for commercialization (Rahman et al., 2023). Industries are reluctant to invest heavily in developing new large-scale manufacturing techniques for nanomaterials without guaranteed profits. This creates a gap between laboratory research and practical industrial applications (AZoNano, 2022).

2.9.4 Integration and Packaging

Integrating nanohybrid biosensors with electronic readout systems and packaging them for practical use can be challenging. Developing robust and reliable packaging methods is essential for ensuring sensor stability and longevity. Effective transition from research to commercialization hinges on scalable manufacturing, which promotes cost reduction and better reproducibility (Akhlaghi et al., 2024).

2.10 CONCLUSION

Nanohybrids have emerged as a revolutionary class of materials in biosensor and bioelectronic applications due to their exceptional physicochemical properties, enhanced sensitivity, and multifunctionality. By integrating various nanomaterials such as metal nanoparticles, carbon-based nanostructures, and conducting polymers, nanohybrids offer synergistic advantages that can improve signal transduction, biocompatibility, and stability in biosensing platforms. The advancements in nanohybrid biosensors have contributed to numerous advances in disease diagnosis, disease control, environmental monitoring and real-time biomolecular detection and showing better performance than their conventional sensor technologies. As such, their application in bioelectronics has created new opportunities for wearable and implantable devices allowing direct connections between biological systems and electronic circuits. Despite these advancements, challenges such as scalability, reproducibility, and long-term stability remain a constant challenge in translating nanohybrid biosensors from laboratory research to daily life and commercial applications. Future research should focus on refining synthesis techniques, enhancing functionalization methods, and incorporating artificial intelligence for smarter data analysis. These efforts will help improve the precision, reliability, and overall stability of these devices. In conclusion, nanohybrids offer tremendous potential to transform the field of biosensors and bioelectronics, paving the way for highly efficient, compact, and affordable diagnostic tools. Ongoing interdisciplinary collaboration and research will be essential to fully realize their promise in real-world biomedical and industrial applications.

REFERENCES

Aich, N., Plazas-Tuttle, J., Lead, J. R., & Saleh, N. B. (2014). A critical review of nanohybrids: Synthesis, applications and environmental implications. *Environmental Chemistry*, *11*(6), 609. https://doi.org/10.1071/en14127

Akhlaghi, A. A., Kaur, H., Adhikari, B. R., & Soleymani, L. (2024). Editors' choice – Challenges and opportunities for developing electrochemical biosensors with commercialization potential in the point-of-care diagnostics market. *ECS Sensors Plus*, *3*(1), 011601. https://doi.org/10.1149/2754-2726/ad304a

Ananikov, V. P. (2019). Organic–Inorganic hybrid nanomaterials. *Nanomaterials*, *9*(9), 1197. https://doi.org/10.3390/nano9091197

Aziz, T., Ullah, A., Fan, H., Jamil, M. I., Khan, F. U., Ullah, R., Iqbal, M., Ali, A., & Ullah, B. (2021). Recent progress in silane coupling agent with its emerging applications. *Journal of Polymers and the Environment*, *29*(11), 3427–3443. https://doi.org/10.1007/s10924-021-02142-1

Batool, R., Rhouati, A., Nawaz, M. H., Hayat, A., & Marty, J. L. (2019). A review of the construction of Nano-Hybrids for electrochemical biosensing of glucose. *Biosensors*, *9*(1), 46. https://doi.org/10.3390/bios9010046

Bhaskar, R., Han, S. S., & Ramasamy, M. S. (2022). Piezoelectric biosensors and nanomaterials-based therapeutics for coronavirus and other viruses: A mini-review. *Current Topics in Medicinal Chemistry*, *23*(2), 115–127. https://doi.org/10.2174/1568026623666221226091907

Boufidis, D., Garg, R., Angelopoulos, E., Cullen, D. K., & Vitale, F. (2025). Bio-inspired electronics: Soft, biohybrid, and "living" neural interfaces. *Nature Communications*, *16*(1). https://doi.org/10.1038/s41467-025-57016-0

Chen, C., & Wang, J. (2020). Optical biosensors: An exhaustive and comprehensive review. *The Analyst*, *145*(5), 1605–1628. https://doi.org/10.1039/c9an01998g

Chen, S., Sun, Y., Fan, X., Xu, Y., Chen, S., Zhang, X., Man, B., Yang, C., & Du, J. (2023). Review on two-dimensional material-based field-effect transistor biosensors: Accomplishments, mechanisms, and perspectives. *Journal of Nanobiotechnology*, *21*(1). https://doi.org/10.1186/s12951-023-01898-z

Cheng, Q., Li, Z., Sun, Y., & Zhang, X. (2019). Controlled synthesis of a core-shell nanohybrid for effective multimodal image-guided combined photothermal/photodynamic therapy of tumors. *NPG Asia Materials*, *11*(1). https://doi.org/10.1038/s41427-019-0164-4

Chi, H., Gu, Y., Xu, T., & Cao, F. (2017, February). Multifunctional organic-inorganic hybrid nanoparticles and nanosheets based on chitosan derivative and layered double hydroxide: Cellular uptake mechanism and application for topical ocular drug delivery. *International Journal of Nanomedicine*, *12*, 1607–1620. https://doi.org/10.2147/IJN.S129311. PMID: 28280329; PMCID: PMC5339005.

Choi, G., Rejinold, N. S., Piao, H., & Choy, J. H. (2021, March). Inorganic-inorganic nanohybrids for drug delivery, imaging and photo-therapy: Recent developments and future scope. *Chemical Science*, *12*(14), 5044–5063. https://doi.org/10.1039/d0sc06724e. PMID: 34168768; PMCID: PMC8179608

Damborský, P., Švitel, J., & Katrlík, J. (2016). Optical biosensors. *Essays in Biochemistry*, *60*(1), 91–100. https://doi.org/10.1042/ebc20150010

Darwish, M. A., Abd-Elaziem, W., Elsheikh, A., & Zayed, A. A. (2024). Advancements in nanomaterials for nanosensors: A comprehensive review. *Nanoscale Advances*, *6*(16), 4015–4046. https://doi.org/10.1039/d4na00214h

Deshmukh, M. A., Park, S., Kang, B., & Ha, T. (2020). Carbon nanohybrids for advanced electronic applications. *Physica Status Solidi (A)*, *217*(17). https://doi.org/10.1002/pssa.202000199

Godja, N., & Munteanu, F. (2024b). Hybrid Nanomaterials: A brief overview of versatile solutions for sensor technology in healthcare and environmental applications. *Biosensors*, *14*(2), 67. https://doi.org/10.3390/bios14020067

Gomez-Romero, P., Pokhriyal, A., Rueda-García, D., Bengoa, L. N., & González-Gil, R. M. (2023). Hybrid materials: A metareview. *Chemistry of Materials*, *36*(1), 8–27. https://doi.org/10.1021/acs.chemmater.3c01878

Gürbüz, B., & Ciftci, F. (2024). Bio-electric-electronics and tissue engineering applications of MXenes wearable materials: A review. *Chemical Engineering Journal*, *489*, 151230. https://doi.org/10.1016/j.cej.2024.151230

Haensch, C., Hoeppner, S., & Schubert, U. S. (2010). ChemInForm Abstract: Chemical modification of self-assembled silane based monolayers by surface reactions. *ChemInform*, *41*(42). https://doi.org/10.1002/chin.201042250

Hao, Q., Lv, H., Ma, H., Tang, X., & Chen, M. (2023). Development of self-assembly methods on quantum dots. *Materials*, *16*(3), 1317. https://doi.org/10.3390/ma16031317

Isaacoff, B. P., & Brown, K. A. (2017). Progress in top-down control of bottom-up assembly. *Nano Letters*, *17*(11), 6508–6510. https://doi.org/10.1021/acs.nanolett.7b04479

Ivashchyshyn, F., Grygorchak, I., Stakhira, P., & Cherpak, V. (2012). Intercalate nanohybrid structure of non-organic/organic semiconductor configuration: Formation, properties and application. *Journal of Experimental Nanoscience*, *9*(7), 678–688. https://doi.org/10.1080/17458080.2012.692487

Jachak, R., Chahande, S., Thaware, J., & Mahakhode, R. (2022). Strategies of nanotechnology as a defense system in plants. In *Elsevier eBooks* (pp. 227–248). https://doi.org/10.1016/b978-0-323-88535-5.00001-9

Jeon, N., Kim, L., Choi, S. G., Lee, H., Min, J. Y., Kim, H. M., Han, E. H., & Lee, E. (2025). Self-assembled peptide-gold nanoparticle 1d nanohybrids functionalized with GHK tripeptide for enhanced wound-healing and photothermal therapy. *ACS Applied Materials & Interfaces*. https://doi.org/10.1021/acsami.4c21924

Jin, W., & Park, D. (2019). Functional layered double hydroxide nanohybrids for biomedical imaging. *Nanomaterials*, *9*(10), 1404. https://doi.org/10.3390/nano9101404

Joudeh, N., & Linke, D. (2022). Nanoparticle classification, physicochemical properties, characterization, and applications: A comprehensive review for biologists. *Journal of Nanobiotechnology*, *20*(1). https://doi.org/10.1186/s12951-022-01477-8

Kang, S. M., You, I., Cho, W. K., Shon, H. K., Lee, T. G., Choi, I. S., Karp, J. M., & Lee, H. (2010). One-Step modification of superhydrophobic surfaces by a Mussel-Inspired polymer coating. *Angewandte Chemie International Edition*, *49*(49), 9401–9404. https://doi.org/10.1002/anie.201004693

Khannyra, S., Luna, M., Gil, M. A., Addou, M., & Mosquera, M. J. (2022). Self-cleaning durability assessment of TiO2/SiO2 photocatalysts coated concrete: Effect of indoor and outdoor conditions on the photocatalytic activity. *Building and Environment*, *211*, 108743. https://doi.org/10.1016/j.buildenv.2021.108743

Komarala, E. P., Tyagi, H., Thiyagarajan, S., Pradhan, L., Aslam, M., & Bahadur, D. (2017). NIR absorbing Au nanoparticle decorated layered double hydroxide nanohybrids for photothermal therapy and fluorescence imaging of cancer cells. *Journal of Materials Chemistry B*, *5*(21), 3852–3861. https://doi.org/10.1039/c7tb00015d

Kulkarni, M. B., Ayachit, N. H., & Aminabhavi, T. M. (2022). Recent advancements in nanobiosensors: Current trends, challenges, applications, and future scope. *Biosensors*, *12*(10), 892. https://doi.org/10.3390/bios12100892

Kumar, M., Gautam, M. K., Singh, K., & Hur, S. H. (2024). A comprehensive review of the MXene-PANI nanohybrids: Preparation, characterization, and electrochemical performances for supercapacitor applications. *Journal of Industrial and Engineering Chemistry*, *142*, 141–156. https://doi.org/10.1016/j.jiec.2024.08.016

Li, Y., Li, N., De Oliveira, N., & Wang, S. (2021). Implantable bioelectronics toward long-term stability and sustainability. *Matter*, *4*(4), 1125–1141. https://doi.org/10.1016/j.matt.2021.02.001

Lin, M., Hong, S., Ding, J., & Liu, C. (2024b). Organic porous materials and their nanohybrids for Next-Generation thermoelectric application. *ACS Applied Materials & Interfaces*. https://doi.org/10.1021/acsami.4c12729

Liu, Z., Lin, C., Hyun, B., Sher, C., Lv, Z., Luo, B., Jiang, F., Wu, T., Ho, C., Kuo, H., & He, J. (2020). Micro-light-emitting diodes with quantum dots in display technology. *Light Science & Applications*, *9*(1). https://doi.org/10.1038/s41377-020-0268-1

Lonkar, S. P., Kutlu, B., Leuteritz, A., & Heinrich, G. (2012). Nanohybrids of phenolic antioxidant intercalated into MgAl-layered double hydroxide clay. *Applied Clay Science*, *71*, 8–14. https://doi.org/10.1016/j.clay.2012.10.009

Mackenzie, J. D., & Bescher, E. P. (2018b). Mechanical properties of organic–inorganic hybrids. In *Springer eBooks* (pp. 1547–1563). https://doi.org/10.1007/978-3-319-32101-1_45

Malik, S., Singh, J., Goyat, R., Saharan, Y., Chaudhry, V., Umar, A., Ibrahim, A. A., Akbar, S., Ameen, S., & Baskoutas, S. (2023). Nanomaterials-based biosensor and their applications: A review. *Heliyon*, *9*(9), e19929. https://doi.org/10.1016/j.heliyon.2023.e19929

Mishra, A., Bhatt, R., Bajpai, J., & Bajpai, A. (2021). Nanomaterials based biofuel cells: A review. *International Journal of Hydrogen Energy*, *46*(36), 19085–19105. https://doi.org/10.1016/j.ijhydene.2021.03.024

Mobin, R., Rangreez, T. A., Chisti, H. T. N., Inamuddin, N., & Rezakazemi, M. (2019). Organic-Inorganic hybrid materials and their applications. In *Polymers and polymeric composites* (pp. 1135–1156). https://doi.org/10.1007/978-3-319-95987-0_33

Mogha, N. K. (2023). *Graphene oxide-based nanohybrids as pesticide biosensors*. IntechOpen.

Naresh, V., & Lee, N. (2021). A review on biosensors and recent development of nanostructured materials-enabled biosensors. *Sensors*, *21*(4), 1109. https://doi.org/10.3390/s21041109

Osaki, S., Saito, M., Nagai, H., & Tamiya, E. (2024). Surface modification of screen-printed carbon electrode through oxygen plasma to enhance biosensor sensitivity. *Biosensors*, *14*(4), 165. https://doi.org/10.3390/bios14040165

Phengdaam, A., Phetsang, S., Jonai, S., Shinbo, K., Kato, K., & Baba, A. (2024). Gold nanostructures/quantum dots for the enhanced efficiency of organic solar cells. *Nanoscale Advances*, *6*(14), 3494–3512. https://doi.org/10.1039/d4na00016a

Purohit, B., Vernekar, P. R., Shetti, N. P., & Chandra, P. (2020). Biosensor nanoengineering: Design, operation, and implementation for biomolecular analysis. *Sensors International*, *1*, 100040.

Radhakrishnan, S., Das, P. P., Alam, A., Dwivedi, S. P., & Chaudhary, V. (2024). Mechanical, thermal, and electrical properties of 2D nanomaterials for advanced applications. *Proceedings of the Institution of Mechanical Engineers Part C Journal of Mechanical Engineering Science*, *238*(17), 8739–8755. https://doi.org/10.1177/09544062241245018

Rahman, M., Islam, K. S., Dip, T. M., Chowdhury, M. F. M., Debnath, S. R., Hasan, S. M. M., Sakib, M. S., Saha, T., Padhye, R., & Houshyar, S. (2023). A review on nanomaterial-based additive manufacturing: Dynamics in properties, prospects, and challenges. *Progress in Additive Manufacturing*, *9*(4), 1197–1224. https://doi.org/10.1007/s40964-023-00514-8

Rando, G., Sfameni, S., Galletta, M., Drommi, D., Cappello, S., & Plutino, M. R. (2022b). Functional nanohybrids and nanocomposites development for the removal of environmental pollutants and bioremediation. *Molecules*, *27*(15), 4856. https://doi.org/10.3390/molecules27154856

Rathinavel, S., Priyadharshini, K., & Panda, D. (2021). A review on carbon nanotube: An overview of synthesis, properties, functionalization, characterization, and the application. *Materials Science and Engineering B*, *268*, 115095. https://doi.org/10.1016/j.mseb.2021.115095

Ren, Y., Zhang, F., Yan, Z., & Chen, P. (2025). Wearable bioelectronics based on emerging nanomaterials for telehealth applications. *Device*, 100676. https://doi.org/10.1016/j.device.2024.100676

Sanchez, C., Belleville, P., Popall, M., & Nicole, L. (2011). Applications of advanced hybrid organic–inorganic nanomaterials: From laboratory to market. *Chemical Society Reviews*, *40*(2), 696. https://doi.org/10.1039/c0cs00136h

Sanchez, C., De A. A. Soler-Illia, G. J., Ribot, F., Lalot, T., Mayer, C. R., & Cabuil, V. (2001). Designed hybrid organic–inorganic nanocomposites from functional nanobuilding blocks. *Chemistry of Materials*, *13*(10), 3061–3083. https://doi.org/10.1021/cm011061e

Sefadi, J. S., & Mochane, M. J. (2021). Multifunctional 3D hybrid nanomaterials for clean energy technologies. In *Springer eBooks* (pp. 1463–1492). https://doi.org/10.1007/978-3-030-40513-7_43

Singh, R., & Bhateria, R. (2020). Core–shell nanostructures: A simplest two-component system with enhanced properties and multiple applications. *Environmental Geochemistry and Health*, *43*(7), 2459–2482. https://doi.org/10.1007/s10653-020-00766-1

Sinha, S., Kim, H., & Robertson, A. (2021). Preparation and application of 0D-2D nanomaterial hybrid heterostructures for energy applications. *Materials Today Advances*, *12*, 100169. https://doi.org/10.1016/j.mtadv.2021.100169

Soto, D., & Orozco, J. (2022b). Hybrid nanobioengineered nanomaterial-based electrochemical biosensors. *Molecules*, *27*(12), 3841. https://doi.org/10.3390/molecules27123841

Sreejith, S., Huong, T. T. M., Borah, P., & Zhao, Y. (2015). Organic-inorganic nanohybrids for fluorescence, photoacoustic, and Raman bioimaging. *Science Bulletin*, *60*(7), 665–678.

Stavrinidou, E., & Proctor, C. M. (2022a). Introduction. In *Introduction to Bioelectronics: Materials, Devices, and Applications* (pp. 1–16). https://doi.org/10.1063/9780735424470_001

Sumitha, & Xavier, T. (2023). Recent advances in electrochemical biosensors – A brief review. *Hybrid Advances*, *2*, 100023. https://doi.org/10.1016/j.hybadv.2023.100023

Thakur, M., Wang, B., & Verma, M. L. (2022). Development and applications of nanobiosensors for sustainable agricultural and food industries. *Environmental Technology & Innovation*, *26*, 102371.

Tian, J., Zhou, L., Zhao, Y., Wang, Y., Peng, Y., & Zhao, S. (2012). Multiplexed detection of tumor markers with multicolor quantum dots based on fluorescence polarization immunoassay. *Talanta*, *92*, 72–77. https://doi.org/10.1016/j.talanta.2012.01.051

Tripathy, N., & Kim, D.-H. (2018). Metal oxide modified ZnO nanomaterials for biosensor applications. *Nano Convergence*, *5*, 27.

Venkadajapathy, V. R. T., & Sivaperumal, S. (2024). Tailoring functional two-dimensional nanohybrids: A comprehensive approach for enhancing photocatalytic remediation. *Ecotoxicology and Environmental Safety*, *275*, 116221. https://doi.org/10.1016/j.ecoenv.2024.116221

Wang, F., Xie, Y., Zhu, W., & Wei, T. (2023). Recent advances in functionalization strategies for biosensor interfaces, especially the emerging Electro-Click: A review. *Chemosensors*, *11*(9), 481. https://doi.org/10.3390/chemosensors11090481

Wang, Z., Hu, T., Liang, R., & Wei, M. (2020b). Application of zero-dimensional nanomaterials in biosensing. *Frontiers in Chemistry*, *8*. https://doi.org/10.3389/fchem.2020.00320

Wikipedia Contributors. (2025, March 18). *Bioelectronics*. Wikipedia. https://en.wikipedia.org/wiki/Bioelectronics

Xu, K., Ko, S. H., & Chen, J. (2024). Advances in wearable and implantable bioelectronics for precision medicine. *Bio-Design and Manufacturing*, *7*(4), 383–387. https://doi.org/10.1007/s42242-024-00302-5

Yoon, J., Lim, J., Shin, M., Lee, S.-N., & Choi, J.-W. (2021). Graphene/MoS_2 nanohybrids for biosensors. *Materials*, *14*(518).

Yüce, M., & Kurt, H. (2017). How to make nanobiosensors: Surface modification and characterisation of nanomaterials for biosensing applications. *RSC Advances*, *7*(78), 49386–49403. https://doi.org/10.1039/c7ra10479k

Zare, E. N., Agarwal, T., Zarepour, A., Pinelli, F., Zarrabi, A., Rossi, F., Ashrafizadeh, M., Maleki, A., Shahbazi, M., Maiti, T. K., Varma, R. S., Tay, F. R., Hamblin, M. R., Mattoli, V., & Makvandi, P. (2021). Electroconductive multi-functional polypyrrole composites for biomedical applications. *Applied Materials Today*, *24*, 101117. https://doi.org/10.1016/j.apmt.2021.101117

Zeng, K., Lin, Y., Liu, S., Wang, Z., & Guo, L. (2024). Applications of piezoelectric biomaterials in dental Treatments: A review of recent advancements and future prospects. *Materials Today Bio*, *29*, 101288. https://doi.org/10.1016/j.mtbio.2024.101288

Zhang, A., & Lieber, C. M. (2015). Nano-bioelectronics. *Chemical Reviews*, *116*(1), 215–257. https://doi.org/10.1021/acs.chemrev.5b00608

Zhang, Q., Wang, Y., Zhang, B., Zhao, K., He, P., & Huang, B. (2017). 3D superelastic graphene aerogel-nanosheet hybrid hierarchical nanostructures as high-performance supercapacitor electrodes. *Carbon*, *127*, 449–458. https://doi.org/10.1016/j.carbon.2017.11.037

Zhang, Y., Chen, H., & Song, Y. (2025). Wearable healthcare monitoring and therapeutic bioelectronics. *Wearable Electronics*. https://doi.org/10.1016/j.wees.2024.12.004

Zhu, S., Sheng, J., Chen, Y., Ni, J., & Li, Y. (2020). Carbon nanotubes for flexible batteries: Recent progress and future perspective. *National Science Review*, *8*(5). https://doi.org/10.1093/nsr/nwaa261

3 Nanohybrids for Disease Diagnosis Applications

P. Paul Vijay, Balla Sai Mrudula, and Srinivas Kunta

3.1 INTRODUCTION

Complex materials made up of both inorganic and organic polymers are known as nanohybrids. Together with organic components, a variety of materials, including silica, alumina, bentonite, and zirconia, aid in the production of nanohybrids. The fundamental idea or process underlying the creation of nanohybrids is understood to be hydrogen bonding or ionic contact between the inorganic component and organic polymer (Chujo, 2007). Several theranostic nanoplatforms have been developed thus far by combining effective therapeutic approaches with high-resolution diagnostic methods that leverage the distinct physicochemical, biological, optical, magnetic, thermal, and radioactive characteristics of nanomaterials (Dai et al., 2017). The current hotspot in this field of study is the development of nanoplatforms with high accuracy, high efficiency, outstanding biocompatibility, and minimally invasive tumor detection and therapy. Self-assembled organic/metal ion nanohybrids, which are made up of two parts – metal ions and organic building blocks – have a number of special qualities that make them ideal for use in the development of tailored nanomedicine to combat cancer. Research on nanomedicine has prepared the way for a significant and promising role in COVID-19 disease diagnosis, treatment, prevention, and vaccine (Vahedifard & Chakravarthy, 2021). Recent developments in nano-biotechnology have revealed amazing potential for conjugate binding between inorganic NPs and polysaccharide polymers. Beneficial capabilities and qualities are produced by improving the engineering of inorganic nanoparticles' surfaces with organic molecules.

3.2 PROPERTIES OF NANOHYBRIDS USED IN MEDICINE AND BIOTECHNOLOGY

The generic fabrication techniques for different metal/organic ion nanohybrids are also provided as a crucial component. In an effort to create novel, adaptable types of self-assembled metal/organic ion nanohybrids, organic molecules have been altered with a variety of unique functional groups to give coordination sites for metal ions due to their positive charge. The types of organic blocks are divided into two categories: biomolecules and synthesized organic molecules. The creation of metal ion-coordinated nanohybrids with a variety of nanostructures and distinctive

DOI: 10.1201/9781003563723-3

optical, electrical, and magnetic properties is made possible by the high designability and controllable production of synthetic organic molecules. N, O, S, P, and other elements that have a significant electron transfer capacity and can give metal ions coordination sites are typically found in eligible organic ligands. In order to create organic/metal ion nanohybrids, a variety of synthetic organic compounds have been used recently. Metallic organic frameworks (MOFs) with a variety of characteristics and special qualities are readily obtainable because of (K. Zhang et al., 2020) the diversity and selectivity of metal ions and organic building blocks. The broad distribution of apertures includes macropores, mesopores, and micropores. Because of their large rigid/flexible skeletons and highly adjustable specific surface areas, MOFs are excellent choices for creating multipurpose diagnostic tools. Novel MOFs with inherent physicochemical characteristics have been created using a variety of functionalized organic compounds. For instance, porphyrins and their derivatives have been employed as photodynamic agents for cancer treatment when they create MOFs by bonding with metal ions (Lu et al., 2015). Zeolitic imidazolate MOFs (ZIF-8) were created using imidazolate-modified organic molecules and Zn^{2+} ions. These MOFs could react to the acidic tumor microenvironment (TME) and breakdown for effective drug release (H. Wang et al., 2019). Meanwhile, MOFs can be equipped with unique features, such Mn^{2+} for MRI6 and Fe^{2+} for cancer chemodynamic treatment (CDT), in conjunction with functional inorganic metal ions (Sun et al., 2019). Typically, biomolecules give organic/metal ion nanohybrids exceptional stability and inherent biocompatibility, particularly in biological systems (Huang et al., 2019). As a class of essential functional macromolecules, proteins take part in a variety of biological processes, including as electron transfer, enzymatic reactions, and metal transport through the ability of coordinated metal ions or metal complexes (C. Ma et al., 2020). Metal coordination in protein scaffolds has produced a variety of protein-based organic/metal ion nanohybrids, also known as artificial metalloproteins, which support the development of novel nanoplatforms for bio-related applications (L. Wang et al., 2018) Immobilized metal ions with imaging properties have been used to create a number of tumor-targeted protein-based nanohybrids that serve as contrast agents for cancer diagnostics. Ferritin and hemoglobin, two proteins with internal gaps, can also be used as templates to build up iron ions and create nanohybrids that can stop free ferric ions from oxidizing (B. Ma et al., 2019). One of the most alluring choices for self-assemblage nanomaterials is DNA, a stunning natural biomolecule with remarkable properties like strong mechanical stiffness of non-single strand, relatively excellent physicochemical stability, and nanometric size. The "Watson–Crick" base-pairing principle is a specific noncovalent hydrogen bonding mechanism that allows a single DNA strand to generate unique double, triple, quadruple, or branched structures (Georgiades et al., 2010). Consequently, it is possible to create programmable self-assembled nanoscale networks. The "metal–base pair" is created when metal ions and/or metal complexes are trapped inside the DNA double helix replace the hydrogen bonding "Watson–Crick" base pairs (B. Liu et al., 2019).Various monovalent and multivalent metal ions, including Ag^{+}, Mn^{2+}, Hg^{2+}, Zn^{2+}, Gd^{3+} , and others, have been used up to this point to create metal ion/DNA nanohybrids by bridging the DNA double helix's skeletons. These nanohybrids have great potential for the development of innovative cancer theranostics systems because of their high rigidity/flexibility, strong stability, superior biocompatibility, and effective tumor-targeting ability.

3.3 VARIOUS METHODS OF SYNTHESIZING NANOHYBRIDS

3.3.1 Physical Techniques to Create Nanoparticles

Radiolytic method: Bimetallic nanoparticles have been synthesized in unique ways from metal clusters produced by the radiation process. Metal ions undergo radiolytic reduction in an aqueous media during a specific process. In order to create NPs using the radiolysis approach, the metal ions are typically reduced using the reducing radicals generated during the process (Redjala et al., 2006).

Sputtering method: In order to produce the desired NPs, this technique uses high energy to blast tiny particles of the material of choice from its surface utilizing gas ions or gaseous plasma over the target metal surfaces (Ferrando et al., 2008; Mujahid et al., 2022). High purity NPs are produced using this method, but the energy required is excessive, and it is challenging to regulate the shape of the NPs that are created throughout the procedure (Sharma et al., 2019).

Sonochemical synthesis: This method relies on the generation of ultrasonic waves within the reaction chamber, which raises the temperature and pressure. At a very fast pace of reaction, it produces minuscule nanoparticles. Small, nanoscale bubbles have formed as a result of the ultrasound, which causes the creation of void NPs (Fujimoto et al., 2001; Patil & Bhanage, 2016; R. Wang et al., 2013; Xu et al., 2013).

3.3.2 Synthesizing of Nanoparticles by Chemical Methods

Hydrothermal method: The hydrothermal method of NP synthesis requires an aqueous solution with a high temperature and high vapor pressure. This technique aids in tracking the development of NPs as well as their physical and chemical characteristics. However, this method's drawbacks include the need for expensive equipment and the creation of high temperatures (Byrappa & Yoshimura, 2001; Gan et al., 2020).

Electrochemical synthesis: Because of the composite reaction, the two main applications related to this NPs manufacturing process are in industries and power. The metal precursor dissolved in the solution at the metallic anode electrode due to a reduction process, and metallic nanoparticles were produced at the cathode.

Chemical Precipitation: By altering the pH, adding a precipitation material or electrooxidizing potential that produces solids, and producing excessively saturated conditions in the solution, the chemical precipitation technique of NPs synthesis renders the soluble components soluble. The primary use of this a single-step technology, which is extensively employed in the water purification process, is the large-scale manufacturing of NPs (Dahman, 2017; Ojovan et al., 2019).

3.3.3 Biological Synthesis of Nanohybrids

Their usage in clinical and biomedical contexts may be severely limited by the costly chemical and physical processes required for the conventional manufacturing of nanoparticles, which frequently include dangerous substances with potential dangers like cytotoxicity, environmental toxicity, and carcinogenicity (Biazar et al., 2011). Consequently, there is currently a lot of interest in creating eco-friendly, durable, biologically compatible, and environmentally acceptable methods for creating nanoparticles (Jain et al., 2011; Kulkarni & Muddapur, 2014). Using an environmentally benign green chemistry-based method, biosynthesis uses both unicellular and multicellular biological entities, including actinomycetes (Ahmad et al., 2003b; Sastry et al., 2003), bacteria (Husseiny et al., 2007; Klaus-Joerger et al., 2001; Lengke & Southam, 2006; Roh et al., 2001), fungi (Ahmad et al., 2003a, 2005; Bhainsa & D'Souza, 2006; Mukherjee et al., 2001), plants (Kumar et al., 2011; Philip, 2010), viruses (Lee et al., 2002), and yeast (Dameron et al., 1989; Gericke & Pinches, 2006; Kowshik et al., 2003). It can be thought of as a bottom-up process whereby the reduction or oxidation of metallic ions is carried out by the enzymes, proteins, and carbohydrates that the microbe secretes, resulting in the formation of nanoparticles (Prabhu & Poulose, 2012). Plant-based nanoparticle synthesis is also a rather straightforward and advantageous method (Iravani, 2011; Thakkar et al., 2010) because it doesn't require any unique, intricate, multi-step processes like isolation, culture preparation, and culture maintenance. Furthermore, it is relatively easy to increase the production of large amounts of nanoparticles through synthesis in plants, which is quicker, more economical, and more straightforward (Bar et al., 2009; Shankar et al., 2004). The decrease and subsequent stabilization of the metallic ions are believed to be greatly facilitated by plant extracts including proteins, carbohydrates, terpenoids, phenolic acids, bioactive alkaloids, and polyphenols (Castro et al., 2011; Marshall et al., 2007).

These active biomolecules vary in quantity and composition among plants, and it is thought that the ensuing interactions with aqueous metal ions are what primarily cause the variety of nanoparticle shapes and sizes that are generated (X. Li et al., 2011). One important strategy to reduce the negative effects of traditional methods of creating nanoparticles is through green synthesis, which is being utilized more and more in both industry and laboratories. When it comes to plant extracts, different plant species have different methods for creating nanoparticles. The diversity of biological phenomena, from microbes to plants, means that a major portion of this topic is yet unknown and unexplored. To assess and comprehend the true plant-dependent mechanisms, more research is required.

3.4 APPLICATIONS OF NANOHYBRIDS IN DIAGNOSING DISEASES

3.4.1 Biosensing

Sensitive physiological species type identification and dynamic monitoring for shifts in their concentrations in vitro or in vivo can help diagnose disease and identify the underlying pathogenic mechanisms. The development of a variety of biosensors that can recognize biomarkers is essential for the creation of biomedicines and illness treatment plans. Because of the exceptional loading capacity, ease of functionalization, outstanding biocompatibility, and stability of the developed organic/metal ion nanohybrids, these nanohybrid-based biosensors demonstrate extraordinary high sensitivity, strong specificity, and low limit of detection.

3.4.2 Detecting Biomacromolecules

Nucleic acids and proteins are crucial regulators of physiological and cellular functions, causing numerous illnesses. Organic/metal ion nanohybrid-based biosensors detect these molecules through chemical bonding, p–p stacking, or electrostatic interactions. For instance, UiO-66 MOF fluorescent nanohybrids customized with three different kinds of DNA hairpin strands may detect numerous DNA molecules in a homogenous solution. Because of UiO-66 MOF's high loading capacity, considerably stronger fluorescence signals were observed when the targets were identified using DNA hairpin probes. The DNA-responsive MOF nanohybrids demonstrated selective discriminating of single-base mismatch and sensitive target detection with a low LOD of 20 fM (J. Li et al., 2017). TK1 and surviving mRNA were quickly and accurately imaged in HepG2 and HL7702 cells using MOF nanohybrids functionalized with DNA amplifiers. particular to metal ions. Due to its high catalytic efficiency, designability, and adaptability, DNAzyme is a novel enzyme-free detection method that has tremendous potential for developing a variety of biosensors for the detection of biomolecules (Meng et al., 2018). MicroRNAs (miRNAs) are a family of endogenous small-molecule RNAs that may be utilized as biomarkers for diagnosis and prognosis.

3.4.3 Detecting Biomicromolecules

In addition to being a crucial energy molecule for cellular metabolism, blood sugar is also believed to be a biomarker for illness detection. A polystyrene electrospun optical fiber membrane doped with an iridium metal ion complex was utilized to produce a quick and incredibly sensitive optical biosensor. Additionally, the nanohybrids were functionalized using glucose oxidases (GOD/EOF). Despite low glucose concentrations, it showed a substantial increase in yellow fluorescence (562 nm) when glucose was present. The sensing platform outperformed existing documented glucose biosensors with a low detection limit of $1.0 \times 10{-}^{10}$ M and a broad concentration range of $3.0 \times 10{-}^{10}$ M to $1.3 \times 10{-}^{10}$ M. One significant class of biomolecules found in living things is H2S. Eosin-Y was used as an indicator in the metal indicator displacement method that created the H2S sensing platform. The high selectivity was confirmed by the unassisted eye by separating biological phosphates, volatile sulfur species, reactive forms of nitrogen, and other anions.

3.4.4 Detection of Metal Ions

As necessary components of the human body, metal ions are crucial for preserving cellular functions and overall health. A surplus of metal ions can be detrimental to one's health, particularly heavy metal ions, which can swiftly build up in the body and impede organ function. Detecting metal ions with high sensitivity and specificity is so crucial. Since some lanthanide-based MOFs may produce strong fluorescent signals with noticeable emission colors, they may find application as chemical detectors for metal ions or tiny organic molecules.

3.4.5 Bio-Imaging

By offering optical support for dynamic, real-time lesion monitoring, bioimaging aids in the early detection of disease. For usage in bioimaging, a variety of imaging methods have been proposed, such as photoacoustic imaging, fluorescence imaging, and positron emission tomography. Organic-metal ion nanohybrids are widely used in bioimaging due to their versatile topologies, easily functionalized architectures, and varied compositions, providing excellent contrast agents for imaging.

Here are some instances of bio-imaging using nanohybrids:

Imaging by Fluorescence: great sensitivity, great stability, and minimal toxicity are only a few of the qualities and advantages that make FLI one of the most important technologies in optical biological imaging (Hilderbrand & Weissleder, 2010).

The remarkable photochemical properties of porphyrins and their analogs, particularly their optical properties, have led to their widespread usage in the construction of various optical devices. Carboxyphenyl porphyrin (TCPP-H2) was encased in zirconium-based nanohybrids (MOF-525) that showed exceptional light stability. Following further irradiation, MOF-525's fluorescence level changed by only 2%, but free porphyrin samples' fluorescence level dropped to 16%. MOF may be far more light stable because of the porphyrin molecules it contains. However, the narrow wavelengths of light used to activate classical porphyrin molecules limited their use in deep tissue bioimaging.

Photoacoustic Imaging: PAI represents one among the non-invasive, non-ionizing hybrid imaging methods that is growing the fastest because it provides superior imaging depth, spatial resolution, and contrast compared to optical imaging (Jiang & Pu, 2017). The remarkable encasing capability of conventional MIL-100 MOF nanohybrids allows for effective transfer of photoacoustic conversion reagents, which in turn effectively loaded curcumin. MOF-based nanohybrids have superior both internal and external loading capabilities because of their porosity and adjustable architectures (Y. Zhang et al., 2018). The MOF surface was then coated with polydopamine-modified hyaluronic acid (HA-PDA) to improve the dispersing and stability of the curcumin-loaded MOF and provide the nanosystem with the ability to target tumors. The multipurpose nanoplatform's great photoacoustic conversion effectiveness was attributed to its two-stage increased photothermal conversion capabilities.

Multimodal Imaging: Comparing multimodal imaging to monomodal bioimaging, the former offers more precision, a more comprehensive evaluation basis, and additional applications for illness identification. Metal ions as well as organic molecules with different functions can self-assemble into a single nanohybrid, which is very advantageous for bioimaging along with multimodal imaging capabilities. A range of photothermal materials based on the synthesis of metal ions and tannic acid (MITA) were proposed by Feng et al. MITA based on FeIII, VIII, and RuIII demonstrated outstanding photothermal conversion efficiency ($\eta = 40\%$). Because MITAs are sticky, a variety of MITA-based nanoplatforms was easily accessible (T. Liu et al., 2018). This study confirmed that nanovesicles are effective for multimodal imaging based on tumor-specific photoactivation, such as T1-weighted MRI, PAI, and photothermal imaging.

3.4.5.1 Metal-Organic Ion Nanohybrids for Cancer Treatment

The creation of innovative nanomedicines for incredibly successful disease treatment is vital and required since healing is regarded as the ultimate goal. Gene therapy, radiation, chemotherapy, gas therapy, photodynamic therapy (PDT), photothermal therapy (PTT), and other therapeutic modalities are currently being extensively researched for the treatment of various diseases (J. Li & Pu, 2020). In the meantime, multimodal therapy approaches have been put forth to improve therapeutic efficacy (J. Li & Pu, 2019). The novel organic-metal ion nanohybrids were studied as a range of biocompatible and highly adaptive medicinal nanoplatforms.

Photodynamic Therapy: As a type of noninvasive phototherapy, PDT has progressively emerged as a substitute for surgery, radiation, and chemotherapy (Lismont et al., 2017). PDT uses light-activated photosensitizers to create highly cytotoxic ROSs, including superoxide anion radical (O2−•), singlet oxygen (1O2), and •OH. These ROSs cause cell death and necrosis, which eradicates malignancies. PDT offers the capacity to be spatiotemporally controlled and has the least invasive characteristics when compared to other conventional treatments like chemotherapy and radiation. Nanotechnology development can improve the efficacy of PDT by precisely delivering photosensitizer molecules to the tumor location, overcoming limitations caused by hydrophobicity, optical stability, and selectivity. Nanohybrids of organic and metal ions can passively gather at the targeted site of action by increasing permeability and retention. They may further actively functionalize with target molecules to target the ideal spot (Zhu et al., 2018).

Photothermal Therapy: PTT, a thermal therapy technique that generates high temperatures by transforming the energy of near-infrared light, has been extensively studied as a potentially useful alternative treatment approach. A key element of PTT is the capacity of photothermal agents to take up photon energy and liberate it via nonradioactive decay, such as heating. When the temperature at the tumor site rises enough, cancer cells undergo irreversible necrosis and apoptosis. PTT targets tumor location, causing harm to healthy tissue. Despite high conversion efficiency, organic or inorganic metal photothermal agents are not commonly used due to their special activity and potential toxicity (Jung et al., 2018). As an alternative, combined metal ion and organic molecule nanoparticles offer benefits including functional controllability and little toxicity (He et al., 2020).

3.4.6 Gene Therapy

Gene therapy is the process of treating diseases brought on by flaws and aberrant genes in target cells by introducing healthy foreign genes. Containing the green fluorescent protein plasmid in the ZIF-8 MOF preserved the functional activity of the genes (Poddar et al., 2019). They were able to stay in the cell for four days because of the gene-loaded nanohybrids. Without any observable cytotoxicity, genes involved in functional activity, intracellular transfer, and trapping were expressed for a relatively long time. This nanoplatform may maintain the functional activity of the DNA plasmid while generating selectivity and durability at the level of in vivo therapies. Despite being widely employed as a practical signal amplification method for biosensing, DNAzymes are a prospective therapeutic agent for cancer gene therapy due to their distinct metal ion-dependent and sequence-specific cleavage characteristics. Wang et al. developed a versatile Zn2+ ion-specific ZIF-8 MOF nanoplatform loaded with DNAzyme for autonomous gene therapy (H. Wang et al., 2019). The efficient intracellular transport of DNAzyme molecules and their pH-responsive release by this nanosystem resulted in DNAzyme-mediated inhibition of EGR-1 and mRNA cleavage-induced gene therapy. Divalent metal ions and DNA or siRNA for nanohybrids must interact with the phosphate backbone of DNA or siRNA for the metal ions to self-assemble. DNA (siRNA)-based nanohybrids are very promising for gene therapy because of the diversity and designability of the DNA or siRNA sequence.

Figure 3.1. **Applications of Nanohybrids in Disease Diagnosis**. Biosensing: At the top of the image, biosensing is shown, which involves using nanohybrids to detect

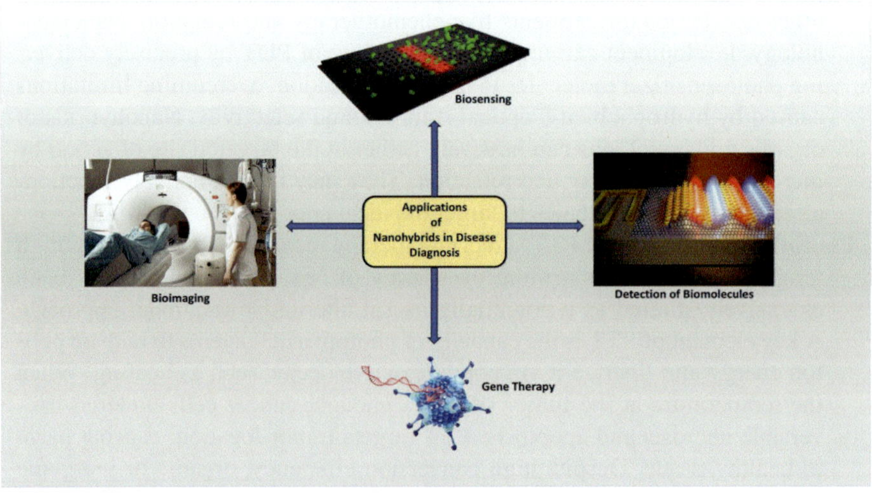

FIGURE 3.1 Illustrates the applications of nanohybrids in disease diagnosis.

and analyze biological molecules and processes. This often appears in the form of a micro-array or chip, where specific reactions can be observed.

Bioimaging: To the left, bioimaging is depicted with a patient undergoing a medical scan, likely a CT or MRI. Nanohybrids can be used as contrast agents to improve the clarity and resolution of these images, helping doctors visualize tissues and diseases more effectively.

Detection of Biomolecules: On the right, the detection of biomolecules is illustrated by a microfluidic device with glowing, colored fluids. Nanohybrids can be engineered to specifically bind to and identify target molecules like proteins or DNA, which is crucial for early disease detection.

Gene Therapy: At the bottom, gene therapy is represented by a viral particle carrying a strand of DNA. Nanohybrids can act as carriers to deliver therapeutic genes into specific cells, offering a way to treat genetic disorders or diseases at the molecular level

REFERENCES

Ahmad, A., Senapati, S., Khan, M. I., Kumar, R., Ramani, R., Srinivas, V., & Sastry, M. (2003a). Intracellular synthesis of gold nanoparticles by a novel alkalotolerant actinomycete, *Rhodococcus* species. *Nanotechnology*, *14*(7), 824–828. https://doi.org/10.1088/0957-4484/14/7/323

Ahmad, A., Senapati, S., Khan, M. I., Kumar, R., & Sastry, M. (2003b). Extracellular biosynthesis of monodisperse gold nanoparticles by a novel extremophilic actinomycete, *Thermomonospora* sp. *Langmuir*, *19*(8), 3550–3553. https://doi.org/10.1021/la026772l

Ahmad, A., Senapati, S., Khan, M. I., Kumar, R., & Sastry, M. (2005). Extra-/intracellular biosynthesis of gold nanoparticles by an alkalotolerant fungus, *Trichothecium* sp. *Journal of Biomedical Nanotechnology*, *1*(1), 47–53. https://doi.org/10.1166/jbn.2005.012

Ai, J., Biazar, E., Jafarpour, M., Montazeri, M., Majdi, A., Aminifard, S., Zafari, M., Akbari, H. R., & Rad, H. G. (2011). Nanotoxicology and nanoparticle safety in biomedical designs. *International Journal of Nanomedicine*, 1117. https://doi.org/10.2147/IJN.S16603

Bar, H., Bhui, D. Kr., Sahoo, G. P., Sarkar, P., De, S. P., & Misra, A. (2009). Green synthesis of silver nanoparticles using latex of Jatropha curcas. *Colloids and Surfaces A: Physicochemical and Engineering Aspects*, *339*(1–3), 134–139. https://doi.org/10.1016/j.colsurfa.2009.02.008

Bhainsa, K. C., & D'Souza, S. F. (2006). Extracellular biosynthesis of silver nanoparticles using the fungus Aspergillus fumigatus. *Colloids and Surfaces B: Biointerfaces*, *47*(2), 160–164. https://doi.org/10.1016/j.colsurfb.2005.11.026

Byrappa, K., & Yoshimura, M. (2001). Hydrothermal technology – Principles and applications. In *Handbook of Hydrothermal Technology* (pp. 1–52). Elsevier. https://doi.org/10.1016/B978-081551445-9.50002-7

Castro, L., Blázquez, M. L., Muñoz, J. A., González, F., García-Balboa, C., & Ballester, A. (2011). Biosynthesis of gold nanowires using sugar beet pulp. *Process Biochemistry*, *46*(5), 1076–1082. https://doi.org/10.1016/j.procbio.2011.01.025

Chujo, Y. (2007). Organic – Inorganic nano-hybrid materials [translated]. *KONA Powder and Particle Journal*, *25*(0), 255–260. https://doi.org/10.14356/kona.2007023

Dahman, Y. (2017). Nanopolymers**by Yaser Dahman, Kevin Deonanan, Timothy Dontsos, and Andrew Iammatteo. In *Nanotechnology and Functional Materials for Engineers* (pp. 121–144). Elsevier. https://doi.org/10.1016/B978-0-323-51256-5.00006-X

Dai, Y., Xu, C., Sun, X., & Chen, X. (2017). Nanoparticle design strategies for enhanced anticancer therapy by exploiting the tumour microenvironment. *Chemical Society Reviews*, *46*(12), 3830–3852. https://doi.org/10.1039/C6CS00592F

Dameron, C. T., Reese, R. N., Mehra, R. K., Kortan, A. R., Carroll, P. J., Steigerwald, M. L., Brus, L. E., & Winge, D. R. (1989). Biosynthesis of cadmium sulphide quantum semiconductor crystallites. *Nature*, *338*(6216), 596–597. https://doi.org/10.1038/338596a0

Ferrando, R., Jellinek, J., & Johnston, R. L. (2008). Nanoalloys: From theory to applications of alloy clusters and nanoparticles. *Chemical Reviews*, *108*(3), 845–910. https://doi.org/10.1021/cr040090g

Fujimoto, T., Terauchi, S., Umehara, H., Kojima, I., & Henderson, W. (2001). Sonochemical preparation of single dispersion metal nanoparticles from metal salts. *Chemistry of Materials*, *13*(3), 1057–1060. https://doi.org/10.1021/cm000910f

Gan, Y. X., Jayatissa, A. H., Yu, Z., Chen, X., & Li, M. (2020). Hydrothermal synthesis of nanomaterials. *Journal of Nanomaterials*, *2020*, 1–3. https://doi.org/10.1155/2020/8917013

Georgiades, S. N., Abd Karim, N. H., Suntharalingam, K., & Vilar, R. (2010). Interaction of metal complexes with G-quadruplex DNA. *Angewandte Chemie International Edition*, *49*(24), 4020–4034. https://doi.org/10.1002/anie.200906363

Gericke, M., & Pinches, A. (2006). Biological synthesis of metal nanoparticles. *Hydrometallurgy*, *83*(1–4), 132–140. https://doi.org/10.1016/j.hydromet.2006.03.019

He, S., Jiang, Y., Li, J., & Pu, K. (2020). Semiconducting polycomplex nanoparticles for photothermal ferrotherapy of cancer. *Angewandte Chemie International Edition*, *59*(26), 10633–10638. https://doi.org/10.1002/anie.202003004

Hilderbrand, S. A., & Weissleder, R. (2010). Near-infrared fluorescence: Application to in vivo molecular imaging. *Current Opinion in Chemical Biology*, *14*(1), 71–79. https://doi.org/10.1016/j.cbpa.2009.09.029

Huang, X., Hu, J., Li, Y., Xin, F., Qiao, R., & Davis, T. P. (2019). Engineering organic/inorganic nanohybrids through RAFT polymerization for biomedical applications. *Biomacromolecules*, *20*(12), 4243–4257. https://doi.org/10.1021/acs.biomac.9b01158

Husseiny, M. I., El-Aziz, M. A., Badr, Y., & Mahmoud, M. A. (2007). Biosynthesis of gold nanoparticles using Pseudomonas aeruginosa. *Spectrochimica Acta Part A: Molecular and Biomolecular Spectroscopy*, *67*(3–4), 1003–1006. https://doi.org/10.1016/j.saa.2006.09.028

Iravani, S. (2011). Green synthesis of metal nanoparticles using plants. *Green Chemistry*, *13*(10), 2638. https://doi.org/10.1039/c1gc15386b

Jain, N., Bhargava, A., Majumdar, S., Tarafdar, J. C., & Panwar, J. (2011). Extracellular biosynthesis and characterization of silver nanoparticles using Aspergillus flavusNJP08: A mechanism perspective. *Nanoscale*, *3*(2), 635–641. https://doi.org/10.1039/C0NR00656D

Jiang, Y., & Pu, K. (2017). Advanced photoacoustic imaging applications of near-infrared absorbing organic nanoparticles. *Small*, *13*(30). https://doi.org/10.1002/smll.201700710

Jung, H. S., Verwilst, P., Sharma, A., Shin, J., Sessler, J. L., & Kim, J. S. (2018). Organic molecule-based photothermal agents: An expanding photothermal therapy universe. *Chemical Society Reviews*, *47*(7), 2280–2297. https://doi.org/10.1039/C7CS00522A

Klaus-Joerger, T., Joerger, R., Olsson, E., & Granqvist, C.-G. (2001). Bacteria as workers in the living factory: Metal-accumulating bacteria and their potential for materials science. *Trends in Biotechnology*, *19*(1), 15–20. https://doi.org/10.1016/S0167-7799(00)01514-6

Kowshik, M., Ashtaputre, S., Kharrazi, S., Vogel, W., Urban, J., Kulkarni, S. K., & Paknikar, K. M. (2003). Extracellular synthesis of silver nanoparticles by a silver-tolerant yeast strain MKY3. *Nanotechnology*, *14*(1), 95–100. https://doi.org/10.1088/0957-4484/14/1/321

Kulkarni, N., & Muddapur, U. (2014). Biosynthesis of metal nanoparticles: A review. *Journal of Nanotechnology*, *2014*, 1–8. https://doi.org/10.1155/2014/510246

Kumar, P., Singh, P., Kumari, K., Mozumdar, S., & Chandra, R. (2011). A green approach for the synthesis of gold nanotriangles using aqueous leaf extract of *Callistemon viminalis*. *Materials Letters*, *65*(4), 595–597. https://doi.org/10.1016/j.matlet.2010.11.025

Lee, S.-W., Mao, C., Flynn, C. E., & Belcher, A. M. (2002). Ordering of quantum dots using genetically engineered viruses. *Science*, *296*(5569), 892–895. https://doi.org/10.1126/science.1068054

Lengke, M., & Southam, G. (2006). Bioaccumulation of gold by sulfate-reducing bacteria cultured in the presence of gold(I)-thiosulfate complex. *Geochimica et Cosmochimica Acta*, *70*(14), 3646–3661. https://doi.org/10.1016/j.gca.2006.04.018

Li, J., Li, D., Yuan, R., & Xiang, Y. (2017). Biodegradable MnO2 nanosheet-mediated signal amplification in living cells enables sensitive detection of down-regulated intracellular microRNA. *ACS Applied Materials & Interfaces*, *9*(7), 5717–5724. https://doi.org/10.1021/acsami.6b13073

Li, J., & Pu, K. (2019). Development of organic semiconducting materials for deep-tissue optical imaging, phototherapy and photoactivation. *Chemical Society Reviews*, *48*(1), 38–71. https://doi.org/10.1039/C8CS00001H

Li, J., & Pu, K. (2020). Semiconducting polymer nanomaterials as near-infrared photoactivatable protherapeutics for cancer. *Accounts of Chemical Research*, *53*(4), 752–762. https://doi.org/10.1021/acs.accounts.9b00569

Li, X., Xu, H., Chen, Z.-S., & Chen, G. (2011). Biosynthesis of nanoparticles by microorganisms and their applications. *Journal of Nanomaterials*, *2011*, 1–16. https://doi.org/10.1155/2011/270974

Lismont, M., Dreesen, L., & Wuttke, S. (2017). Metal-organic framework nanoparticles in photodynamic therapy: Current status and perspectives. *Advanced Functional Materials*, *27*(14). https://doi.org/10.1002/adfm.201606314

Liu, B., Zhang, J., & Li, L. (2019). Metal–DNA coordination-driven self-assembly: A conceptual methodology to expand the repertoire of DNA nanobiotechnology. *Chemistry – A European Journal*, *25*(59), 13452–13457. https://doi.org/10.1002/chem.201902501

Liu, T., Zhang, M., Liu, W., Zeng, X., Song, X., Yang, X., Zhang, X., & Feng, J. (2018). Metal ion/tannic acid assembly as a versatile photothermal platform in engineering multimodal nanotheranostics for advanced applications. *ACS Nano*, *12*(4), 3917–3927. https://doi.org/10.1021/acsnano.8b01456

Lu, K., He, C., & Lin, W. (2015). A chlorin-based nanoscale metal–organic framework for photodynamic therapy of colon cancers. *Journal of the American Chemical Society*, *137*(24), 7600–7603. https://doi.org/10.1021/jacs.5b04069

Ma, B., Wang, S., Liu, F., Zhang, S., Duan, J., Li, Z., Kong, Y., Sang, Y., Liu, H., Bu, W., & Li, L. (2019). Self-assembled copper–amino acid nanoparticles for in situ glutathione "AND" H_2O_2 sequentially triggered chemodynamic therapy. *Journal of the American Chemical Society*, *141*(2), 849–857. https://doi.org/10.1021/jacs.8b08714

Ma, C., Malessa, A., Boersma, A. J., Liu, K., & Herrmann, A. (2020). Supercharged proteins and polypeptides. *Advanced Materials*, *32*(20). https://doi.org/10.1002/adma.201905309

Marshall, A. T., Haverkamp, R. G., Davies, C. E., Parsons, J. G., Gardea-Torresdey, J. L., & van Agterveld, D. (2007). Accumulation of gold nanoparticles in *Brassic Juncea*. *International Journal of Phytoremediation*, *9*(3), 197–206. https://doi.org/10.1080/15226510701376026

Meng, X., Zhang, K., Dai, W., Cao, Y., Yang, F., Dong, H., & Zhang, X. (2018). Multiplex microRNA imaging in living cells using DNA-capped-Au assembled hydrogels. *Chemical Science*, *9*(37), 7419–7425. https://doi.org/10.1039/C8SC02858C

Mujahid, M. H., Upadhyay, T. K., Khan, F., Pandey, P., Park, M. N., Sharangi, A. B., Saeed, M., Upadhye, V. J., & Kim, B. (2022). Metallic and metal oxide-derived nanohybrid as a tool for biomedical applications. *Biomedicine & Pharmacotherapy*, *155*, 113791. https://doi.org/10.1016/j.biopha.2022.113791

Mukherjee, P., Ahmad, A., Mandal, D., Senapati, S., Sainkar, S. R., Khan, M. I., Parishcha, R., Ajaykumar, P. V., Alam, M., Kumar, R., & Sastry, M. (2001). Fungus-mediated synthesis of silver nanoparticles and their immobilization in the mycelial matrix: A novel biological approach to nanoparticle synthesis. *Nano Letters*, *1*(10), 515–519. https://doi.org/10.1021/nl0155274

Ojovan, M. I., Lee, W. E., & Lee, W. E. (2019). Treatment of radioactive wastes. In *An Introduction to Nuclear Waste Immobilisation* (pp. 231–269). Elsevier.

Patil, A. B., & Bhanage, B. M. (2016). Sonochemistry: A greener protocol for nanoparticles synthesis. In *Handbook of Nanoparticles* (pp. 143–166). Springer International Publishing. https://doi.org/10.1007/978-3-319-15338-4_4

Philip, D. (2010). Green synthesis of gold and silver nanoparticles using Hibiscus rosa sinensis. *Physica E: Low-Dimensional Systems and Nanostructures*, *42*(5), 1417–1424. https://doi.org/10.1016/j.physe.2009.11.081

Poddar, A., Conesa, J. J., Liang, K., Dhakal, S., Reineck, P., Bryant, G., Pereiro, E., Ricco, R., Amenitsch, H., Doonan, C., Mulet, X., Doherty, C. M., Falcaro, P., & Shukla, R. (2019). Encapsulation, visualization and expression of genes with biomimetically mineralized zeolitic imidazolate framework-8 (ZIF-8). *Small*, *15*(36). https://doi.org/10.1002/smll.201902268

Prabhu, S., & Poulose, E. K. (2012). Silver nanoparticles: Mechanism of antimicrobial action, synthesis, medical applications, and toxicity effects. *International Nano Letters*, *2*(1), 32. https://doi.org/10.1186/2228-5326-2-32

Redjala, T., Remita, H., Apostolescu, G., Mostafavi, M., Thomazeau, C., & Uzio, D. (2006). Bimetallic Au-Pd and Ag-Pd clusters synthesised by γ or electron beam radiolysis and study of the reactivity/structure relationships in the selective hydrogenation of buta-1,3-diene. *Oil & Gas Science and Technology – Revue de l'IFP*, *61*(6), 789–797. https://doi.org/10.2516/ogst:2006019

Roh, Y., Lauf, R. J., McMillan, A. D., Zhang, C., Rawn, C. J., Bai, J., & Phelps, T. J. (2001). Microbial synthesis and the characterization of metal-substituted magnetites. *Solid State Communications*, *118*(10), 529–534. https://doi.org/10.1016/S0038-1098(01)00146-6

Sastry, M., Kumar, R., Ahmad, A., & Khan, M. I. (2003). Biosynthesis of metal nanoparticles using fungi and actinomycete. *Current Science*, *85*(2), 162–170.

Shankar, S. S., Rai, A., Ahmad, A., & Sastry, M. (2004). Rapid synthesis of Au, Ag, and bimetallic Au core–Ag shell nanoparticles using Neem (Azadirachta indica) leaf broth. *Journal of Colloid and Interface Science*, *275*(2), 496–502. https://doi.org/10.1016/j.jcis.2004.03.003

Sun, L., Xu, Y., Gao, Y., Huang, X., Feng, S., Chen, J., Wang, X., Guo, L., Li, M., Meng, X., Zhang, J., Ge, J., An, X., Ding, D., Luo, Y., Zhang, Y., Jiang, Q., & Ning, X. (2019). Synergistic amplification of oxidative stress–mediated antitumor activity via liposomal dichloroacetic acid and MOF-Fe2+. *Small*, *15*(24). https://doi.org/10.1002/smll.201901156

Thakkar, K. N., Mhatre, S. S., & Parikh, R. Y. (2010). Biological synthesis of metallic nanoparticles. *Nanomedicine: Nanotechnology, Biology and Medicine*, *6*(2), 257–262. https://doi.org/10.1016/j.nano.2009.07.002

Vahedifard, F., & Chakravarthy, K. (2021). Nanomedicine for COVID-19: The role of nanotechnology in the treatment and diagnosis of COVID–19. *Emergent Materials*, *4*(1), 75–99. https://doi.org/10.1007/s42247-021-00168-8

Wang, H., Chen, Y., Wang, H., Liu, X., Zhou, X., & Wang, F. (2019). DNAzyme-loaded metal–organic frameworks (MOFs) for self-sufficient gene therapy. *Angewandte Chemie International Edition*, *58*(22), 7380–7384. https://doi.org/10.1002/anie.201902714

Wang, L., Liang, K., Jiang, X., Yang, M., & Liu, Y. (2018). Dynamic protein–metal ion networks: A unique approach to injectable and self-healable metal sulfide/protein hybrid hydrogels with high photothermal efficiency. *Chemistry – A European Journal*, *24*(25), 6557–6563. https://doi.org/10.1002/chem.201705841

Wang, R., Hughes, T., Beck, S., Vakil, S., Li, S., Pantano, P., & Draper, R. K. (2013). Generation of toxic degradation products by sonication of Pluronic® dispersants: Implications for nanotoxicity testing. *Nanotoxicology*, *7*(7), 1272–1281. https://doi.org/10.3109/17435390.2012.736547

Xu, H., Zeiger, B. W., & Suslick, K. S. (2013). Sonochemical synthesis of nanomaterials. *Chemical Society Reviews*, *42*(7), 2555–2567. https://doi.org/10.1039/C2CS35282F

Zhang, K., Zhao, N., & Xu, F. (2020). Self-assembled organic/metal ion nanohybrids for theranostics. *VIEW*, *1*(2). https://doi.org/10.1002/viw2.17

Zhang, Y., Wang, L., Liu, L., Lin, L., Liu, F., Xie, Z., Tian, H., & Chen, X. (2018). Engineering metal–organic frameworks for photoacoustic imaging-guided chemo-/photothermal combinational tumor therapy. *ACS Applied Materials & Interfaces*, *10*(48), 41035–41045. https://doi.org/10.1021/acsami.8b13492

Zhu, H., Li, J., Qi, X., Chen, P., & Pu, K. (2018). Oxygenic hybrid semiconducting nanoparticles for enhanced photodynamic therapy. *Nano Letters*, *18*(1), 586–594. https://doi.org/10.1021/acs.nanolett.7b04759

4 Nanohybrids for Cancer Therapeutic Applications

Kalyani Chepuri, Vadakavila Geethikalal, Chittepu Pranitha, Kathuroju Harikrishna, Siddhartha Palasala, Suchitra Nakka, and Thulasi Gandamalla

4.1 INTRODUCTION

Despite advances in medicine, cancer remains the second leading health issue worldwide, with roughly 19.1 to 20 million new cases diagnosed annually. Tragically, this results in about ten million deaths each year, underscoring the urgent need for improved treatments and early detection methods. This burden is expected to rise significantly by 2050, with projections indicating up to 30 million new cases annually. Developing nations, particularly those facing socio-economic challenges, are disproportionately affected due to limited access to healthcare, lack of awareness, and insufficient treatment options (Bizuayehu et al. 2024).

Common cancers include breast and cervical cancers in women, leukemia and lymphoma in children, and lung and prostate cancers in men. Early diagnosis, effective screening programs, and targeted therapies are essential to combating the rising cancer burden. Additionally, lowering exposure to risk factors like smoking and unhealthy eating habits can aid in the prevention of numerous cancer types. Efforts toward improving healthcare infrastructure and increasing access to affordable treatments are critical in the global fight against cancer

Despite conventional treatments like surgery, chemotherapy, and radiation, these methods have significant constraints like side effects, drug resistance, and incomplete tumor removal, leading to recurrence and reduced efficacy. This drives the need for innovative approaches to improve cancer treatment. Nanotechnology has emerged as a groundbreaking advancement in oncology, with the potential to transform how cancer is diagnosed and treated. Among its many innovations, nanohybrids – combinations of organic and inorganic materials – stand out as versatile and powerful tools in cancer management. Nanohybrids offer unique advantages due to their multifunctionality, precision, and ability to overcome the limitations of traditional treatments (X. Wang et al. 2021). Their ability to integrate therapeutic and diagnostic capabilities has led to the development of advanced "theranostics," which enable simultaneous cancer imaging and treatment. This dual functionality enhances

DOI: 10.1201/9781003563723-4

efficiency, reduces treatment timelines, and provides a more comprehensive approach to managing the disease.

Nanohybrids are essential in delivering drugs specifically to target areas, presenting a major benefit over traditional chemotherapy, which impacts both cancerous and healthy cells indiscriminately. These are devised to specifically target tumor cells through mechanisms like enhanced permeability and retention (EPR), allowing for more effective accumulation at tumor sites. Additionally, ligand-mediated targeting enhances the precision of drug delivery by guiding nanohybrids to attack cancer cells with specific molecular markers. This approach not only minimizes adverse effects on healthy tissues but also ensures the improved therapeutic outcomes. By minimizing off-target effects and concentrating on the tumor, nanohybrids improve the general well-being of patients receiving cancer treatment.

Nanohybrids enhance the solubility and bioavailability of hydrophobic drugs like Paclitaxel, ensuring effective delivery directly to tumor cells. They address drug resistance, a major challenge in cancer therapy, by enabling controlled and sustained release of anticancer agents. This enhances efficacy, reduces treatment frequency, and improves patient compliance. Acting as multifunctional platforms, nanohybrids can deliver chemotherapy drugs and genetic materials like siRNA, boosting cancer cell targeting. Compatible with advanced photothermal (PTT) and photodynamic (PDT) therapies, they utilize light energy for localized tumor regression and produce reactive oxygen species (ROS) to initiate cancer cell apoptosis, minimizing healthy tissue damage (Liang et al. 2020).

Emerging designs with stimuli-responsive features allow nanohybrids to adapt to changes in the tumor microenvironment, such as pH, hypoxia conditions, and oxidative stress, increasing their functionality. However, challenges remain in ensuring biocompatibility, large-scale production, and regulatory approval. Despite these obstacles, nanohybrids are transforming oncology by offering targeted, precise, and multifunctional solutions to overcome the limitations of traditional therapies. With their potential to advance drug delivery, imaging, and combination treatments, they promise to reduce cancer mortality and improve patient outcomes, representing a significant leap in cancer care (Z. Cheng et al. 2021).

4.2 NANOHYBRIDS

Nanohybrids are engineered materials created by combining organic polymers with inorganic compounds like silica, alumina, and zirconia. These hybrid materials capitalize on the unique properties of both organic and inorganic components, offering enhanced stability, versatility, and functionality. For the precise and strong integration of both organic and inorganic materials, the production process relies on precise interactions like hydrogen bonding, ionic bonding, and covalent bonding. The organic polymers provide flexibility, biocompatibility, and modification ease, while inorganic compounds enhance mechanical strength, conductivity, and specialized properties like magnetism or optics. In cancer treatment, nanohybrids can be designed for targeted drug delivery, improving therapy precision and reducing side effects.

4.2.1 Classification of Nanohybrids

Nanohybrids can be divided into two categories based on the nature of the interaction between the organic and inorganic components.

4.2.1.1 Class I Hybrids

Class I hybrids are defined by weak interactions between two phases, such as van der Waals forces, hydrogen bonds, or weak electrostatic interactions.

4.2.1.2 Class II Hybrids

Class II hybrids are distinguished by strong interactions, including covalent and ionic bonds. These materials possess unique properties, making them highly valuable in diverse fields such as medicine, electronics, energy, and environmental science (N. Zhao et al. 2019).

4.2.2 Types of Nanohybrids Used in Cancer Therapy

The combination of therapeutic modalities and enhanced treatment efficacy of nanohybrids has significantly increased their use in cancer therapies. Their precise targeted delivery and biocompatibility make nanohybrids highly effective in improving cancer treatment outcomes (W. Zhang et al. 2023). Various types of nanohybrids have been developed for different cancers, incorporating diverse components and unique capabilities to address the limitations of traditional treatments. They are tabulated in Table 4.1.

4.3 MECHANISM OF ACTION OF NANOHYBRIDS IN CANCER TREATMENT

Nanohybrids are transforming cancer therapy by enhancing targeted drug delivery, minimizing harm to healthy cells, and increasing drug concentration at tumors. They leverage passive targeting via the EPR effect and active targeting through ligand-based precision delivery to cancer cells. Nanohybrids can also address drug resistance by carrying multiple therapeutic agents and delivering genes that suppress resistance mechanisms. Some nanohybrids can generate heat to eliminate resistant cells or enhance the efficacy of chemotherapy. Additionally, they can modify the tumor microenvironment, such as normalizing blood vessels or modulating immune responses to reduce resistance. These versatile strategies significantly enhance the precision and effectiveness of cancer therapies, making nanohybrids a powerful tool in combating cancer and improving treatment outcomes (W. Zhang et al. 2023).

4.3.1 Targeted Drug Delivery and Tumor Localization

Targeted drug delivery directs therapeutics to tumors while minimizing harm to healthy tissues, enhancing efficacy and reducing side effects. It operates via passive and active targeting: passive targeting exploits the enhanced permeability and retention (EPR) effect for nanoparticle accumulation in tumors, while active targeting

TABLE 4.1
Classification, Composition, and Applications of Nanohybrids

Type of Nanohybrid	Composition	Uses	References
Dendrimer-gold nanohybrids	Poly(amidoamine) dendrimers combined with gold nanoparticles (AuNPs)	Used for gene delivery, immunotherapy, and combination therapies such as gene/photothermal and gene/chemotherapy	(J. Li, Shen, and Shi 2020)
Naphthalene diimide-based nanohybrids	Organic naphthalene diimide-based molecules combined with inorganic $CoFe_2O_4$	A multifunctional platform for photothermal, photodynamic, and sonodynamic therapies, guided by photoacoustic imaging	(G. Chen et al. 2024)
Polycation-carbon nanohybrids	Carbon nanoparticles with polycationic gene vectors	Used in gene and photothermal therapy, nanohybrids also have capabilities for drug delivery and NIR-II responsive therapy	(N. Zhao et al. 2020)
Gold-nanoparticle hybrid nanostructure	Gold nanoparticles hybridized with liposomes or polymers	Used in chemotherapy, photothermal therapy, and radiotherapy, nanohybrids also hold potential for imaging applications	(Ali et al. 2022)
Oncocyte membrane-camouflaged nanohybrids	Core components include therapeutic agents like chemotherapeutic drugs encapsulated in nanoparticles, while the outer layer consists of cell membranes, often from cancer cells, enabling evasion of the host's immune surveillance	Enhanced drug delivery, synergistic therapies, immune modulation	(F. Zhang et al. 2022)

uses ligand- or antibody-functionalized carriers to selectively bind cancer cell receptors for precise drug delivery.

Accurate tumor localization is essential for the effectiveness of targeted drug delivery, guaranteeing that therapeutic agents are precisely delivered to the intended sites. This involves identifying the exact location and extent of the tumor. Imaging techniques, such as MRI, CT scans, and PET scans, provide detailed visuals of tumors and surrounding tissues, aiding in treatment planning and monitoring. Tumor-specific biomarkers, detectable in blood, urine, or tissue, help identify and track the presence of cancer cells. Additionally, engineered nanoparticles, sometimes tagged with imaging agents, enhance both imaging and drug delivery, improving tumor visibility during scans. Solid tumors often develop drug resistance due to various mechanisms, including alternative drug export pumps, changes in gene expression, and alterations in metabolic pathways. The tumor microenvironment also influences the effectiveness of drug delivery (Tredan et al. 2007).

Nano-sized agents present several benefits over conventional drugs, such as high capacity for loading, resistance to degradation, targeted delivery, and controlled release. These agents take advantage of the enhanced permeability and retention (EPR) effect, which allows them to accumulate in tumors. However, while the EPR effect provides some benefits, it often requires strategies to temporarily enhance its efficiency for better drug uptake in tumors. The EPR effect is a phenomenon that aids nano-sized drugs in reaching tumors more effectively. When injected into the bloodstream, these drugs travel through tiny blood vessels, particularly capillaries, to reach the tumor. In normal tissues, capillaries are tightly sealed and well-supported, making it difficult for drugs to penetrate. However, tumor blood vessels are leaky and poorly supported, with large gaps and less structural integrity, which allows drugs to easily pass through. Tumors require a continuous supply of nutrients and oxygen for growth, prompting them to recruit new blood vessels or modify existing ones. These abnormal blood vessels, being poorly formed and lacking proper support, allow nanoparticles to slip through and accumulate in the tumor, aided by poor lymphatic drainage (Nakamura et al. 2016).

4.3.2 Nanohybrids-Mediated Drug Release Mechanism

Nanohybrids-mediated drug release mechanisms play a pivotal role in advancing drug delivery, providing a versatile solution to various medical challenges. These systems combine different nanomaterials to enhance drug delivery efficiency, control release rates, and improve biocompatibility. Drug release from nanohybrids can be controlled through diffusion, solvent interaction, chemical reactions, or stimuli-responsive mechanisms, such as pH changes, temperature shifts, or enzymatic activity. This ensures that drugs are released precisely when and where they are needed (Patra et al. 2018).

Targeted delivery is a major advantage of nanohybrids, allowing therapeutic agents to be directed specifically to disease sites, such as cancer cells. This minimizes side effects and maximizes treatment effectiveness. By modifying the surface of nanoparticles, they can either actively target specific cell receptors or passively accumulate in tumor tissues through the enhanced permeability and retention (EPR) effect.

Nanohybrids also address drug resistance in cancer therapy by bypassing drug efflux transporters and targeting defective apoptotic pathways, ensuring effective eradication of cancer cells. The protein corona effect – where nanoparticles form a layer of biomolecules upon entering the body – can influence drug release behavior by altering the nanoparticles' physicochemical properties and their interaction with target cells. Enhanced stability and biocompatibility of nanohybrids further contribute to their effectiveness, ensuring that drugs remain stable and active for longer durations while minimizing adverse reactions. As research progresses, the applications of nanohybrids in drug delivery continue to expand, offering promising solutions for targeted, controlled, and efficient treatments across various medical fields. Future developments may include multifunctional nanohybrids capable of simultaneously diagnosing and treating conditions, personalized medicine approaches, and advanced stimuli-responsive systems, paving the way for more precise and efficient healthcare (Y. Chen et al. 2020).

4.3.3 Cellular Uptake and Internalization of Nanohybrid Based Drugs

Delivering drug molecules precisely and safely to specific cell types in therapeutic amounts remains a significant challenge in drug delivery. One effective strategy to achieve this is through the usage of nanomedicines or nanoparticulate agents. The main goals of nanomedicine development are to enhance drug formulations with targeted delivery, controlled release, reduced toxicity, and the ability to bypass biological barriers. Achieving this requires navigating endocytic pathways like caveolae-mediated endocytosis and micropinocytosis, along with intracellular trafficking, which are influenced by particle size, shape, surface charge, lipophilicity, nanocarrier type, and cell type. Computational studies have shown that nanoparticle endocytosis occurs through membrane-particle adhesion, elastic deformation of the cell membrane, and receptor diffusion to the membrane surface, all of which depend on these factors (Sahay, Alakhova, and Kabanov 2010).

To design effective nanomedicine, it's crucial to understand both endocytosis and intracellular trafficking pathways to ensure that drugs reach the desired cell types at effective therapeutic concentrations. Endocytosis is crucial for particle internalization and supports key physiological and biochemical functions, including debris clearance, cell motility, immune surveillance, receptor regulation, membrane remodeling, neurotransmission, and cellular communication. The regulation of endocytosis and intracellular trafficking is influenced by numerous associated proteins, like coat proteins, adaptors, retrieval proteins, scission proteins, Rab GTPases, and soluble N-ethylmaleimide-sensitive factor attachment protein receptors (SNAREs) (Donahue, Acar, and Wilhelm 2019).

Endocytosis, an active transport mechanism crucial for nanomedicines, enables precise particle delivery to cells, while facilitated diffusion passively moves molecules via transport proteins. Attached particles can bypass cytoplasmic barriers, reaching the perinuclear region and reducing opsonization risk. Clathrin- and caveolae-mediated pathways, associated with acidic and neutral pH environments, provide opportunities for tailored drug delivery. Most nanocarriers enter cells via endocytosis, categorized into phagocytosis and pinocytosis.

Phagocytosis enables phagocytes to ingest large particles (> 500 nm) for pathogen clearance and debris removal. Circulating phagocytes detect nanoparticles, binding them via receptors such as Toll-like, mannose/lectin, and scavenger receptors. The plasma membrane engulfs nanoparticles into phagosomes, which then fuse with lysosomes for acidic degradation. Pinocytosis, another endocytic pathway, includes clathrin mediated and caveolae-mediated endocytosis. Understanding these processes ensures the effective design and implementation of nanomedicines for therapeutic applications, offering precise control over the delivery, internalization, and distribution of drugs within targeted cells (W. Zhang et al. 2023).

4.4 THERAPEUTIC APPLICATIONS OF NANOHYBRIDS IN CANCER

Despite the availability of multiple treatment approaches, including surgery, chemotherapy, and immunotherapy, these methods often come with adverse side effects, such as cytotoxic effects on healthy cells. In some severe cases, cancer cells become resistant to chemotherapeutic drugs, and many treatments fail to precisely target and deliver drugs to the tumor microenvironment, particularly to the stroma cells (mother cells), which play a pivotal role in cancer growth.

Nanohybrids, which combine nanoscale materials with organic or inorganic components, offer a promising solution. These multifunctional systems are designed for therapeutic applications, leveraging nanotechnology to enhance drug delivery and collectively minimizing damage to non-cancerous cells. Nanotechnology enables the efficient and targeted delivery of drugs using various nanocarriers, thus improving treatment outcomes (Kumar et al. 2022).

4.4.1 Nanohybrids in Chemotherapy

Recent advancements in nanotechnology have enhanced drug delivery precision, reducing toxicity and ensuring stability. Nanohybrids and carbon nanotubes (CNTs) are emerging as effective carriers for targeted drug delivery to tumors. These nanocarriers offer controlled release, targeted delivery, and biocompatibility. By functionalizing nanohybrids with ligands or antibodies, they ensure precise targeting of tumor sites. The enhanced permeability and retention (EPR) effect, driven by enzyme secretion like metalloproteinases, allows the nanoparticles to accumulate in tumors due to their nature of leaky blood vessels and poor lymphatic drainage. Nanohybrids also improve the solubility of hydrophobic chemotherapy drugs, enhancing absorption and therapeutic effectiveness. For example, Paclitaxel's low solubility is improved by encapsulation in lipid-polymer nanoparticles, reducing toxicity and improving its therapeutic index. Overall, nanohybrids improve drug solubility, targeted delivery, and sustained retention, making them a promising tool for enhancing chemotherapy efficacy and safety.

Nanohybrids are specifically designed to control drug release in response to the tumor environment. Tumors typically have an acidic microenvironment, which allows nanohybrids made from polymers that dissolve in acidic conditions to release their therapeutic payload. Additionally, these nanohybrids can be equipped with enzyme-sensitive linkers that respond to tumor-associated enzymes such as metalloproteinases (MMPs) and urokinase-type plasminogen activators (uPAs) (Prakash et al. 2011). Another advantage is the slightly elevated temperatures (hyperthermia) in tumor tissues, which can trigger temperature-sensitive polymers in nanohybrids to release the drug. These nanohybrids can also be activated externally by heat sources like near-infrared (NIR) lasers, which specifically target and release the drug within the tumor without affecting adjacent healthy tissues.

NIR radiation can penetrate deeply into tissues, selectively heating the nanohybrids within the tumor while sparing the surrounding healthy tissue. Notable examples of temperature-sensitive nanohybrids include NIR-responsive nanohybrids made of carbon nanotubes or gold nanoparticles encased in a polymer shell (Mehrotra and Pal 2024). Another example is poly (N-isopropylacrylamide) (PNIPAM)-based nanohybrids, a temperature-sensitive polymer that becomes hydrophobic above a critical temperature (around 32°C), causing it to collapse and release the drug (Mi 2020).

4.4.1.1 Nanohybrid-Based Chemotherapeutic Agents

Nanohybrid-based chemotherapeutic agents are emerging as a promising approach to improve cancer treatment by enhancing drug delivery, reducing side effects, and overcoming challenges such as drug resistance. One particularly innovative strategy involves utilizing bacteria, such as *Salmonella* and *Escherichia coli*, to deliver therapeutic agents directly to tumor sites. These bacteria are naturally capable of migrating toward tumors, especially to areas that are hypoxic and necrotic, guided by chemotactic signals in the tumor microenvironment. This characteristic makes them ideal candidates for targeted drug delivery systems.

By combining these bacteria with nano-drugs or cytokines like tumor necrosis factor-alpha (TNF-α), the antitumor effects can be significantly boosted. For example, nanoliposomes containing the chemotherapeutic agent Doxorubicin (DOX) have been successfully loaded into *Salmonella*, which then migrates efficiently to tumor sites. Tumors are typically characterized by a low pH and high glucose levels, which contrast sharply with the normal tissues. This metabolic difference is exploited by the bacteria, which preferentially accumulate in these areas, improving the efficacy of nanoparticle delivery.

This combination of bacteria and nanohybrids can enhance the precision of drug delivery by targeting the tumor microenvironment directly, reducing the risk of systemic toxicity and minimizing the side effects often associated with traditional chemotherapy. Moreover, the bacteria can help overcome the challenge of drug resistance by ensuring that therapeutic agents reach the tumor site more effectively, even in difficult-to-target areas. This approach represents an exciting avenue for cancer therapy, offering improved treatment outcomes and reduced complications for patients (Y. Chen et al. 2020).

4.4.1.2 Overcoming Drug Resistance with Nanohybrids

Cancer cells often develop resistance to drugs by limiting drug delivery and effectiveness, especially on stroma cells. Proteins like P-glycoprotein help pump drugs out of tumor cells, which eventually decrease the intracellular drug concentration. Mutations in target proteins (e.g., tyrosine kinase receptors) reduce drug binding, while the tumor microenvironment (TME) creates barriers, such as hypoxia and dense extracellular matrix, preventing drug penetration and aiding cancer cell survival. Additionally, gene expression changes without DNA sequence alterations can activate survival pathways or suppress drug sensitivity genes.

Nanohybrids present an innovative approach to combat drug resistance by improving targeted drug delivery, enhancing drug accumulation, and minimizing off target effects. Surface modifications, such as attaching antibodies, enable specific binding to tumor markers, facilitating precise and controlled drug release at the tumor site. Additionally, incorporating multiple therapeutic agents within a single nanohybrid system allows for synergistic effects that can overcome resistance mechanisms. For instance, gold-silver nanohybrids combining photothermal therapy with chemotherapy have shown enhanced therapeutic outcomes in cancers like breast cancer. Beyond traditional therapies, nanohybrids can also deliver genetic agents, such as siRNA or CRISPR-Cas9, directly into cancer cells to alter their genetic makeup, potentially reducing resistance to existing treatments. This approach not only boosts the efficacy of chemotherapy but also offers a route to personalized cancer treatment by targeting the underlying genetic factors contributing to resistance (Lin et al. 2016).

4.4.2 Nanohybrids in Gene Therapy and RNA Interference

Gene therapy and RNA interference (RNAi) in nanohybrid systems offer efficient, stable, and targeted delivery of nucleic acids like DNA, mRNA, siRNA, and miRNA. Gene therapy aims to replace or repair defective genes, while RNAi silences specific genes to modify cellular functions. Nanohybrids improve the stability of nucleic acids and ensure their accurate delivery to target tissues or cells, protecting them from degradation. By incorporating surface modifications, nanohybrids minimize off-target effects, enhancing the precision and effectiveness of gene therapy and RNAi. This advancement strengthens the potential of these therapies in treating various diseases, including cancer (X. Cheng, Xie, and Sun 2023).

4.4.2.1 DNA/RNA Delivery Systems Using Nanohybrids

Gene therapy holds great potential in cancer treatment by targeting or replacing defective genes to correct underlying issues. However, conventional genetic vectors often face issues such as instability, degradation, and eliciting an immune response, limiting their therapeutic effectiveness. Nanohybrids help overcome these challenges by offering enhanced structural stability, especially with inorganic components like gold and silica. These materials can be easily functionalized with antibodies or peptides to target specific cancer cell markers such as HER2 and EGFR, improving their interaction with tumor cell receptors.

Several delivery systems have shown promising results in clinical trials for genetic disorders and also even for the several types of cancer. A notable example is the CALAA-01 gene delivery system, which targets ribonucleotide reductase (RRM2) in melanoma cells and demonstrated successful siRNA delivery with antiproliferative effects during phase-1 clinical trials (Davis et al. 2010). Additionally, PEI-based gene delivery systems combined with Polyethyleneimine-cholesterol (PEG-PEI-cholesterol) have shown enhanced cytokine expression, particularly interleukin-12, for ovarian cancer immunotherapy. Future clinical trials will likely focus on combination therapies, integrating chemotherapy, radiotherapy, photodynamic therapy, and immunotherapy, to maximize therapeutic efficacy and overcome resistance mechanisms (J. Chen et al. 2016).

4.4.2.2 CRISPR/Cas9-Based Nanohybrids for Gene Editing

CRISPR/Cas9 is an innovative approach to cancer treatment, focusing on targeting and modifying genetic mutations that drive cancer development. By using a single guide RNA (sgRNA), Cas9 endonuclease is directed to specific target sites, inducing precise double-strand breaks in DNA and enabling site-specific genomic modifications.

Traditional gene transformation methods, such as microinjections or viral vectors, have limitations, including immune responses, off-target effects, and high production costs. These challenges have been addressed by nanotechnology-based non-viral vectors, such as polymers, lipids, and mesoporous and metal-organic frameworks. These carriers offer low immunogenicity, high biocompatibility, and efficient drug delivery, making them promising for cancer treatment. Polymer-based nanohybrids, including micelles, dendrimers, vesicles, and hydrogels, are particularly effective for drug delivery. Micelles, with both hydrophobic and hydrophilic components, protect drug delivery systems from the immune response. They are particularly useful for delivering hydrophobic anti-cancer drugs like calprotectin and paclitaxel (PTX), improving drug stability and enhancing anti-cancer effects (Xu et al. 2021).

4.4.3 Nanohybrids in Immunotherapy

Nanohybrids in immunotherapy represent a key advancement in cancer treatment, utilizing the unique properties of nanomaterials to enhance immune responses against tumors. These innovations address the limitations of traditional immunotherapy, such as poor tumor penetration and immune evasion by cancer cells. Nanohybrids are designed to alter the tumor microenvironment and boost immune function by supporting the host defense mechanism. For example, recent breakthroughs in nanotechnology have resulted in synthesizing improved advancements in CAR-T cells therapy, which exhibit reduced toxicity to healthy cells while improving anti-tumor activity (Y. Wang, Barrett, and Hu 2024).

4.4.3.1 Nanohybrids for Antigen Delivery and Vaccination

Nanohybrids enhance the delivery and presentation of antigens to the host immune system by leveraging nanoparticle properties like surface charge, efficient antigen encapsulation, and lymph node targeting. For instance, manganese oxide nanoparticles combined with cationic polymers can load model antigens like ovalbumin to form MPO nano-vaccines. These vaccines offer personalized tumor treatment by releasing tumor-associated antigens through immunogenic cell death (ICD). MPO vaccines have proven effective in eliciting robust T-cell immune responses to inhibit B16-OVA melanoma that expresses ovalbumin. Additionally, they hold promise as personalized cancer vaccines by generating autologous antigen depots, activating potent anti-tumor immunity, and reversing immunosuppression (X. Zhao et al. 2023).

Various nanohybrids, including biodegradable, pH-responsive, and PLGA nanoparticles, have been developed for precise antigen delivery, helping convert non-responsive tumors into responsive ones by modulating the immune system environment (Liu, Zhang, and Xu 2019).

4.4.3.2 Nanohybrids for Immune Checkpoint Inhibition

Ligands such as PD-L1 are overexpressed by cancer cells, which binds to PD-1 receptors on T cells, inhibiting T cell activity and preventing the immune system from attacking the tumor (Hanahan and Weinberg 2011). Nanohybrids can enhance immune response by incorporating immune checkpoint inhibitors, such as anti-PD-L1 antibodies, which block the pathways that tumors use to evade immune detection. By combining multiple anti-cancer agents, nanohybrids can increase drug accumulation in cancer cells, promoting apoptosis and improving anti-tumor activity compared to single-agent therapies. For example, combining cisplatin with immune checkpoint inhibitors in nanohybrids can enhance drug accumulation and anti-tumor effects (N. Wang et al. 2018). Nanohybrids improve cancer immunotherapy by ensuring precise targeting, enhancing delivery, and reducing side effects typically involved with traditional treatments like chemotherapy.

4.4.4 Nanohybrids for Photothermal and Photodynamic Therapy

Photothermal therapy (PTT) and photodynamic therapy (PDT) are innovative cancer treatments that utilize light to target and destroy cancer cells. PTT converts light energy into heat, inducing localized hyperthermia that ultimately leads to cancer cell death (C. Li et al. 2022). PDT, on the contrary, relies on photosensitizers that produce reactive oxygen species (ROS), which can eventually initiate the apoptotic pathways in cancer cells. PDT also activates immune responses, such as T cell and dendritic cell activation, triggering immunogenic cell death (Hou et al. 2020). The combination of PTT and PDT with nanohybrids has shown improved therapeutic outcomes compared to individual therapies. Nanohybrids enhance treatment efficacy and address the constraints of traditional therapies. For example, integrating gold nanoparticles with graphene quantum dots generates singlet oxygen, boosting phototherapeutic outcomes (Soleimany et al. 2023). Additionally, the combination of iron oxide nanoflowers with copper sulfide shells, along with magnetic hyperthermia, enhances both photothermal and photodynamic effects (Q. Cheng et al. 2019). Combination therapy with nanohybrid and photothermal therapy for cancer treatment is depicted in Figure 4.1.

4.4.5 Nanohybrids in Combination Therapy

Combination therapy leverages the synergistic effects of multiple therapeutic agents to combat cancer, potentially minimizing drug resistance, enhancing anti-tumor effects, and reducing tumor progression. For example, a combination of methotrexate, 6-mercaptopurine, vincristine, and prednisone has been proven effective in treating acute lymphocytic leukemia in children, reducing tumor burden and recurrence risk (Mokhtari et al. 2017). However, combining multiple drugs can increase toxicity and affect targeted delivery (Lopez and Banerji 2017).

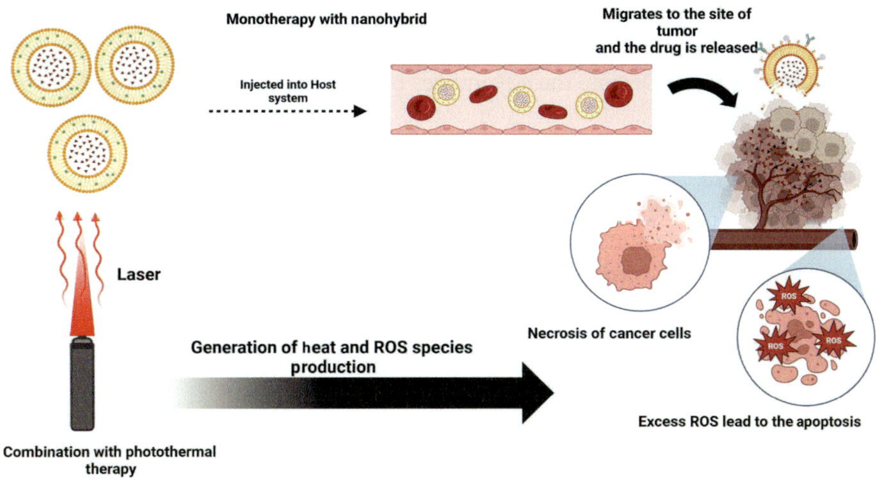

FIGURE 4.1 Combination therapy with nanohybrid and photothermal therapy for cancer treatment.

Nanohybrid-based delivery systems offer a promising solution by enhancing drug efficacy and limiting side effects, especially in cancer chemotherapy. Various nanomaterials, such as liposomes and polymeric nanomaterials, have been utilized for their ability to safely preserve drugs, provide controlled release, and ensure precise targeting. For instance, layered double hydroxide (LDH) nanomaterials have shown potential for delivering anionic anticancer drugs like methotrexate (MTX) and 5-fluorouracil (5-FU), which typically struggle with low affinity for negatively charged cell membranes. When MTX is incorporated into ZnAl-LDH through ion exchange, it can be efficiently internalized by cancer cells via clathrin-mediated endocytosis, resulting in enhanced anti-cancer efficacy. These MTX/LDH nanohybrids can overcome drug resistance in cancer cells, a significant challenge in chemotherapy, and improve precise drug release, boosting anti-cancer effects (Kim et al. 2014).

4.4.5.1 Multi-Modal Therapy with Nanohybrids

Multimodal treatments, such as combining chemotherapy and radiotherapy, have been explored to overcome tumor resistance. These therapies can effectively target tumors that resist traditional monotherapies. However, the downside is the high dosage and radiation exposure, which can lead to toxicity, damage to healthy cells, and suppression of the immune system. Nanoparticle-based delivery systems can address this issue by targeting tumors specifically through the enhanced permeability and retention (EPR) effect, minimizing harm to healthy tissues.

For example, gold nanoparticle (GNP) hybrids have been widely investigated for their ability to perform photothermal therapy (PTT), chemotherapy, radiotherapy, and imaging simultaneously. GNPs leverage their localized surface plasmon resonance (LSPR) properties to transform near-infrared (NIR) light into heat energy, enabling non-invasive tumor regression through hyperthermia.

Gold nanoparticle liposome hybrids loaded with chemotherapeutic drugs like doxorubicin (DOX) allow for temperature-triggered drug release, enhancing the synergy between PTT and chemotherapy, and leading to tumor eradication. Surface modifications with folic acid or antibodies improve targeting capabilities, minimizing off-target effects. Despite the advantages of GNP-based nanohybrids, challenges remain, such as accumulation in vital organs like the liver and spleen, which may cause systemic toxicity. Ongoing research is focused on overcoming these issues by using biodegradable and biocompatible polymers, like chitosan, to prevent toxicity. Additionally, maintaining nanohybrid quality and functionality for clinical use remains a significant challenge. Further research is required to overcome these limitations and minimize complications (Ali et al. 2022).

4.5 ADVANCEMENTS AND EMERGING TRENDS IN NANOHYBRIDS FOR CANCER TREATMENT

Advancements in nanohybrids for cancer treatment focus on enhancing targeted drug delivery, overcoming resistance, and improving treatment efficacy through combination therapies and precision targeting as shown in Figure 4.2. Emerging trends

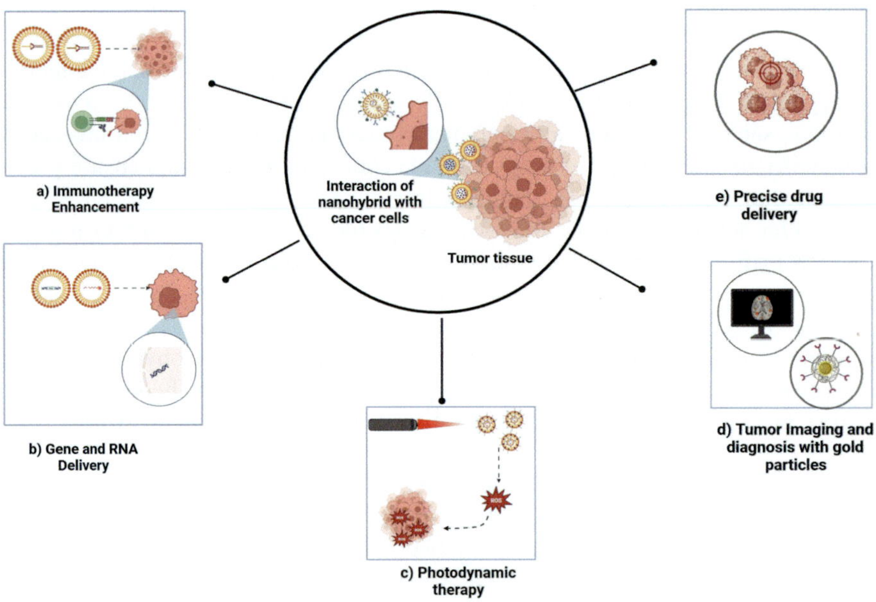

FIGURE 4.2 Advancements in nanohybrids for cancer therapy. (a) Immunotherapy enhancement: Nanohybrids can stimulate the immune system to recognize and attack cancer cells more effectively. (b) Gene and RNA delivery: These nanocarriers facilitate the targeted delivery of genetic material, such as RNA, to modify or suppress cancer cell functions. (c) Photodynamic therapy: Nanohybrids enhance the effectiveness of light-activated treatments to destroy cancer cells with minimal damage to surrounding tissues. (d) Tumor imaging and diagnosis with gold particles: Gold-based nanohybrids aid in imaging and diagnosing tumors with high precision, improving early detection and monitoring. (e) Precise drug delivery: Nanohybrids ensure targeted and controlled release of therapeutic agents directly to tumor sites, reducing side effects and improving efficacy.

include integrating nanohybrids with immunotherapy, gene editing tools like CRISPR-Cas9, and photothermal/photodynamic therapies for more effective and less toxic cancer treatments.

4.5.1 Tumor-Specific Targeting Strategies

Tumor-specific targeting delivers therapeutic agents precisely to cancer cells, minimizing damage to non-cancerous tissues. Passive targeting leverages tumor environment properties, while active targeting uses specific molecules for precision. Both approaches have unique benefits and challenges, with ongoing research enhancing their efficacy in cancer treatment (Dhilip Kumar and Abrahamse 2022).

4.5.1.1 Passive Targeting Mechanism

This strategy leverages the enhanced permeability and retention (EPR) effect, wherein nanomaterials accumulate in the tumor due to their leaky vasculature and poor lymphatic drainage. Examples include fully pegylated dendrimers, Doxil (pegylated liposomal doxorubicin), and Abraxane (albumin-based paclitaxel). However, passive targeting is less specific and may inadvertently affect healthy tissues, causing side effects.

4.5.1.2 Active Targeting Mechanism

The active targeting mechanism involves functionalizing nanomaterials with ligands or antibodies that can bind specifically to cancer cell receptors, increasing drug concentration at tumor sites. This approach offers greater precision, reducing side effects. Examples include MM-302 (HER2 receptor-targeting doxorubicin), BIND-014 (PSMA-targeting docetaxel), and MBP-426 (TfR-targeting oxaliplatin). However, active targeting involves complex design and production processes and may provoke immune responses against the targeting ligands.

4.5.2 Ligand-Based Targeting

Ligand-based targeting exploits specific receptors on cancer cells to deliver therapeutic agents directly.

4.5.2.1 RGD Peptides

The RGD (Arg-Gly-Asp) peptide binds to the $\alpha v\beta 3$ integrin receptor, commonly overexpressed in tumors. Modified nanocarriers with RGD peptides, including cyclic variants like c(RGDyK), enhance targeting and therapeutic delivery by improving receptor affinity and stability.

4.5.2.2 EGFR Antibody Targeting

The epidermal growth factor receptor (EGFR) is overexpressed in various types of cancers that majorly contribute to tumor progression. Cetuximab, a monoclonal antibody, inhibits EGFR signaling, reducing cancer cell proliferation. Cetuximab-modified nanocarriers, such as camptothecin-loaded nanoparticles, enhance targeting precision and tumor suppression, improving therapeutic outcomes.

4.5.3 Smart Nanohybrids

Smart nanoparticles represent a breakthrough in cancer therapy, responding to specific stimuli (e.g., pH, temperature, or enzymes) for achieving controlled drug release and targeted delivery. This approach minimizes the side effects and enhances treatment precision and efficacy (Sun et al. 2023).

4.5.4 Multifunctional Nanohybrids

Hybrid nanostructures (HNSs) integrate diagnostic and therapeutic capabilities, broadening their application beyond oncology to neurodegenerative and cardiovascular diseases. Examples include lipid-polymer nanoparticles for Alzheimer's treatment, biomimetic nanomaterials for cardiovascular conditions, and boron nitride nanotubes (BNNTs) for Parkinson's disease. These versatile systems enable the targeted drug delivery, enhanced diagnostic precision, and improved treatment outcomes, driving innovative solutions across diverse medical fields (Harun-Ur-Rashid and Jahan 2024).

4.5.5 Emerging Trends

With the continuous advancement of nanotechnology, its application in tumor treatment is evolving at an accelerated pace, promising transformative breakthroughs in oncology. The future of nanomaterials in cancer therapy is expected to focus on a variety of exciting developments that combine scientific innovation with clinical precision. A major area of focus is developing multifunctional integrated nanomaterials. These nanomaterials will combine diagnostic, therapeutic, and monitoring capabilities into a single platform. By offering real-time monitoring and treatment capabilities, these nanomaterials will not only allow for precise targeting of tumors but will also help monitor the effectiveness of treatment, enabling a dynamic and adaptive approach to therapy. Such integrated systems will help minimize side effects by ensuring that curative agents are delivered only to cancer cells while sparing surrounding healthy tissues.

Another promising aspect is the development of smart nanomaterials that can respond to environmental stimuli like pH, temperature, or enzyme activity. These stimuli-responsive nanomaterials will revolutionize the way drugs are delivered to tumor sites, ensuring that drugs are released only under distinct conditions, such as when they encounter the tumor acidosis or hypothermia. This selective drug release will significantly improve therapeutic outcomes by maximizing the concentration of drugs at the tumor site while minimizing systemic exposure and side effects. Moreover, nano biomaterials with outstanding biocompatibility and biodegradability are being explored for their potential applications in drug delivery and immunotherapy. These materials ensure that the nanocarriers do not trigger harmful immune responses and are safely broken down in the body after they have delivered their payload. This is crucial for the development of sustainable cancer therapies that are safe for long-term use (Srinivasan, Rajabi, and Mousa 2015).

The usage of nanomaterials in individualized tumor therapy is also set to expand. By analyzing the genomic, proteomic, and metabolomic profiles of a patient's tumor, personalized treatments can be designed. Nanomaterials play a crucial role by enabling precise and tailored drug delivery, which can adapt according to the distinct characteristics of each tumor. This innovative approach holds the promise of maximizing therapeutic efficacy and minimizing adverse effects (Shi et al. 2022).

In addition, the integration of nanoscience with emerging fields like gene editing and cell therapy presents groundbreaking opportunities for cancer treatment. Techniques like CRISPR-Cas9 could be paired with nanomaterials to deliver gene-editing tools directly to cancer cells, allowing for the altering the genetic mutations or the targeting of specific oncogenes. Similarly, nanomaterials could be used to improve cell-based therapies, such as CAR-T cells, by enhancing the delivery and efficacy of these therapies in the tumor microenvironment. Collectively, these advancements demonstrate the immense potential of nanotechnology to revolutionize cancer treatment.

By combining diagnostic, therapeutic, and monitoring functions, and by leveraging cutting-edge innovations like gene editing and cell therapies, nanomaterials will enable more precise, efficient, and personalized oncology treatments. These trends not only hold the promise of overcoming the limitations of current cancer therapies but also pave the way for highly effective, individualized treatments that offer hope for improved patient outcomes (Yang, Li, and Xie 2023).

4.6 PRECLINICAL AND CLINICAL STUDIES

In vitro models play a role in the evaluating nanohybrids for cancer therapy, as they provide crucial insights into the cytotoxicity, prodrug conversion efficiency, and therapeutic impact of these novel systems before proceeding to more complex in vivo studies. Cancer cell cultures are commonly used for these assessments, with well-established cell lines such as MCF-7 (breast cancer), MIA PaCa-2 (pancreatic cancer), and A549 (lung cancer). In 2D cell cultures, nanohybrids are tested for their effects on cell viability, proliferation, and the production of ROS. For example, enzyme nanohybrids that combine horseradish peroxidase (HRP) with magnetic nanoparticles were tested on MIA PaCa-2 cells to investigate the cytotoxic effects triggered by an alternating magnetic field (AMF) and the subsequent prodrug conversion process. This in vitro setup allowed the researchers to quantify the effects of the magnetic field-triggered activation of HRP, which generated ROS, leading to cancer cell death (Ravi, Kaviya, and Paramesh 2016).

3D spheroid models provide an additional layer of complexity and realism by replicating the three-dimensional architecture and microenvironment of solid tumors. These models are increasingly used to assess nanohybrid penetration and their effectiveness in mimicking real tumor conditions. For instance, gold nanohybrids functionalized with photosensitizers were tested in MCF-7 spheroids to evaluate their performance in photothermal and photodynamic therapy (PTT and PDT). These therapies rely on the ability of nanohybrids to convert light into heat or generate ROS, thereby killing tumor cells. Testing in spheroids provides a more accurate representation of how these nanohybrids would behave in vivo, especially regarding penetration through dense tumor tissue.

Beyond in vitro studies, in vivo models are essential for testing the biodistribution, therapeutic efficacy, and safety of nanohybrids. Xenograft models, in which human cancer cells are incorporated into immunocompromised mice, allow researchers to simulate a human-like tumor environment for assessing the therapeutic potential of nanohybrids. For instance, MIA PaCa-2 pancreatic tumors in mice were treated with enzyme nanohybrids combined with 3IAA and AMF exposure, leading to a prominent reduction in the size of tumor growth. These studies demonstrated the ability of the nanohybrids to localize the therapeutic effects to the tumor site, with minimal impact on healthy tissues (Torres-Herrero et al. 2023).

In addition, syngeneic models, where tumors are extracted from the same genetic lineage as the host, are used to assess immune responses in immunocompetent mice. For example, iron oxide-silica nanohybrids were tested in syngeneic melanoma mouse models to explore their combined immunotherapy and hyperthermia effects. These models are crucial for evaluating how nanohybrids interact with the host's immune system and the tumor microenvironment, providing valuable insights into their potential for combination therapies such as immunotherapy and hyperthermia (Balivada et al. 2010).

Orthotopic models, where cancer cells are implanted in their organ of origin, closely mimic the natural tumor microenvironment, offering an additional layer of realism. For example, nanohybrids loaded with cisplatin were used in orthotopic ovarian cancer models to study intraperitoneal drug release and efficacy. This model allows for the precise evaluation of how nanohybrids perform in the same anatomical and physiological conditions as human cancers, providing more reliable data for clinical translation. Together, these in vitro and in vivo models offer a comprehensive platform to study the therapeutic potential, safety, and effectiveness of nanohybrids in cancer treatment, providing essential data to inform the development of next-generation cancer therapies (Z. Zhao, Simms, and Steinmetz 2022).

Case Study: Remote Activation of Enzyme Nanohybrids for Cancer Prodrug Therapy Controlled by Magnetic Heating

A groundbreaking case study explores the usage of enzyme nanohybrids (nHs) for directed enzyme prodrug therapy (DEPT) in cancer treatment, focusing on pancreatic cancer. These nanohybrids consist of magnetic nanoparticles (MNPs) co-encapsulated with horseradish peroxidase (HRP) within a biomimetic silica matrix. The unique feature of these nanohybrids is their ability to be activated remotely by magnetic heating, offering a targeted approach for cancer treatment without affecting the surrounding healthy tissues. HRP converts prodrug indole-3-acetic acid (3IAA) into cytotoxic radicals, which selectively target tumor cells.

In vitro experiments with MIA PaCa-2 human pancreatic cancer cells demonstrated that incubating the cells with the nanohybrids and 3IAA, followed by exposure to an AMF, resulted in significant cytotoxicity. This was evidenced by a marked decrease in cell viability and an increase in ROS production, which are key factors in inducing cancer cell death.

The ability to selectively activate the therapeutic enzyme at the tumor site is a major advantage of this system, as it minimizes the off-target effects associated with traditional therapies. In vivo studies using mouse models of pancreatic cancer showed that intratumoral injection of the nanohybrids, followed by intraperitoneal administration of 3IAA and AMF exposure, led to significant tumor growth reduction. The results also highlighted the effective biodistribution of the nanohybrids, as they localized to the tumor site and triggered the desired therapeutic effects with minimal systemic toxicity. These findings underscore the potential of enzyme nanohybrids for remotely controlled, localized cancer treatment, offering a promising strategy for targeted therapy that avoids the complications associated with conventional chemotherapy.

This case study exemplifies the versatility and potential of nanohybrids in cancer treatment, demonstrating their ability to integrate multiple functions – such as targeted drug delivery, remote activation, and minimal toxicity – into a single system, offering a novel approach to cancer therapy (Torres-Herrero et al. 2023).

4.7 CHALLENGES

The application of nanomaterials in oncology, while promising, is accompanied by a range of significant challenges that must be overcome to unlock their full potential in cancer treatment. One of the primary issues is the inadequate conversion efficiency of nanoparticles, particularly those used in therapies like photothermal and photodynamic treatments. In some cases, nanoparticles struggle to effectively convert light energy into localized heat, limiting their capacity to induce the desired thermal ablation of tumor cells. This inefficiency hinders the therapeutic efficacy of such treatments and calls for innovations that can enhance the energy conversion efficiency of nanoparticles, especially in clinical settings (Cui et al. 2023).

Biocompatibility and toxicity are also pressing concerns, especially with metal-based plasmonic nanoparticles, which are commonly used in cancer treatment. These nanoparticles, while effective in certain applications, may suffer from stability issues and potential toxicity, which could limit their clinical usability. The safety of nanomaterials is heavily dependent on their biodistribution, metabolism, and excretion within the body, as improper accumulation in organs or tissues can lead to adverse effects. Additionally, long-term studies on the toxicity and immunogenicity of nanomaterials are limited; necessitating further research to evaluate the long-term effects of these materials on the human body and ensure their safety for clinical use (Roshani et al. 2023).

The preparation and quality control of nanomaterials present another significant challenge. The therapeutic efficacy of nanohybrids depends on the refinement of production methods to improve the stability, bioactivity, and drug-loading capacity of nanoparticles. Despite promising laboratory results, these materials often face issues in scaling up for clinical use. The translation from laboratory to clinical application is complicated by the need for reproducible, standardized production techniques that ensure consistent quality, efficacy, and safety of the nanomaterials. Extensive clinical trials are crucial to assess the effectiveness and safety of these materials in practical clinical settings. However, these trials can be both time consuming and resource intensive.

Furthermore, the interaction between nanomaterials and the tumor microenvironment plays a key role in determining their therapeutic outcomes. Nanoparticles often have to navigate complex biological barriers to reach tumor sites, and the tumor microenvironment itself may influence the nanoparticles' behavior, including their uptake by cancer cells. A deeper understanding of these interactions is crucial for designing nanoparticles that can precisely target tumors and deliver therapeutic agents effectively, minimizing off-target effects. Research in this area is essential to optimize targeting strategies and enhance the precision of nanomaterials in oncology. Interdisciplinary collaboration among materials scientists, biologists, and medical professionals is crucial to driving innovations and addressing these challenges. However, nanoparticle size, shape, and composition can exhibit significant heterogeneity, which leads to inconsistent performance and unpredictable therapeutic outcomes. This variability complicates the clinical application of nanomaterials and underscores the need for further research into their consistent fabrication and controlled performance (Torres-Herrero et al. 2023).

Additionally, the scalability and manufacturing of nanomaterials pose logistical and financial hurdles. High-quality, cost-effective production methods are required to ensure that nanomaterials can be produced on a large scale for clinical usage while ensuring safety, biocompatibility, and efficacy. These challenges also involve important ethical concerns, particularly regulation and approval of new nanomaterials for medical use. Regulatory bodies need to establish clear and comprehensive guidelines to address safety, efficacy, and ethical considerations in the use of nanomaterials in cancer therapy.

Ultimately, to realize the full potential of nanomaterials in oncology, comprehensive research, interdisciplinary collaboration, and the establishment of clear regulatory frameworks are essential. Addressing these multifaceted challenges will be key to ensuring that nanomaterials can safely and effectively contribute to the advancement of cancer therapies, providing personalized, targeted treatments that improve patient outcomes (Yang, Li, and Xie 2023).

4.8 CONCLUSION

Nanohybrids represent a transformative and innovative approach in the field of cancer therapeutics by offering precise and targeted treatment methods. By combining both organic and inorganic materials, these hybrid systems enhance drug delivery and precision, minimizing the cytotoxic effects of high doses of chemotherapeutic drugs and addressing the limitations of traditional therapies such as radiotherapy and chemotherapy. Utilizing mechanisms like EPR and ligand-mediated targeting, these systems ensure localized delivery of therapeutic agents to the tumor site, thereby improving treatment outcomes. The usage of nanohybrids in combination therapies such as PTT, PDT, and gene therapy enhances the therapeutic efficacy and reduces the cytotoxic effects. Nanohybrids have the unique response to stimuli like pH and temperature (hypoxia) conditions in the tumor microenvironment with greater adaptability. This ensures the precise and controlled drug release and improvement of the survival rate.

Despite their innovative and promising approaches toward the cancer therapy, there are some challenges like long-term biocompatibility of nanohybrids, regulatory approval, etc. Advancements in the advanced technologies like CRISPR-Cas9 and immunomodulation are exploring the new pathways and horizons of nanohybrid applications that can regulate the toxicity effects of multidrug therapies and also tackle the issues like multi drug resistance.

Preclinical and clinical studies ensure the efficacy and safety of nanohybrids, highlighting the ability of these delivery systems to penetrate into the tumor microenvironment, which eventually leads to the greater therapeutic value and minimizes the systemic toxicity. Integration of diagnosis and therapy into a single nanohybrid system promises a future of real-time, patient-specific cancer care.

In summary, nanohybrids stand at the forefront of innovative approaches toward the cancer treatment, addressing the precise targeting, effective drug dosage, and personalized therapies. Interdisciplinary principles of medicine and nanotechnology do not improve the survival rate of the individual, but do improve the quality life of the individual who is suffering from the cancer. With continuous research, advancements, and collaborations between the fields of nanotechnology and medicine, these approaches explore the landscape of cancer therapy, offering and aid in gaining the upper hand in battling against cancer, which is one of humanity's greatest health challenges.

REFERENCES

Ali, Amaal Abdulraqeb, Waad H. Abuwatfa, Mohammad H. Al-Sayah, and Ghaleb A. Husseini. 2022. "Gold-Nanoparticle Hybrid Nanostructures for Multimodal Cancer Therapy." *Nanomaterials* 12 (20): 3706. https://doi.org/10.3390/nano12203706.

Balivada, Sivasai, Raja Shekar Rachakatla, Hongwang Wang, Thilani N. Samarakoon, Raj Kumar Dani, Marla Pyle, Franklin O. Kroh, et al. 2010. "A/C Magnetic Hyperthermia of Melanoma Mediated by Iron(0)/Iron Oxide Core/Shell Magnetic Nanoparticles: A Mouse Study." *BMC Cancer* 10 (1): 119. https://doi.org/10.1186/1471-2407-10-119.

Bizuayehu, Habtamu Mellie, Kedir Y. Ahmed, Getiye Dejenu Kibret, Abel F. Dadi, Sewunet Admasu Belachew, Tanmay Bagade, Teketo Kassaw Tegegne, et al. 2024. "Global Disparities of Cancer and Its Projected Burden in 2050." *JAMA Network Open* 7 (11): e2443198. https://doi.org/10.1001/jamanetworkopen.2024.43198.

Chen, Gongning, Fu Yang, Danping Wu, Jun Yang, Xiaojuan Hu, Longcai Liu, Yehui Kang, et al. 2024. "Naphthalene Diimide-Based Polycyclic Conjugated Molecule Composite CoFe2 O4 Nanohybrids for Photoacoustic Imaging-Mediated Photo-/Sonic Therapy." *Advanced Healthcare Materials* 13 (27): 2401074. https://doi.org/10.1002/adhm.202401074.

Chen, Jie, Zhaopei Guo, Huayu Tian, and Xuesi Chen. 2016. "Production and Clinical Development of Nanoparticles for Gene Delivery." *Molecular Therapy – Methods & Clinical Development* 3: 16023. https://doi.org/10.1038/mtm.2016.23.

Chen, Yuhao, Meng Du, Jinsui Yu, Lang Rao, Xiaoyuan Chen, and Zhiyi Chen. 2020. "Nanobiohybrids: A Synergistic Integration of Bacteria and Nanomaterials in Cancer Therapy." *BIO Integration* 1 (1). https://doi.org/10.15212/bioi-2020-0008.

Cheng, Qian, Zi-Hao Li, Yun-Xia Sun, and Xian-Zheng Zhang. 2019. "Controlled Synthesis of a Core-Shell Nanohybrid for Effective Multimodal Image-Guided Combined Photothermal/Photodynamic Therapy of Tumors." *NPG Asia Materials* 11 (1): 63. https://doi.org/10.1038/s41427-019-0164-4.

Cheng, Xiaoxiao, Qirong Xie, and Yang Sun. 2023. "Advances in Nanomaterial-Based Targeted Drug Delivery Systems." *Frontiers in Bioengineering and Biotechnology* 11 (April): 1177151. https://doi.org/10.3389/fbioe.2023.1177151.

Cheng, Zhe, Maoyu Li, Raja Dey, and Yongheng Chen. 2021. "Nanomaterials for Cancer Therapy: Current Progress and Perspectives." *Journal of Hematology & Oncology* 14 (1): 85. https://doi.org/10.1186/s13045-021-01096-0.

Cui, Ximin, Qifeng Ruan, Xiaolu Zhuo, Xinyue Xia, Jingtian Hu, Runfang Fu, Yang Li, Jianfang Wang, and Hongxing Xu. 2023. "Photothermal Nanomaterials: A Powerful Light-to-Heat Converter." *Chemical Reviews* 123 (11): 6891–952. https://doi.org/10.1021/acs.chemrev.3c00159.

Davis, Mark E., Jonathan E. Zuckerman, Chung Hang J. Choi, David Seligson, Anthony Tolcher, Christopher A. Alabi, Yun Yen, Jeremy D. Heidel, and Antoni Ribas. 2010. "Evidence of RNAi in Humans from Systemically Administered siRNA via Targeted Nanoparticles." *Nature* 464 (7291): 1067–70. https://doi.org/10.1038/nature08956.

Dhilip Kumar, Sathish Sundar, and Heidi Abrahamse. 2022. "Recent Advances in the Development of Biocompatible Nanocarriers and Their Cancer Cell Targeting Efficiency in Photodynamic Therapy." *Frontiers in Chemistry* 10 (August): 969809. https://doi.org/10.3389/fchem.2022.969809.

Donahue, Nathan D., Handan Acar, and Stefan Wilhelm. 2019. "Concepts of Nanoparticle Cellular Uptake, Intracellular Trafficking, and Kinetics in Nanomedicine." *Advanced Drug Delivery Reviews* 143 (March): 68–96. https://doi.org/10.1016/j.addr.2019.04.008.

Hanahan, Douglas, and Robert A. Weinberg. 2011. "Hallmarks of Cancer: The Next Generation." *Cell* 144 (5): 646–74. https://doi.org/10.1016/j.cell.2011.02.013.

Harun-Ur-Rashid, Mohammad, and Israt Jahan. 2024. "Innovative Hybrid Nanostructures: Pioneering Advances in Modern Therapy." *Frontiers in Nanotechnology* 6 (August): 1458894. https://doi.org/10.3389/fnano.2024.1458894.

Hou, Yun-Jing, Xin-Xin Yang, Rui-qi Liu, Di Zhao, Che-Xu Guo, An-Chao Zhu, Mei-Na Wen, Zhao Liu, Guo-fan Qu, and Hong-Xue Meng. 2020. "Pathological Mechanism of Photodynamic Therapy and Photothermal Therapy Based on Nanoparticles." *International Journal of Nanomedicine* 15 (September): 6827–38. https://doi.org/10.2147/IJN.S269321.

Kim, Tae-Hyun, Gyeong Jin Lee, Joo-Hee Kang, Hyoung-Jun Kim, Tae-il Kim, and Jae-Min Oh. 2014. "Anticancer Drug-Incorporated Layered Double Hydroxide Nanohybrids and Their Enhanced Anticancer Therapeutic Efficacy in Combination Cancer Treatment." *BioMed Research International* 2014: 1–11. https://doi.org/10.1155/2014/193401.

Kumar, Arun, Mirkomil Sharipov, Abbaskhan Turaev, Shavkatjon Azizov, Ismatdjan Azizov, Edwin Makhado, Abbas Rahdar, Deepak Kumar, and Sadanand Pandey. 2022. "Polymer-Based Hybrid Nanoarchitectures for Cancer Therapy Applications." *Polymers* 14 (15): 3027. https://doi.org/10.3390/polym14153027.

Li, Chaowei, Yue Cheng, Dawei Li, Qi An, Wei Zhang, Yu Zhang, and Yijun Fu. 2022. "Antitumor Applications of Photothermal Agents and Photothermal Synergistic Therapies." *International Journal of Molecular Sciences* 23 (14): 7909. https://doi.org/10.3390/ijms23147909.

Li, Jin, Mingwu Shen, and Xiangyang Shi. 2020. "Poly(Amidoamine) Dendrimer-Gold Nanohybrids in Cancer Gene Therapy: A Concise Overview." *ACS Applied Bio Materials* 3 (9): 5590–605. https://doi.org/10.1021/acsabm.0c00863.

Liang, Chen, Xinglin Zhang, Zhichao Wang, Wenjun Wang, Mengsu Yang, and Xiaochen Dong. 2020. "Organic/Inorganic Nanohybrids Rejuvenate Photodynamic Cancer Therapy." *Journal of Materials Chemistry B* 8 (22): 4748–63. https://doi.org/10.1039/D0TB00098A.

Lin, Gan, Peng Mi, Chengchao Chu, Jun Zhang, and Gang Liu. 2016. "Inorganic Nanocarriers Overcoming Multidrug Resistance for Cancer Theranostics." *Advanced Science* 3 (11): 1600134. https://doi.org/10.1002/advs.201600134.

Liu, Jianping, Run Zhang, and Zhi Ping Xu. 2019. "Nanoparticle-Based Nanomedicines to Promote Cancer Immunotherapy: Recent Advances and Future Directions." *Small* 15 (32): 1900262. https://doi.org/10.1002/smll.201900262.

Lopez, Juanita S., and Udai Banerji. 2017. "Combine and Conquer: Challenges for Targeted Therapy Combinations in Early Phase Trials." *Nature Reviews Clinical Oncology* 14 (1): 57–66. https://doi.org/10.1038/nrclinonc.2016.96.

Mehrotra, Neha, and Kaushik Pal. 2024. "Tumor Targeted Nanohybrid for Dual Stimuli Responsive and NIR Amplified Photothermal/Photo-Induced Thermodynamic/Chemodynamic Combination Therapy." *Biomedical Materials* 19 (3): 035019. https://doi.org/10.1088/1748-605X/ad330f.

Mi, Peng. 2020. "Stimuli-Responsive Nanocarriers for Drug Delivery, Tumor Imaging, Therapy and Theranostics." *Theranostics* 10 (10): 4557–88. https://doi.org/10.7150/thno.38069.

Mokhtari, Reza Bayat, Tina S. Homayouni, Narges Baluch, Evgeniya Morgatskaya, Sushil Kumar, Bikul Das, and Herman Yeger. 2017. "Combination Therapy in Combating Cancer." *Oncotarget* 8 (23): 38022–43. https://doi.org/10.18632/oncotarget.16723.

Nakamura, Yuko, Ai Mochida, Peter L. Choyke, and Hisataka Kobayashi. 2016. "Nanodrug Delivery: Is the Enhanced Permeability and Retention Effect Sufficient for Curing Cancer?" *Bioconjugate Chemistry* 27 (10): 2225–38. https://doi.org/10.1021/acs.bioconjchem.6b00437.

Patra, Jayanta Kumar, Gitishree Das, Leonardo Fernandes Fraceto, Estefania Vangelie Ramos Campos, Maria Del Pilar Rodriguez-Torres, Laura Susana Acosta-Torres, Luis Armando Diaz-Torres, et al. 2018. "Nano Based Drug Delivery Systems: Recent Developments and Future Prospects." *Journal of Nanobiotechnology* 16 (1): 71. https://doi.org/10.1186/s12951-018-0392-8.

Prakash, Satya, Meenakshi Malhotra, Wei Shao, Catherine Tomaro-Duchesneau, and Sana Abbasi. 2011. "Polymeric Nanohybrids and Functionalized Carbon Nanotubes as Drug Delivery Carriers for Cancer Therapy." *Advanced Drug Delivery Reviews* 63 (14–15): 1340–51. https://doi.org/10.1016/j.addr.2011.06.013.

Ravi, Maddaly, S. R. Kaviya, and V. Paramesh. 2016. "Culture Phases, Cytotoxicity and Protein Expressions of Agarose Hydrogel Induced Sp2/0, A549, MCF-7 Cell Line 3D Cultures." *Cytotechnology* 68 (3): 429–41. https://doi.org/10.1007/s10616-014-9795-z.

Roshani, Mohammad, Arya Rezaian-Isfahni, Mohammad Hassan Lotfalizadeh, Negar Khassafi, Mohammad Hassan Jafari Najaf Abadi, and Majid Nejati. 2023. "Metal Nanoparticles as a Potential Technique for the Diagnosis and Treatment of Gastrointestinal Cancer: A Comprehensive Review." *Cancer Cell International* 23 (1): 280. https://doi.org/10.1186/s12935-023-03115-1.

Sahay, Gaurav, Daria Y. Alakhova, and Alexander V. Kabanov. 2010. "Endocytosis of Nanomedicines." *Journal of Controlled Release* 145 (3): 182–95. https://doi.org/10.1016/j.jconrel.2010.01.036.

Shi, Zhiyuan, Jianzhong Zheng, Wenbin Tang, Yang Bai, Lei Zhang, Zuodong Xuan, Huimin Sun, and Chen Shao. 2022. "Multifunctional Nanomaterials for Ferroptotic Cancer Therapy." *Frontiers in Chemistry* 10 (March): 868630. https://doi.org/10.3389/fchem.2022.868630.

Soleimany, Amir, Sepideh Khoee, Sofia Dias, and Bruno Sarmento. 2023. "Exploring Low-Power Single-Pulsed Laser-Triggered Two-Photon Photodynamic/Photothermal Combination Therapy Using a Gold Nanostar/Graphene Quantum Dot Nanohybrid." *ACS Applied Materials & Interfaces* 15 (17): 20811–21. https://doi.org/10.1021/acsami.3c03578.

Srinivasan, Mathangi, Mehdi Rajabi, and Shaker Mousa. 2015. "Multifunctional Nanomaterials and Their Applications in Drug Delivery and Cancer Therapy." *Nanomaterials* 5 (4): 1690–703. https://doi.org/10.3390/nano5041690.

Sun, Leming, Hongmei Liu, Yanqi Ye, Yang Lei, Rehmat Islam, Sumin Tan, Rongsheng Tong, Yang-Bao Miao, and Lulu Cai. 2023. "Smart Nanoparticles for Cancer Therapy." *Signal Transduction and Targeted Therapy* 8 (1): 418. https://doi.org/10.1038/s41392-023-01642-x.

Torres-Herrero, Beatriz, Ilaria Armenia, Maria Alleva, Laura Asín, Sonali Correa, Cecilia Ortiz, Yilian Fernández-Afonso, et al. 2023. "Remote Activation of Enzyme Nanohybrids for Cancer Prodrug Therapy Controlled by Magnetic Heating." *ACS Nano* 17 (13): 12358–73. https://doi.org/10.1021/acsnano.3c01599.

Tredan, O., C. M. Galmarini, K. Patel, and I. F. Tannock. 2007. "Drug Resistance and the Solid Tumor Microenvironment." *JNCI Journal of the National Cancer Institute* 99 (19): 1441–54. https://doi.org/10.1093/jnci/djm135.

Wang, Na, Zhigang Wang, Zoufeng Xu, Xianfeng Chen, and Guangyu Zhu. 2018. "A Cisplatin-Loaded Immunochemotherapeutic Nanohybrid Bearing Immune Checkpoint Inhibitors for Enhanced Cervical Cancer Therapy." *Angewandte Chemie International Edition* 57 (13): 3426–30. https://doi.org/10.1002/anie.201800422.

Wang, Xiangdong, Zhongning Liu, Ronghua Jin, Bolei Cai, Shiyu Liu, Yongkang Bai, and Xin Chen. 2021. "Multifunctional Hierarchical Nanohybrids Perform Triple Antitumor Theranostics in a Cascaded Manner for Effective Tumor Treatment." *Acta Biomaterialia* 128 (July): 408–19. https://doi.org/10.1016/j.actbio.2021.04.019.

Wang, Yixin, Allie Barrett, and Quanyin Hu. 2024. "Nanotechnology-Assisted CAR -T-Cell Therapy for Tumor Treatment." *WIREs Nanomedicine and Nanobiotechnology* 16 (5): e2005. https://doi.org/10.1002/wnan.2005.

Xu, Xiaoyu, Chang Liu, Yonghui Wang, Oliver Koivisto, Junnian Zhou, Yilai Shu, and Hongbo Zhang. 2021. "Nanotechnology-Based Delivery of CRISPR/Cas9 for Cancer Treatment." *Advanced Drug Delivery Reviews* 176 (September): 113891. https://doi.org/10.1016/j.addr.2021.113891.

Yang, Hongmei, Chen Li, and Qiang Xie. 2023. "Advances in the Use of Nanomaterials in Tumour Therapy: Challenges and Prospects." *Cancer Insight* 2 (2): 37–48. https://doi.org/10.58567/ci02020004.

Zhang, Feifei, Chenglong Xin, Zhichao Dai, Heli Hu, Qi An, Fei Wang, Zunfu Hu, Yunqiang Sun, Lu Tian, and Xiuwen Zheng. 2022. "Oncocyte Membrane-Camouflaged Multi-Stimuli-Responsive Nanohybrids for Synergistic Amplification of Tumor Oxidative Stresses and Photothermal Enhanced Cancer Therapy." *ACS Applied Materials & Interfaces* 14 (36): 40633–44. https://doi.org/10.1021/acsami.2c11200.

Zhang, Wei, Lu Chen, Xianbin Zhang, Peng Gong, Xiyu Wang, Zhiying Xu, Ganyu Nie, and Lu Xu. 2023. "Functionalized Nanohybrids with Rod Shape for Improved Chemo-Phototherapeutic Effect against Cancer by Sequentially Generating Singlet Oxygen and Carbon Dioxide Bubbles." *Biomaterials Science* 11 (20): 6894–905. https://doi.org/10.1039/D3BM00541K.

Zhao, Nana, Weili Fan, Xiaoyi Zhao, Yanjun Liu, Yang Hu, Feng Duan, and Fu-Jian Xu. 2020. "Polycation–Carbon Nanohybrids with Superior Rough Hollow Morphology for the NIR-II Responsive Multimodal Therapy." *ACS Applied Materials & Interfaces* 12 (10): 11341–52. https://doi.org/10.1021/acsami.9b22373.

Zhao, Nana, Liemei Yan, Xiaoyi Zhao, Xinyan Chen, Aihua Li, Di Zheng, Xin Zhou, Xiaoguang Dai, and Fu-Jian Xu. 2019. "Versatile Types of Organic/Inorganic Nanohybrids: From Strategic Design to Biomedical Applications." *Chemical Reviews* 119 (3): 1666–762. https://doi.org/10.1021/acs.chemrev.8b00401.

Zhao, Xiaoyi, Jiatong Zhang, Beibei Chen, Xiaokang Ding, Nana Zhao, and Fu-Jian Xu. 2023. "Rough Nanovaccines Boost Antitumor Immunity Through the Enhancement of Vaccination Cascade and Immunogenic Cell Death Induction." *Small Methods* 7 (5): 2201595. https://doi.org/10.1002/smtd.202201595.

Zhao, Zhongchao, Andrea Simms, and Nicole F. Steinmetz. 2022. "Cisplatin-Loaded Tobacco Mosaic Virus for Ovarian Cancer Treatment." *Biomacromolecules* 23 (10): 4379–87. https://doi.org/10.1021/acs.biomac.2c00831.

5 Nanohybrids for Inflammatory Disease Therapeutic Applications

Kalyani Chepuri, Chittepu Pranitha, Kathuroju Harikrishna, Vadakavila Geethikalal, Himabindu Kurra, Joshika Rerelly, Shreyas Sadineni, and Madeeha Owais

5.1 INTRODUCTION

Inflammation is the immune system's initial response to infections and tissue injury (Liu et al. 2024). Pro-inflammatory cytokines like IL-1, IL-6, TNF-α, and IFN-γ promote immune responses, whereas anti-inflammatory cytokines like TGF-β, IL-4, and IL-10 limit excessive inflammation to maintain immunological balance. Stress, aging, and genetic susceptibility can all disrupt this balance, leading to tissue damage and persistent inflammation. It was also asserted that persistent inflammation disrupts cellular functions vital for preserving tissue strength and slowing disease progression (Park et al. 2020; Janakiraman et al. 2018). Early identification and therapy are necessary for managing inflammatory diseases and minimizing systemic damage. Accurate diagnosis of inflammation involves blood tests and imaging. Markers like IL-6 support early detection, while imaging methods such as CT and MRI provide visual insights, each with specific advantages and limitations (Liu et al. 2024; Hosseinikhah et al. 2021).

Inflammatory diseases are treated via gene therapies, pharmaceutical drugs, and drugs that comprise proteins or peptides. NSAIDs, such as aspirin and ibuprofen, reduce inflammation by blocking the formation of prostaglandins; nevertheless, they can also cause bleeding in the gastrointestinal tract and cardiac problems (Stiller and Hjemdahl 2022). Despite decreasing immune activity, long-term use of corticosteroids, such as dexamethasone, can lead to risks such osteoporosis and diabetes (Tu et al. 2022). Gene therapy provides promise for conditions including arthritis and cystic fibrosis, despite challenges like immunogenicity and instability (Wang et al. 2020). Better delivery methods are required due to the volatility and high production costs of protein-based therapies and peptide drugs, even though they target specific inflammatory pathways (Cao et al. 2021).

DOI: 10.1201/9781003563723-5

Nanotechnology has tremendously changed the way that inflammatory illnesses are diagnosed and treated. Nano-drug delivery systems (nano-DDSs) employ nanoparticle (NP) properties like surface charge, size, shape, and surface alterations to boost efficacy. Nanotechnology is the breakthrough of contemporary medicine, offering cutting-edge instruments for precise health evaluation and intervention. In particular, nanoparticles are of great interest for inflammatory diseases since they reinforce the stability, bioavailability, and targeted delivery of therapeutics. NPs can pass biological barriers; PEGylation boosts circulation and immune evasion qualities while mannose ligands guarantee targeting only specific cells. Nanohybrids offer enhanced versatility by integrating therapeutic and diagnostic features. This comprehensive approach to inflammation allows for more effective and safer management, paving the way for next-generation therapies (Jeong and Park 2021; Wang et al. 2021).

Nano-DDSs improve pharmacokinetics, bioavailability, and drug solubility to provide customized and effective treatment. By facilitating controlled drug release, co-delivery of many drugs, and real-time biosensing, these devices offer synergistic benefits and combat resistance (Brusini, Varna, and Couvreur 2020). Nanoprobes and nano sensors enhance the imaging, detection, and monitoring of inflammatory lesions. At the same time, customized nano-DDSs reduce off-target toxicity and extend drug circulation. Examples include surface-engineered liposomes, curcumin-loaded solid lipid nanoparticles, and metallic and polymeric nanoparticles based on NSAIDs, including hyaluronic-gold-tocilizumab NPs and chitosan-dexamethasone (CS-Dex) NPs (Schiavi et al. 2020). Functionalizing NPs with antibodies improves treatment outcomes and also lowers the side effects by specifically targeting macrophages, which cause inflammation (Feng and Guo 2020; J. Wu et al. 2020; Aden et al. 2019).

Nanohybrids improve target specificity and allow for regulated drug release and solubilizing hydrophobic drugs; they offer special promise for the treatment of inflammatory diseases. Advanced molecular imaging, like MRI, which can differentiate between healthy and diseased cells, is also supported by these techniques. Inflammatory tissues can be effectively repaired by using nanohybrids such as superparamagnetic iron oxide nanoparticles (SPIONs), gold nanoparticles, and chitosan-glyco nanoparticles (Zhao et al. 2021). Because of their exceptional biocompatibility, SPIONs are especially well suited for repeated therapeutic and diagnostic applications (Zhang et al. 2020). Nanohybrids enhance resolution and precise inflammation detection when combined with drugs like dexamethasone (Brusini, Varna, and Couvreur 2020). These developments show how revolutionary nanotechnology can be used in the treatment of inflammatory illnesses.

This chapter gives insights into the therapeutic applications of nanohybrids in inflammatory diseases. It also explores the types and characteristics of nanohybrids, targeting mechanisms, and modulation of inflammation. Nanohybrids offer precise drug delivery, better bioavailability, and lower toxicity compared to conventional therapies. Challenges such as biocompatibility and scalability are discussed, alongside promising AI-based delivery innovations. Emphasis is placed on the need for research to fully realize their therapeutic potential in better managing inflammatory diseases.

5.2 NANOHYBRIDS

Nanohybrids are an intriguing class of materials that blend multiple nanomaterials to achieve enhanced properties and multifunctionality. These materials consist of organic and inorganic components bonded together at the nanoscale, either covalently or non-covalently. The resulting material is not merely a simple mixture of its components but a synergistic material with unique properties and performance, determined by the interface of the components at the molecular or supramolecular level. Its functionality is linked to the improvement of physicochemical properties. The primary goal of creating nanohybrids is to modify material properties such as size, composition, structure, and surface chemistry, resulting in improved performance for various applications (Idris et al. 2023).

5.2.1 Classification of Nanohybrids

Nanohybrids are classified based on the types of parent materials used (Figure 5.1). The main types of nanohybrids are:

Carbon-carbon nanohybrids (CCNHs): These nanohybrids consist of various forms of carbon nanomaterials combined together. Carbon-based nanohybrids consist of combinations of three primary carbon nanostructures: zero-dimensional fullerenes, one-dimensional carbon nanotubes (CNTs), and two-dimensional graphene and carbon nanohorns (CNHs) (Vizuete et al. 2012).

Carbon–metal nanohybrids (CMNHs): These nanohybrids are formed by combining carbon nanomaterials with metal nanomaterials. The metallic nanomaterials can be noble metals like Ag, Au, Pt, Ru, and Rh and lanthanide series metals like La, Sc, and Gd. CMNHs also include metal oxide nanomaterials such as ZnO, TiO_2, SiO_2, Fe_3O_4 and CuO, semiconducting quantum dots like CdSe and CdTe, and ligand-based metallic compounds like ferrocene (B. Wu et al. 2011).

Metal–metal nanohybrids (MMNHs): These nanohybrids are formed by combining different metal nanomaterials. When metals and metal oxides are combined to form multi-metallic ensembles, they are known as metal-metal nanohybrids. These metals can be categorized by their functionalities, such as plasmonic (Au, Ag, Pt) (Anker et al. 2008), magnetic $\left(Fe_3O_4, Fe_2O_3\right)$ (Pankhurst et al. 2003), semiconducting oxides $\left(TiO_2\right)$ (Kamat 2002), and quantum dots (CdSe, CdTe, ZnO, ZnS, PbS) (Alivisatos 1996), etc.

Organic molecule-coated nanohybrids (OMCNHs): Organic molecule-coated nanohybrids are materials that blend multiple nanomaterials to achieve enhanced properties and multifunctionality. These materials are composed of organic and inorganic components that are bonded together at the nanoscale, either covalently or noncovalently. This combination creates a synergistic effect that enhances their properties, making them highly effective for various applications (Zeb and Riaz 2022).

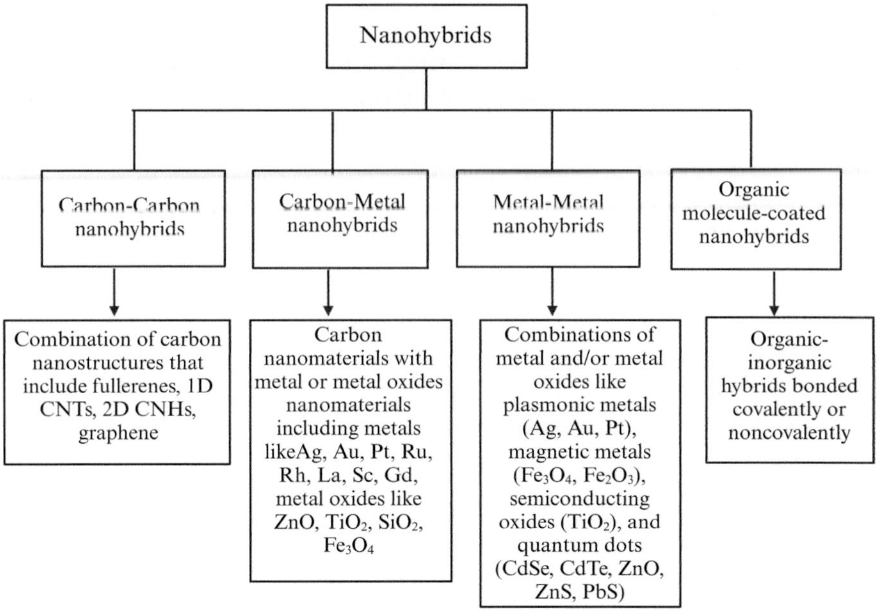

FIGURE 5.1 Classification of nanohybrids.

The nanohybrids that combine nanoparticles or other nanoscale materials with biopolymers (organic), which are naturally occurring polymers obtained from renewable resources, are called biopolymer-based nanohybrids. Biopolymers used in the production of bio nanocomposites include cellulose, alginate, chitosan, starch, polylactic acid (PLA), polyhydroxyalkanoates (PHA), and polyhydroxybutyrate (PHB) (Shaikh et al. 2024).

5.2.2 Structural and Functional Characteristics of Nanohybrids

Nanohybrids are engineered by integrating various nanomaterials to enhance properties and multifunctionality. The design process for these materials requires meticulous attention to synthesis methods and the interactions among their components. The following are some key structural features of nanohybrids:

- Composition: Nanohybrids are composite materials made up of two components at the nanoscale or molecular level, typically with one being inorganic and the other organic. Unlike traditional macroscopic composites, which mix components at the micrometer or millimeter scale, nanohybrids achieve a more homogeneous material with properties that lie between the original phases or even exhibit entirely new characteristics (Kickelbick 2006).
- Bonding: The components of nanohybrids are bound to each other at the nanoscale through different types of interactions such as covalent bonds, hydrogen bonds, van der Waals forces, ionic bonds, etc. These interactions

are essential for preserving the structural integrity and functional properties of nanohybrids (Idris et al. 2023).

- Morphology: The morphology of nanohybrids can vary significantly based on the synthesis method and the components involved. Typical morphologies include core-shell structures, layered structures, and dispersed nanoparticles within a matrix. The morphology directly influences their functional properties, application-specific design, and stability (Tanveer et al. 2022).
- Interface: The interface in nanohybrids is the boundary where the organic and inorganic components converge. This interface is pivotal in defining the properties of nanohybrids, influencing their mechanical, thermal, and electrical characteristics (Vargas-Bernal 2020).

Nanohybrids possess a variety of functional characteristics that make them extremely versatile and valuable for numerous applications. They often show enhanced properties including increased mechanical strength, thermal stability, electrical conductivity, and chemical reactivity (Idris et al. 2023). Due to the combination of different materials, nanohybrids can perform multiple functions simultaneously, acting as catalysts, sensors, and drug delivery systems. They are effective in environmental remediation, removing pollutants from water and air due to their high surface area and reactivity (Kickelbick 2006). In energy storage and conversion, nanohybrids are used in batteries, super capacitors, and fuel cells to enhance efficiency and performance. In the biomedical field, nanohybrids are utilized for drug delivery, diagnostics, and therapeutics due to their biocompatibility and functional versatility. These functional characteristics make nanohybrids valuable in a wide range of industries, from environmental science to medicine and energy (Aich et al. 2014).

5.3 MECHANISM OF ACTION OF INFLAMMATORY DISEASES

Although inflammation plays a significant role in the host's defenses against injury and infectious pathogens, it also plays a role in the pathophysiology of numerous chronic illnesses. Many organ disorders are caused by acute and chronic inflammation, which is influenced by interactions between cells in the innate immune system, adaptive immune system, and inflammatory mediators. Tissue damage, oxidative stress, extracellular matrix remodeling, angiogenesis, and fibrosis are all caused by a coordinated set of similar effector mechanisms of inflammation in a variety of target tissues (Libby 2008).

5.3.1 Pathophysiology of Inflammatory Disease

Inflammation is a process involving the selective and sequential migration of blood cells into tissues, followed by local activation and interaction with resident tissue cells. In some diseases, inflammatory mediators are absent, while others exhibit only a few aspects of classic inflammatory processes. In Alzheimer's disease, a persistent monocytic cell called a microglial cell expresses pro-inflammatory mediators and plays a significant role in innate immune responses. The innate and adaptive immune systems' signals converge on two prototypical cell types: epithelial cells and mesenchymal cells of damaged organs. These signals coordinate various tissue reactions, including angiogenesis, extracellular matrix remodeling, cellular proliferation or death, and the recruitment of leukocytes involved in chronic inflammation. In some organs, helper T-cells and mononuclear phagocytes are abundant in chronic inflammation lesions. Epithelial cells in atherosclerosis, enterocytes in inflammatory bowel disease, and glomerular or tubular epithelial cells in renal disease are implicated. Different mesenchymal cell types are involved in inflammatory and immunological systems (Libby 2008).

5.3.1.1 Inflammasomes

Inflammasome involvement is an additional mechanism of inflammation. At the post-translational level, inflammasome complexes and associated integral receptor proteins play crucial roles in controlling inflammation and the innate immune response. However, despite their protective effect, autoimmune and autoinflammatory disorders in humans appear to be influenced by gain of function mutations in inflammasome component genes and abnormal activation of inflammation proteins. The ability of number of receptor proteins to form inflammasomes has been established throughout the last 20 years. However, only a small number of these inflammasome complexes have had their precise activation and regulatory mechanisms thoroughly described (Bulté et al. 2023).

5.3.1.2 Oxidative Stress

The imbalance between the body's generation of free radicals and antioxidants' ability to neutralize them is known as oxidative stress. Damage to organs and tissues is one of the issues that oxidative stress can cause in the body. Free radicals are dangerous substances that are created by bodily biological functions including breathing and food digestion. They can harm the body by damaging DNA, obstructing the production of energy, and stopping regular cell division. They may also encourage inflammation (Gambini and Stromsnes 2022).

5.3.2 Cellular and Molecular Targets of Nanohybrids

Nanohybrids majorly work on different cellular and molecular components of the body to reduce the inflammation; they can either directly act on the cells that are causing the inflammation (like in the case of macrophages the nanohybrids can inhibit their function) and suppressing the keratinocytes or else they can influence molecules to act on the reduction of the inflammation like reducing the proinflammatory cytokines and increasing the anti-inflammatory cytokines.

5.3.2.1 Cellular Targets

Nanohybrids designed for treating inflammation caused by various conditions target different cells to reduce inflammation. Key cellular targets include macrophages and keratinocytes, which are crucial in the inflammation process.

5.3.2.1.1 Macrophages

Macrophages are a type of white blood cells that play an important role in our immune system and participate in the process of phagocytosis, antigen presentation, and importantly inflammation. Lipid-latex (LiLa) hybrid nanoparticles have been developed to target macrophages involved in inflammation. The lipids provide colloidal stability and targeting capabilities, while the latex core serves as a model hydrophobic polymeric template. Coating LiLa with phosphatidylserine (PtdSer) and the oxidized cholesterol ester product cholesterol-9-carboxynonanoate (9-CCN) allows for targeted treatment of inflammatory conditions. Macrophages effectively phagocytize these lipids, known as "eat-me" signals, which are commonly used in the theranostic nanocarriers. LiLa particles are very versatile, which is appropriate for high-throughput nanoparticle screening. LiLa's selectivity for imaging pro-inflammatory macrophages was tested using two disease models: experimental atherosclerosis and diet-induced obesity. The potential of LiLa nanoparticles as effective theranostics for inflammation highlights their adaptability and suitability for high-throughput screening (Bagalkot et al. 2015).

5.3.2.1.2 Keratinocytes

These are the cells present in the outer layer of the skin and act as a barrier and these cells also have a role in immune function where they have the ability to produce cytokines (pro inflammatory). Psoriasis is an autoimmune skin condition involving immune cells and keratinocytes. A new treatment for psoriatic inflammation has been developed using lipid-polymer nanohybrids and anti-Dsg3 antibodies. These nanocarriers, with a small, easy-to-prepare monovalent antibody, target keratinocytes and suppress cytokine/chemokine upregulation. They also inhibit keratinocyte-released chemokines, preventing neutrophil migration. The nanocarriers reduced psoriasis symptoms in a mouse model treated with IMQ. The active targeted nanocarriers inhibited cytokine and chemokine synthesis, stopping keratinocyte growth and restoring skin barrier function. This treatment is more effective than previous antibody fragments and is more easily prepared (Lin et al. 2021).

5.3.2.2 Molecular Targets

Numerous molecular mediators can be targeted by nanohybrids. The development of more potent treatments for inflammatory illnesses may be possible by engineering nanohybrids to interact with particular targets, including cytokines, enzymes, immune cells, and inflammatory signaling molecules. This can improve therapeutic outcomes and minimize adverse effects.

5.3.2.2.1 Cytokines

Cytokines are small protein molecules that are produced from different types of cells like macrophages, dendritic cells, T-cells, keratinocytes etc., which act in regulation of the signaling pathways, immune response and inflammation. If pro-inflammatory cytokines can be inhibited among all the cytokines present, inflammation at the site can be reduced. The study found that chitosan nanoparticles (CNs), AMP microcin J25 (MccJ25) Conjugates (CNs-MccJ25) effectively inhibited the inflammatory response by downregulating pro-inflammatory cytokines such as NO, TNF-α, IL-6, and IL-1β, thereby decreasing their secretion and expression (Haitao et al. 2022).

5.3.3 Nanohybrid-Mediated Modulation of Inflammatory Pathways

Nanohybrids interact with immune cells to modulate inflammatory pathways by influencing cytokines, chemokines, and other signaling molecules. These interactions can either promote or suppress inflammation, depending on the desired therapeutic outcome. The tunable size, shape, surface charge, and functionalization of nanohybrids allow for precise control over their biological interactions. This enables targeted treatment of diseases where inflammation is central. Figure 5.2 depicts the role of nanohybrids in modulating inflammatory pathways by various mechanisms.

5.3.3.1 Remodeling ECM

Organic nanomaterials plays an important part in combating inflammation by preventing oxidation and supporting tissue regeneration. A dynamic nanohybrid peptide hydrogel (NHPH) was developed to influence the inflammatory environment of the intervertebral disc (IVD) and enhanced regeneration (Conley et al. 2023). NHPH demonstrated enzyme-like properties after self- and differentiation agents, remodeled the extracellular matrix, and scavenged reactive oxygen species (Liu et al. 2024).

5.3.3.2 Polarization to M2 Macrophages

Macrophages, a major part of the peripheral immune response, play a crucial regulatory role in this process. Macrophages can be categorized as M1 or M2 based on their secreted products and activation pathways. M2 macrophages secrete anti-inflammatory and tissue repair cytokines, while M1-type macrophages cause excessive fibrosis and healing disorders by secreting pro-inflammatory cytokines. A change in macrophage polarization from M1 to M2 influences the inflammatory response surrounding biomaterials, establishing a microenvironment that promotes tissue regeneration. A nano-hybrid QCS-GO was created using covalent grafting of QCS and GO, modified with PDA to create QCS-GO-PDA. The findings showed that 5QCS-1GO-PDA can induce M2-type macrophage polarization, promote tissue regeneration, and remove reactive oxygen species (ROS) (Xue et al. 2022).

5.3.3.3 Reducing Proinflammatory Cytokines

High levels of oxidative stress in inflammatory lung diseases cause cells to become inflamed or apoptose, leading to alveolar collapse and hypoxia. When dexamethasone binds to the glucocorticoid receptor in the cytoplasm of cells, it induces the production of annexin I and mitogen-activated protein kinase (MAPK) phosphatase, which in turn suppresses the expression of cytosolic phospholipase A 2a and reduces the production of inflammatory mediators such as leukotrienes. Additionally, it suppresses NF-kB transcription, which lowers the synthesis of cell adhesion proteins like ICAM-1 and pro-inflammatory cytokines including IL-1b, IL-6, and TNF-a. Nanohybrids composed of phospholipids 1,2-dipalmitoyl sn-glycerol-3-phosphatidylcholine (DPPC) and 1-palmitoyl-2-oleoyl-sn-glycerol-3 phosphoglycerol ammonium salt (POPG) at 9: 1 w/w ratio along with surface active polymeric anti-oxidant D-a-tocopheryl polyethylene glycol 1000 succinate (TPGS) and an anti-inflammatory drug dexamethasone disodium phosphate (DXP) were developed. These nanohybrids act to reduce inflammation at the lungs (Shah et al. 2015).

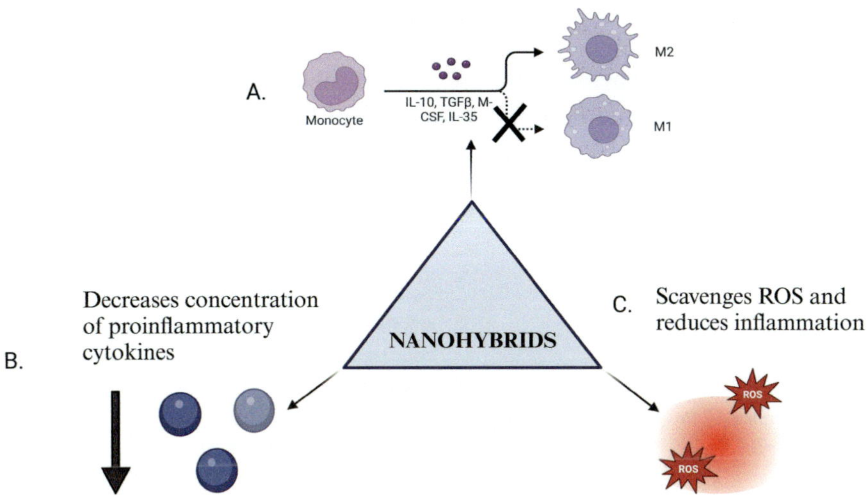

FIGURE 5.2 Mechanisms of nanohybrids in modulating inflammatory pathways by (a) promoting the polarization of monocytes into M2 macrophages (anti-inflammatory), (b) decreasing the concentration of pro-inflammatory cytokines, and (c) removing ROS to reduce inflammation.

5.3.4 Immune System Interactions and Nanohybrids

The immune system is closely related to nanomedicine, which uses materials at the nanoscale for treatment and medication delivery. The immune system recognizes nanomedicines because they have physicochemical traits in common with infections, such as their small size and surface features. Both the innate and adaptive immune systems are impacted by them. Table 5.1 summarizes the effects of nanohybrids on both innate and adaptive immune responses, emphasizing their influence on various components of the immune system.

5.3.4.1 Effects of the Innate Immune System

- Phagocytosis: The interaction between nanomedicines and monocytes and macrophages plays a vital role in determining their biological fate, even when the nanomaterials' diameter is below the optimal range for phagocytosis. These cells can engulf the nanomedicine, aiding in its distribution. Steric protection on the surface of liposomes and polymer nanoparticles reduces unwanted distribution to the liver and spleen, enhancing blood circulation.
- Complement System Activation: Nanomedicine can activate the complement system, leading to enhanced clearance of unexpected inflammatory responses. This complement cascade produces opsonins, cytokines, and terminal lytic complexes. Cytokines C3a, C4a, and C5a attract macrophages and mast cells, which then eliminate antigens identified by C1q, C4b, C3b, or other C3 fragments (iC3b and C3c). Complement proteins can also

TABLE 5.1
The Impact of Nanohybrids on Innate and Adaptive Immunity, and Their Influence on Different Components of the Immune System

Immune System	Component of Immune System	Influence of Nanohybrid	References
Innate immune system	Phagocytosis	Helps in delivery of nanomedicine.	(Viana et al. 2021; Du et al. 2020)
	Complement system activation	Triggered by the nanomedicine and clears inflammation	
	Cytokines	Reduces proinflammatory cytokines	
Adaptive immune system	Presentation of antigens	Phagocytose nanoparticles and helps in immunological memory	
	Antibody formation	Increases production of antibodies	

participate in the adaptive humoral response beyond these direct effects. After administering nanomedicine and incubating it for a while, it was observed that the concentration of complement proteins decreased, resulting in a reduction of inflammatory macrophages.

- Release of Cytokines: When nanomedicines interact, they trigger the release of cytokines, which in turn affect immune responses. Certain nanohybrids can reduce proinflammatory cytokines to minimize inflammation. Cytokines present in the environment impact NK cells. For proper priming of NK cell functions, nearby macrophages or dendritic cells need to release IL-15, IL-12, and IL–18. Consequently, NK cells influence their environment by producing anti-inflammatory IL-10 and pro-inflammatory interferon-g (IFN-g) and TNFa. Importantly, when NK cells lyse target cells, free antigens are released, which dendritic cells can then absorb and present, ultimately contributing to the adaptive immune response (Viana et al. 2021). Studies have reported that selenium-based nanoparticles may enhance NK cell activity. These nanoparticles not only improve NK cell function but also increase IL-17 and IFN-γ, triggering non-specific humoral and cell-mediated immune responses (Murugan et al. 2022).

5.3.4.2 Effects of the Adaptive Immune System

- Presentation of Antigens: Dendritic cells and macrophages have the ability to phagocytose nanoparticles, which expose T cells to antigens and may affect immunological memory. Antigen-presenting cells (APCs), such as dendritic cells, macrophages, and B lymphocytes, help the adaptive immune response by delivering antigens to T lymphocytes.

- Antibody formation: The formation of antibodies, including anti-PEG antibodies, can affect the effectiveness and safety of certain nanomedicines, especially those with repeating patterns like PEGylated nanoparticles. Examples of PEGylated colloids include polymer nanoparticles, lipid complexes of proteins, viruses, and nucleic acids. The physicochemical properties of the nanomedicines appear to influence the synthesis of anti-PEG IgM (Viana et al. 2021).

5.4 THERAPEUTIC APPLICATIONS OF NANOHYBRIDS IN INFLAMMATORY DISEASES

Evidence is mounting that chronic inflammation plays a major role in the onset and progression of many diseases with major health and socioeconomic consequences, including cancer and autoimmune, cardiovascular, and musculoskeletal conditions. To effectively treat and resolve chronic inflammatory conditions, it is imperative to create medicines that can overcome the primary drawbacks of currently employed techniques, including non-target activity and partial modulation of the complicated inflammatory pathways (Almeida et al. 2024). The following describes the therapeutic applications of nanohybrids in various inflammatory diseases.

5.4.1 Rheumatoid Arthritis

A series of chronic inflammatory processes are underpinned by rheumatoid arthritis (RA), a systemic autoimmune disease. Despite many advances in current therapeutic strategies, the response rate to effective RA treatments has remained low over the past few decades. This is mostly due to poor accumulation in the inflamed joints and associated off-target side effects. Recently, there has been a lot of interest in employing nanotechnology to develop tailored drug delivery systems since it can help increase the effectiveness of RA therapy (H. Yu et al. 2022).

One such nanomedicine used to treat RA is HA@RFM@PB@SE nanoparticles (HRPS NPs) which is a nanohybrid system. In order to create multifunctional HA@RFM@PB@SE nanoparticles (HRPS NPs), *Schisandra lactone E* (SE, also known as xuetongsu), an anti-RA compound that was isolated from Tujia ethnomedicine, is loaded into Prussian blue nanoparticles (PB NPs). The RBC-RAFLS hybrid membrane is then camouflaged onto PB@SE NPs (PS NPs) using HA modification. PB NPs modified with RFM, owing to the homing effects of the parental cells, are excellent decoys for targeting inflammatory mediators of arthritis. Additionally, RFM's encapsulation on PB@SE NPs increased blood circulation duration and enhanced targeting capability, resulting in the best possible SE accumulation in arthritic rat paws. The exceptional efficacy of HRPS NPs for synergistic chemo-photothermal treatment of RA without adverse effects on healthy tissues was shown by in vitro and in vivo assays

Investigation into the molecular mechanisms revealed partial suppression of the NF-κB signaling pathway and matrix metalloproteinase expression, leading to a significant prevention of synovial hyperplasia and bone degradation. The nano-drug delivery method demonstrated targeted accumulation at arthritic sites, controlled release behavior, and systemic immune management, enhancing therapeutic efficacy

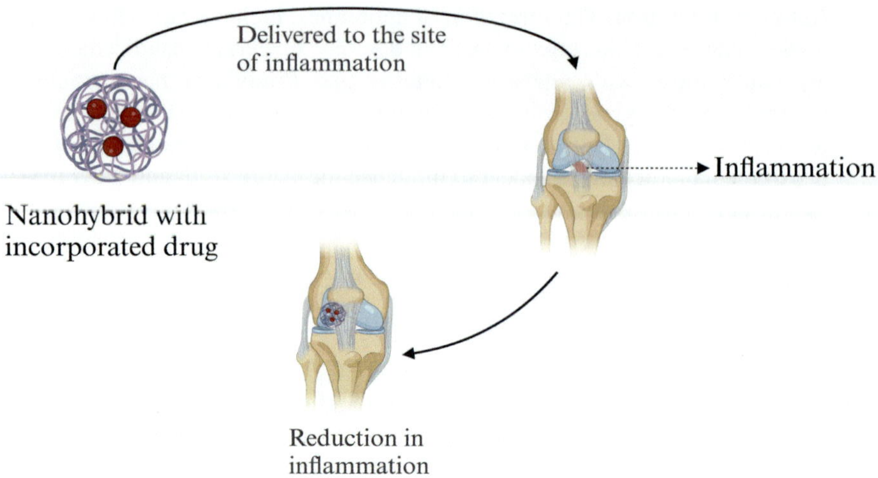

FIGURE 5.3 Drug-loaded nanohybrid targeting inflammatory sites.

and clinical outcomes without compromising safety (H. Yu et al. 2022). Figure 5.3 illustrates a nanohybrid incorporated with a drug designed for targeted delivery to the site of inflammation. At the site, the nanohybrid releases the drug, which acts to reduce inflammation and alleviate pain.

5.4.2 Inflammatory Bowel Disease (IBD)

Recurrent intestinal inflammation is a hallmark of inflammatory bowel disease (IBD), a chronic disorder. Ulcerative colitis and Crohn's disease are the two primary phenotypic expressions of the ailment, which is categorized based on severity. The disease's etiology is unclear, although it is anticipated that genetic predisposition, environmental variables like bacterial pathogens, and a dysregulated immune response would interact. The goal of IBD treatment is to stop the disease's progression and lessen the intensity and scope of symptoms. Corticosteroids, immunosuppressive medicines, and 5-aminosalicylates (5-ASAs) have been the mainstay medications. The traditional medication delivery routes include parenteral, oral, and rectal; oral administration is the most commonly used of these (Piotrowska et al. 2023). To get over a number of therapeutic roadblocks and deliver drugs locally to target tissues, innovative drug delivery methods have been developed. These innovative approaches include lipid-based vesicular systems, prodrug systems, different nano-drug delivery techniques, enteric-coated microneedle pills, hybrid drug delivery systems, and biological drug delivery systems. Hybrid drug delivery systems, which combine the benefits of multiple carriers into one, have enormous potential despite being challenging to develop.

One such system is the Cur-HA NPs, (hydroxyapatite (HA)) which has been shown to increase cellular contact and uptake of curcumin, suggesting it could be useful for oral medication administration to treat local colonic illness. Encapsulation of curcumin with bovine b-lactoglobulin has also been shown to enhance curcumin's aqueous solubility, while succinylated-b-lactoglobulin inhibits its release in gastric juices. Curcumin has high medical value, including anti-inflammatory by stimulating leukocytes, reducing the expression of proinflammatory molecules, and blocking the creation of interleukin 2 (IL-2) and IL–12. By negating the side effects, we can directly target the drug at the location of the disease using the Cur-HA NPs hybrid system (Piotrowska et al. 2023).

5.4.3 Asthma and Chronic Obstructive Pulmonary Disease (COPD)

Nowadays, medications used for the treatment of respiratory conditions are mostly injected intravenously, taken orally, or nebulized into the body for therapeutic effects. Because of its many benefits, including higher patient agreement, low cost, convenience of administration, non-invasiveness, and safety, oral administration is the most popular method of administering most medications' absorption, however, this can be a complicated process that can be influenced by numerous factors, including the physiology of the gastrointestinal tract (GIT), dosage form, and physicochemical characteristics of medication. Only particular kinds of molecules can pass through the GIT since it has multiple absorption barriers that keep foreign compounds from entering the body (Guo et al. 2023).

5.4.3.1 Application of Poly (Lactic-co-Glycolic Acid): Micro/ Nano Particles (PLGA M/NPS) in COPD

Commonly used therapeutic drugs include glucocorticoids, expectorants, bronchodilators (including β1 adrenergic agonists, anticholinergics, and theophyllines), and others. In recent decades, it has been demonstrated that there are numerous strategies to activate macrophages. These activations may promote the reduction of inflammation and facilitate tissue repair in addition to the conventional pro-inflammatory activation that sets off host defense reactions. Activating macrophages through certain pathways may therefore have therapeutic applications in promoting the reduction of inflammation. Through the activation of macrophages through endosomal/phagosomal CD14 and Toll-like receptors 1 and 2, the anti-inflammatory properties of the small heat-shock protein alpha B-crystallin (HSPB5) were recognized (Van Noort et al. 2013).

HSPB5 was encapsulated in porous PLGA MPs to treat COPD. HSPB5-loaded PLGA MPs were found to be selectively absorbed by alveolar macrophages upon intratracheal administration. Through the activation of an immune-regulatory macrophage response through TLR1/2 and CD14, a crucial co-receptor, the anti-inflammatory impact was associated with a considerable reduction in neutrophil and lymphocyte infiltration in the lungs (Guo et al. 2023).

5.4.4 Cardiovascular Inflammation (e.g., Atherosclerosis)

One of the primary causes of cardiovascular disease, a major cause of death worldwide, is atherosclerosis (AS), which is mostly brought on by inflammation and altered immune system processes. The main objective in contemporary medicine is to create carriers that accurately convey therapeutic drugs to the target locations in order to reduce potential side effects and improve lesion treatment. Stimuli-responsive nano-based drug delivery systems (NDDSs) have shown promise in treating AS because of their low toxicity, AS microenvironment response, accurate placement, and real-time monitoring (Song et al. 2022).

The development of stable, intravenously injectable ticagrelor-loaded and DSPE-PEG2000 integrated PtCe bimetallic raspberry-like nanoparticles, which is a hybrid model DSPE-PEG2000Tica-PtCe NRs (DPTP NRs), aims to address platelet agglutination and inflammation in atherosclerosis. Because of its rough surface and capacity to trap, the DPTP NRs improve ticagrelor's loading efficiency and maintain its activity throughout biological transport. In an intravital setting, PtCe NRs can quickly reduce H_2O_2 levels by breaking down endogenous H_2O_2. Additionally, the nanosystem reduces oxidized low-density lipoprotein (oxLDL), inhibits the growth of foam cells, and increases superoxide dismutase to counterbalance O_2 stress from Pt alone. Additionally, the DPTP NRs lower the incidence of plaque and platelet aggregation (Wang et al. 2021).

5.4.5 Neurological Inflammation (e.g., Multiple Sclerosis)

Myelin sheath loss is a hallmark of multiple sclerosis (MS), a neurological condition. Multiple sclerosis is a neurodegenerative and neuroinflammatory illness brought on by aberrant immune responses. The release of cytokines (macrophages, T-cells, and others) and antibodies (plasma cells) by immune cell infiltration in the central nervous system may ultimately cause the myelin sheath to degrade. The loss of the myelin coating would cause the impacted neurons to malfunction in sending electrical impulses, which would result in sensory and motor impairments because the sheath could shield nerve fibers from the external environment. Because the blood-brain barrier (BBB) exists, treating MS is associated with limited treatment efficacy and the incidence of adverse effects because of ineffective targeting (Zeng et al. 2020).

Recently, nanomedicines have been used to deliver MS therapeutic agents to the lesions in order to get around these problems with conventional MS therapy methods. These nano-based therapies have shown good results and have emerged as another promising MS therapy approach with superior therapeutic results due to their deep BBB penetration and targeted targeting. Nanomedicines based on fullerene: Along with graphite, diamond, and amorphous carbon, fullerenes have been one of the most researched carbon allotropes since its discovery. They have a hollow region inside their cage-like nanostructure where various atoms, ions, or clusters could be embedded (Zeng et al. 2020).

5.4.5.1 Fullerene Hybrid

Fullerenes are extensively used in the domains of photovoltaics, drug delivery, and biosensing when they are combined with various compounds and groups. More significantly, fullerenes may potentially provide neuroprotection by eliminating oxidative free radicals and minimizing axon cellular damage. A nanocarbon hybrid comprising reduced graphene oxide (rGO), β-cyclodextrin (β-CD), and azobenzene-functionalized C 60 (azo-C60) was created by Hu et al. These nanohybrids have greater effectiveness in nitric oxide (NO) scavenging when it is activated by UV light, preventing oxidative damage.

These fullerene structures could shield and even repair cell damage brought on by oxidative free radicals by implementing these nanomedicines into cellular and animal models. This would improve the symptoms and possibly lower the incidence; functionalized fullerenes might be a strong antioxidant since, even at low dosages, they are efficient at scavenging free radicals and protecting neurons, which indicates that their toxicity may be low. Fullerenes may therefore be a good option for treating MS and when designed as a nanohybrid can result in significant reduction of symptoms (Zeng et al. 2020).

5.5 ADVANTAGES AND CHALLENGES OF NANOHYBRIDS IN INFLAMMATORY DISEASE TREATMENT

Nanohybrids represent a significant advancement in nanotechnology, enhancing drug delivery, stability, and controlled release, which makes them highly effective in treating inflammatory diseases. However, they also pose challenges such as complex manufacturing processes, biocompatibility and safety concerns, regulatory hurdles, and potential toxicity. Addressing these challenges is essential for their successful application in medical treatments.

Some of the advantages of nanohybrids in inflammatory disease treatment include the following.

5.5.1 Enhanced Targeting and Bioavailability

Enhanced targeting and bioavailability are essential features of nanohybrids in medical treatments, especially for inflammatory diseases. By designing nanohybrids to deliver drugs directly to the inflamed sites, therapeutic agents can be precisely concentrated where they are most needed. This targeted approach enhances the treatment's efficacy while minimizing systemic side effects, as the drugs are less likely to impact healthy tissues (Salah et al. 2022). Additionally, nanohybrids can boost the bioavailability of drugs, meaning a larger proportion of the drug enters the bloodstream and remains active. Many drugs face challenges with solubility and stability, which can limit their effectiveness. Nanohybrids address these issues, ensuring a higher percentage of the drug reaches the target site in its active form. This enhancement can result in more effective treatments with lower doses, thereby reducing the risk of side effects and improving patient outcomes. The enhanced targeting and bioavailability provided by nanohybrids make them a promising tool for treating inflammatory diseases, offering more precise and effective therapeutic options (Zhuo, Zhao, and Zhang 2024).

5.5.2 Controlled Release and Sustained Drug Delivery

Controlled release can be done by nanohybrids using a variety of processes, including carrier material swelling, degradation, and diffusion. For instance, by regulating the crystallite size of the polymer matrix, which produces a complex pathway for the drug to diffuse through, biodegradable polymer-based nanohybrids can offer sustained drug release. The medication will remain effective for a longer period of time because of this gradual and regulated release, which enhances patient compliance and results (Shukla and Maiti 2019). Additionally, controlled release systems can be customized to respond to specific stimuli in the biological environment, such as changes in the pH or the presence of certain enzymes. This enables precise control over the drug release, ensuring it is delivered exactly when and where it is needed (Agrawal et al. 2022).

The challenges associated with the use of nanohybrids in inflammatory disease treatment can be complex manufacturing processes, biocompatibility, potential toxicity and safety concerns, regulatory hurdles, and stability issues in biological environments.

5.5.3 Biocompatibility Concerns and Toxicity Concerns

Nanohybrids need to be meticulously designed to prevent immune reactions. This requires choosing materials that are known for their biocompatibility and employing surface modifications to minimize potential immunogenicity. However, the biocompatibility of nanohybrids can differ based on their composition and specific application, making thorough testing crucial (Jin et al. 2020). Toxicity is a significant concern with nanohybrids. The materials used in these hybrids can sometimes be harmful to cells or tissues, particularly if they accumulate in the body over time. For example, combining multiple nanomaterials can change their physicochemical properties, potentially leading to unexpected toxicological effects. Research has shown that the toxicity of nanohybrids can be affected by factors such as particle size, shape, surface charge, and the presence of reactive surface groups. Therefore, it is essential to conduct thorough toxicity assessments to ensure the safety of nanohybrids before they are used in clinical settings (Saleh et al. 2014).

5.5.4 Scale-Up and Manufacturing Challenges

Nanohybrids manufacturing and scaling up pose a number of difficulties that must be overcome for successful large-scale production.

- Complexity of Processes: The synthesis of nanohybrids often involves intricate processes that are challenging to replicate on a large scale. Maintaining the precise conditions necessary for nanohybrid formation can be difficult when transitioning from laboratory to industrial production.
- Consistency and Quality Control: Ensuring consistency and quality of nanohybrids in large batches is a major challenge. Variations in particle size, shape, and composition can affect nanohybrid performance, making it important to implement rigorous quality control measures.
- Cost of Production: The expense of raw materials and the complexity of manufacturing processes can make producing nanohybrids costly. Scaling up production demands substantial investment in specialized equipment and facilities.

- Environmental and safety concerns: Producing nanohybrids can present environmental and safety risks. Proper handling, disposal, and recycling of nanomaterials are crucial to minimizing their impact on the environment and human health (Hecht 2022).

5.5.5 Regulatory and Clinical Challenges

Nanohybrids offer significant potential for medical applications, but they encounter considerable regulatory and clinical challenges that must be addressed to ensure their safe and effective use.

- Complex approval processes: The approval process for nanohybrids can be prolonged and complex due to strict regulatory requirements. Agencies such as the FDA and EMA demand comprehensive data on the safety, efficacy, and quality of nanohybrids, which can delay their market entry. There are no standardized protocols for characterization and testing of nanohybrids, which makes it difficult to compare study results and complicates the regulatory approval process (Gottardo et al. 2021).
- Clinical trial design and patient safety and monitoring: Designing clinical trials for nanohybrids is intricate. It requires careful consideration of dosage, delivery methods, and potential side effects. Furthermore, the unique properties of nanohybrids may require innovative trial designs and endpoints. Monitoring the safety and efficacy of nanohybrids in patients is essential. This requires regular assessments to identify any adverse effects and ensure that the nanohybrids are functioning as intended (Debnath et al. 2024).

5.6 EMERGING TRENDS AND FUTURE DIRECTIONS

Nanohybrids are at the forefront of revolutionizing the treatment of inflammatory diseases. By merging the precision of nanotechnology with the therapeutic power of hybrid formulations, they provide targeted, controlled, and highly effective treatment solutions (Oshi et al. 2022).

5.6.1 Emerging Trends in Nanohybrids for Therapeutic Applications in Inflammatory Diseases

5.6.1.1 Smart Nanohybrids for Targeted Therapy

Smart nanohybrids are increasingly being employed for focused therapy of inflammatory diseases, resulting in precise medicine administration with minimum side effects. These nanohybrids combine nanoparticles like liposomes with metals or other functional components to enhance medicine stability, bioavailability, and targeted administration. They may be designed to respond to a variety of stimuli, including pH, temperature, light, and magnetic fields, resulting in regulated medication release at disease locations. For example, pH-responsive nanocarriers exploit the acidic milieu of inflamed tissues to promote medication release at the target region. Ligands such as folate, peptides, and glycoproteins (e.g., transferrin) are employed to increase the explicitness of nanohybrids by binding to upregulated receptors on inflammatory tissues or cells. These ligands improve cellular uptake, directing therapeutic agents to the site of inflammation. Magnetic nanoparticles can also aid in localized drug delivery via magnetic fields, enhancing the accumulation of drugs in the affected area (Debnath et al. 2024). Nanohybrids, such as DNA-functionalized gold-loaded liposomes, provide additional benefits such as regulated and reversible drug release, improved stability, and decreased leakage. The combination of these qualities enables extremely selective targeting, enhanced therapeutic results, and reduced side effects, making smart nanohybrids a potential method in the treatment of inflammatory illnesses (Alwattar et al. 2021).

5.6.1.2 Role of Artificial Intelligence in Nanohybrid Design

AI can analyze large datasets to speculate nanostructure behavior and custom synthesize drugs to specific patient profiles, resulting in improved outcomes while reducing adverse effects. AI's integration with contemporary synthesis technologies, including microfluidic devices and self-assembly processes, allows for exact control of nanostructure size, shape, and composition. This improves their ability and efficacy in delivering medicines to inflamed regions. AI also makes it possible to employ theranostic nanostructures, which have the ability to channel therapeutic chemicals, target particular disease areas, and track treatment outcomes in real time. This provides a holistic strategy for managing health issues. AI's role in personalizing treatments ensures that drugs are delivered specifically to the disease site, improving the targeting efficiency and minimizing side effects (Rashid et al. 2024).

5.6.1.3 Clinical Trials and Translational Research in Inflammatory Diseases

This variant emphasizes the need of homogeneous nanoparticle formulations that allow for consistent therapeutic responses. Clinical trials have extra challenges because of limited light penetration in tissues when applying photothermal treatment (PPTT) to treat deep inflammatory lesions. Researchers are investigating the use of longer wavelength light and enhanced light-scattering nanoparticles to improve light penetration and therapeutic effectiveness. However, the translation of nanoparticle-based therapeutics into clinical applications is hampered by issues like agglomeration and potential toxicity, which must be addressed before they can be utilized broadly to treat inflammatory illnesses. As research progresses, the emphasis moves toward developing nanoparticles for effective pharmaceutical delivery while avoiding side effects in clinical trials. Improved manufacturing techniques that result in homogenous particles may enable more consistent therapeutic effects, boosting nanomedicine in the treatment of inflammatory illnesses. The variability in nanoparticle size, shape, and composition is a serious issue, as it impacts their consistency and efficacy in treating illnesses like rheumatoid arthritis and inflammatory bowel disease. Variations in nanoparticle characteristics, such as those reported in gold-silicon (Au-Si) hybrids, might have an influence on their therapeutic powers, resulting in uneven clinical outcomes (Debnath et al. 2024).

5.6.2 Future Perspectives and Potential Innovations

The future of nanomedicine, especially concerning inorganic nanostructures (NPS), looks promising due to advancements in hybrid systems and multifunctional materials. Notably, theranostic gadgets that combine diagnostic and therapeutic functions are gaining popularity, enabling real-time monitoring and personalized treatment. Polydopamine-based nanostructures have the potential to improve targeting while reducing side effects, particularly in cancer and neurological disorders (Liu et al. 2024). Furthermore, biodegradable materials and novel hybrid technologies are being studied for their lower toxicity and environmental impact, which will improve nanoparticle stability and therapeutic efficacy (S. Yu et al. 2025).

Boron neutron capture therapy (BNCT) is an example of an emerging approach, since novel boron-based nanomedicines such as layered double hydroxide (LDH)-BSH hybrids improve cancer treatment selectivity and effectiveness. However, concerns about the toxicity and long-term stability of inorganic nanoparticles, such as quantum dots (QDs), persist. Surface protection strategies and safety measures need to be further developed before they can be used in clinical applications (S. Yu et al. 2025). Furthermore, combining artificial intelligence (AI) with nanomedicine is projected to enhance therapy customization, improve results, and reduce side effects (Liu et al. 2024).

The goal of future research should be to enhance the biocompatibility and stability of inorganic nanoparticles while also understanding their in vivo metabolism. Additionally, emphasis should be placed on increasing the synthesis of multifunctional materials that offer both diagnostic and therapeutic benefits for individualized treatments. Efforts in these areas could lead to breakthroughs in cancer therapy, immunotherapy, and beyond, ushering in a new era of medical innovation.

5.7 CONCLUSION

This chapter comprehensively explores the therapeutic applications of nanohybrids in inflammatory diseases, highlighting their types, structural and functional characteristics, cellular and molecular targets, and mechanisms for modulating inflammatory pathways. Nanohybrids overcome the limitations of conventional therapies by introducing a transformative approach with sophisticated drug delivery techniques that reduce systemic toxicity, increase target selectivity, and improve bioavailability. Mechanistic insights reveal their role in cytokine modulation, extracellular matrix remodeling, and immune cell polarization, thus underscoring their multifaceted therapeutic potential. The future scope of nanohybrids in personalized and precision medicine has been further enhanced by emerging technologies, such as AI-driven nanostructure design and theranostic applications. Challenges associated with scaling nanohybrids to clinical applications include concerns related to biocompatibility, toxicity, and regulatory hurdles. The integration of novel synthesis methods along with AI-guided designs has the potential to address most of these current limitations, enabling safer therapeutic options and enhanced efficacy.

In conclusion, the concept of nanohybrids offers a paradigmatic shift in treating inflammatory diseases due to the exceptional accuracy and control offered by the delivery system. While traditional anti-inflammatory therapies are hampered by off-target effects and systemic toxicity, nanohybrids allow for targeted delivery, sustained release, and enhanced bioavailability. Successful applications in diseases such as inflammatory bowel disease, rheumatoid arthritis, and neurological inflammation speak to their clinical promise. However, widespread adoption is contingent upon overcoming scalability, safety, and regulatory approval challenges. As research continues to advance, the integration of AI and emerging theranostic technologies will further refine their therapeutic potential, ensuring personalized treatments that are both effective and safe. With continued innovation, nanohybrids stand to revolutionize inflammatory disease management, offering hope for more precise, tailored, and patient-centric care.

REFERENCES

Aden, Konrad, Ateequr Rehman, Silvio Waschina, Wei-Hung Pan, Alesia Walker, Marianna Lucio, Alejandro Mena Nunez, et al. 2019. "Metabolic Functions of Gut Microbes Associate with Efficacy of Tumor Necrosis Factor Antagonists in Patients With Inflammatory Bowel Diseases." *Gastroenterology* 157 (5): 1279–92.e11. https://doi.org/10.1053/j.gastro.2019.07.025.

Agrawal, Yogeeta O., Muzammil Husain, Kiran D. Patil, Vishal Sodgir, Tulshidas S. Patil, Vinit V. Agnihotri, Hitendra S. Mahajan, Charu Sharma, Shreesh Ojha, and Sameer N. Goyal. 2022. "Verapamil Hydrochloride Loaded Solid Lipid Nanoparticles: Preparation, Optimization, Characterisation, and Assessment of Cardioprotective Effect in Experimental Model of Myocardial Infarcted Rats." *Biomedicine & Pharmacotherapy* 154 (October): 113429. https://doi.org/10.1016/j.biopha.2022.113429.

Aich, Nirupam, Jaime Plazas-Tuttle, Jamie R. Lead, and Navid B. Saleh. 2014. "A Critical Review of Nanohybrids: Synthesis, Applications and Environmental Implications." *Environmental Chemistry* 11 (6): 609. https://doi.org/10.1071/EN14127.

Alivisatos, A. P. 1996. "Semiconductor Clusters, Nanocrystals, and Quantum Dots." *Science* 271 (5251): 933–37. https://doi.org/10.1126/science.271.5251.933.

Almeida, Ana F., Margarida S. Miranda, Rui L. Reis, Manuela E. Gomes, and Márcia T. Rodrigues. 2024. "Using Hybrid Nanoplatforms to Combine Traditional Anti-Inflammatory Drug Delivery with RNA-Based Therapeutics for Macrophage Reprograming." *International Journal of Molecular Sciences* 25 (19): 10693. https://doi.org/10.3390/ijms251910693.

Alwattar, Jana K., Amina T. Mneimneh, Kawthar K. Abla, Mohammed M. Mehanna, and Ahmed N. Allam. 2021. "Smart Stimuli-Responsive Liposomal Nanohybrid Systems: A Critical Review of Theranostic Behavior in Cancer." *Pharmaceutics* 13 (3): 355. https://doi.org/10.3390/pharmaceutics13030355.

Anker, Jeffrey N., W. Paige Hall, Olga Lyandres, Nilam C. Shah, Jing Zhao, and Richard P. Van Duyne. 2008. "Biosensing with Plasmonic Nanosensors." *Nature Materials* 7 (6): 442–53. https://doi.org/10.1038/nmat2162.

Bagalkot, Vaishali, Marcus A. Badgeley, Thomas Kampfrath, Jeffrey A. Deiuliis, Sanjay Rajagopalan, and Andrei Maiseyeu. 2015. "Hybrid Nanoparticles Improve Targeting to Inflammatory Macrophages through Phagocytic Signals." *Journal of Controlled Release* 217 (November): 243–55. https://doi.org/10.1016/j.jconrel.2015.09.027.

Brusini, Romain, Mariana Varna, and Patrick Couvreur. 2020. "Advanced Nanomedicines for the Treatment of Inflammatory Diseases." *Advanced Drug Delivery Reviews* 157: 161–78. https://doi.org/10.1016/j.addr.2020.07.010.

Bulté, Dimitri, Chiara Rigamonti, Alessandro Romano, and Alessandra Mortellaro. 2023. "Inflammasomes: Mechanisms of Action and Involvement in Human Diseases." *Cells* 12 (13): 1766. https://doi.org/10.3390/cells12131766.

Cao, Shu-jun, Zhi-qiang Lv, Su Guo, Guo-ping Jiang, and Hong-ling Liu. 2021. "An Update – Prolonging the Action of Protein and Peptide Drugs." *Journal of Drug Delivery Science and Technology* 61 (February): 102124. https://doi.org/10.1016/j.jddst.2020.102124.

Conley, Brian M., Letao Yang, Basanta Bhujel, Jeffrey Luo, Inbo Han, and Ki-Bum Lee. 2023. "Development of a Nanohybrid Peptide Hydrogel for Enhanced Intervertebral Disc Repair and Regeneration." *ACS Nano* 17 (4): 3750–64. https://doi.org/10.1021/acsnano.2c11441.

Debnath, Monalisha, Sujit Kumar Debnath, Mangal Vishnu Talpade, Shweta Bhatt, Prem Prakash Gupta, and Rohit Srivastava. 2024. "Surface Engineered Nanohybrids in Plasmonic Photothermal Therapy for Cancer: Regulatory and Translational Challenges." *Nanotheranostics* 8 (2): 202–18. https://doi.org/10.7150/ntno.92639.

Du, Wei, Chen Chen, Peng Sun, Shengchang Zhang, Jing Zhang, Xiaoyu Zhang, Ying Liu, et al. 2020. "Eliciting an Immune Hot Tumor Niche with Biomimetic Drug-Based Multi-Functional Nanohybrids Augments Immune Checkpoint Blockade-Based Breast Cancer Therapy." *Nanoscale* 12 (5): 3317–29. https://doi.org/10.1039/C9NR09835F.

Feng, Naibo, and Fengjin Guo. 2020. "Nanoparticle-siRNA: A Potential Strategy for Rheumatoid Arthritis Therapy?" *Journal of Controlled Release* 325 (September): 380–93. https://doi.org/10.1016/j.jconrel.2020.07.006.

Gambini, Juan, and Kristine Stromsnes. 2022. "Oxidative Stress and Inflammation: From Mechanisms to Therapeutic Approaches." *Biomedicines* 10 (4): 753. https://doi.org/10.3390/biomedicines10040753.

Gottardo, Stefania, Agnieszka Mech, Jana Drbohlavová, Aleksandra Małyska, Søren Bøwadt, Juan Riego Sintes, and Hubert Rauscher. 2021. "Towards Safe and Sustainable Innovation in Nanotechnology: State-of-Play for Smart Nanomaterials." *NanoImpact* 21 (January): 100297. https://doi.org/10.1016/j.impact.2021.100297.

Guo, Xiaoping, Xu Zuo, Zhengjie Zhou, Yinuo Gu, Haoyu Zheng, Xinlei Wang, Guoqiang Wang, Caina Xu, and Fang Wang. 2023. "PLGA-Based Micro/Nanoparticles: An Overview of Their Applications in Respiratory Diseases." *International Journal of Molecular Sciences* 24 (5): 4333. https://doi.org/10.3390/ijms24054333.

Haitao, Yu, Chen Yifan, Sun Mingchao, and Han Shuaijuan. 2022. "A Novel Polymeric Nanohybrid Antimicrobial Engineered by Antimicrobial Peptide MccJ25 and Chitosan Nanoparticles Exerts Strong Antibacterial and Anti-Inflammatory Activities." *Frontiers in Immunology* 12 (January): 811381. https://doi.org/10.3389/fimmu.2021.811381.

Hecht, Jeff. 2022. "Nanomaterials Pave the Way for the next Computing Generation." *Nature* 608 (7922): S2–3. https://doi.org/10.1038/d41586-022-02147-3.

Hosseinikhah, Seyedeh Maryam, Mahmood Barani, Abbas Rahdar, Henning Madry, Rabia Arshad, Vahideh Mohammadzadeh, and Magali Cucchiarini. 2021. "Nanomaterials for the Diagnosis and Treatment of Inflammatory Arthritis." *International Journal of Molecular Sciences* 22 (6): 3092. https://doi.org/10.3390/ijms22063092.

Idris, Mustapha Omenesa, Mohamad Nasir Mohamad Ibrahim, Akil Ahmad, and Mohammed B. Alshammari. 2023. "Synthesis and Characterization of Nanohybrid Materials." In *Nanohybrid Materials for Treatment of Textiles Dyes*, edited by Akil Ahmad, Mohammad Jawaid, Mohamad Nasir Mohamad Ibrahim, Asim Ali Yaqoob, and Mohammed B. Alshammari, 61–74. Smart Nanomaterials Technology. Singapore: Springer Nature Singapore. https://doi.org/10.1007/978-981-99-3901-5_4.

Janakiraman, Kumar, Venkateshwaran Krishnaswami, Vijaya Rajendran, Subramanian Natesan, and Ruckmani Kandasamy. 2018. "Novel Nano Therapeutic Materials for the Effective Treatment of Rheumatoid Arthritis-Recent Insights." *Materials Today Communications* 17 (December): 200–13. https://doi.org/10.1016/j.mtcomm.2018.09.011.

Jeong, Moonkyoung, and Ji-Ho Park. 2021. "Nanomedicine for the Treatment of Rheumatoid Arthritis." *Molecular Pharmaceutics* 18 (2): 539–49. https://doi.org/10.1021/acs.molpharmaceut.0c00295.

Jin, Wenji, Dongki Lee, Yukwon Jeon, and Dae-Hwan Park. 2020. "Biocompatible Hydrotalcite Nanohybrids for Medical Functions." *Minerals* 10 (2): 172. https://doi.org/10.3390/min10020172.

Kamat, Prashant V. 2002. "Photophysical, Photochemical and Photocatalytic Aspects of Metal Nanoparticles." *The Journal of Physical Chemistry B* 106 (32): 7729–44. https://doi.org/10.1021/jp0209289.

Kickelbick, Guido, ed. 2006. *Hybrid Materials: Synthesis, Characterization, and Applications*. 1st ed. Wiley. https://doi.org/10.1002/9783527610495.

Libby, Peter. 2008. "Inflammatory Mechanisms: The Molecular Basis of Inflammation and Disease." *Nutrition Reviews* 65 (June): S140–46. https://doi.org/10.1111/j.1753-4887.2007.tb00352.x.

Lin, Zih-Chan, Tsong-Long Hwang, Tse-Hung Huang, Kohei Tahara, Jiří Trousil, and Jia-You Fang. 2021. "Monovalent Antibody-Conjugated Lipid-Polymer Nanohybrids for Active Targeting to Desmoglein 3 of Keratinocytes to Attenuate Psoriasiform Inflammation." *Theranostics* 11 (10): 4567–84. https://doi.org/10.7150/thno.56995.

Liu, Yuting, Ziqi Lin, Yuting Wang, Liuhui Chen, Yuequan Wang, and Cong Luo. 2024. "Nanotechnology in Inflammation: Cutting-Edge Advances in Diagnostics, Therapeutics and Theranostics." *Theranostics* 14 (6): 2490–2525. https://doi.org/10.7150/thno.91394.

Murugan, Dhanashree, Vasanth Murugesan, Balaji Panchapakesan, and Loganathan Rangasamy. 2022. "Nanoparticle Enhancement of Natural Killer (NK) Cell-Based Immunotherapy." *Cancers* 14 (21): 5438. https://doi.org/10.3390/cancers14215438.

Oshi, Murtada A., Adnan Haider, Muhammad Irfan Siddique, Alam Zeb, Syed Babar Jamal, Atif Ali Khan Khalil, and Muhammad Naeem. 2022. "Nanomaterials for Chronic Inflammatory Diseases: The Current Status and Future Prospects." *Applied Nanoscience* 12 (11): 3097–110. https://doi.org/10.1007/s13204-021-02019-8.

Pankhurst, Q. A., J. Connolly, S. K. Jones, and J. Dobson. 2003. "Applications of Magnetic Nanoparticles in Biomedicine." *Journal of Physics D: Applied Physics* 36 (13): R167–81. https://doi.org/10.1088/0022-3727/36/13/201.

Park, Jun-Young, Song Kwon, Sang-Hyun Kim, Youn Joo Kang, and Dongwoo Khang. 2020. "Triamcinolone–Gold Nanoparticles Repolarize Synoviocytes and Macrophages in an Inflamed Synovium." *ACS Applied Materials & Interfaces* 12 (35): 38936–49. https://doi.org/10.1021/acsami.0c09842.

Piotrowska, Marta, Julia B. Krajewska, Marcin Talar, Olga Długosz, Marcin Banach, and Jakub Fichna. 2023. "Anti-Inflammatory Properties of Curcumin and Silver (I) Nanocomplexes in Inflammatory Bowel Disease: In Vitro and in Vivo Examination." *Journal of Drug Delivery Science and Technology* 86 (September): 104723. https://doi.org/10.1016/j.jddst.2023.104723.

Rashid, Adib Bin, Mahima Haque, S. M. Mohaimenul Islam, and K. M. Rafi Uddin Labib. 2024. "Nanotechnology-Enhanced Fiber-Reinforced Polymer Composites: Recent Advancements on Processing Techniques and Applications." *Heliyon* 10 (2): e24692. https://doi.org/10.1016/j.heliyon.2024.e24692.

Salah, Mai, Marwa A. Sallam, Mona A. Abdelmoneem, Mohamed Teleb, Kadria A. Elkhodairy, Adnan A. Bekhit, Asmaa F. Khafaga, Ahmed E. Noreldin, Ahmed O. Elzoghby, and Sherine N. Khattable 2022. "Sequential Delivery of Novel Triple Drug Combination via Crosslinked Alginate/Lactoferrin Nanohybrids for Enhanced Breast Cancer Treatment." *Pharmaceutics* 14 (11): 2404. https://doi.org/10.3390/pharmaceutics14112404.

Saleh, Navid, A. Afrooz, Joseph Bisesi, Nirupam Aich, Jaime Plazas-Tuttle, and Tara Sabo-Attwood. 2014. "Emergent Properties and Toxicological Considerations for Nanohybrid Materials in Aquatic Systems." *Nanomaterials* 4 (2): 372–407. https://doi.org/10.3390/nano4020372.

Schiavi, Simona, Mario Ocampo-Pineda, Muhamed Barakovic, Laurent Petit, Maxime Descoteaux, Jean-Philippe Thiran, and Alessandro Daducci. 2020. "A New Method for Accurate in Vivo Mapping of Human Brain Connections Using Microstructural and Anatomical Information." *Science Advances* 6 (31): eaba8245. https://doi.org/10.1126/sciadv.aba8245.

Shah, Apurva R., Tejashree Hagawane, Nilima Kshirsagar, and Rinti Banerjee. 2015. "Surface-Active Drug Loaded Lipopolymeric Nanohybrid Aerosol Therapy: Potential Non-Invasive Way to Mitigate Lipopolysaccharide Mediated Inflammation in Murine Lungs." *RSC Advances* 5 (13): 9683–94. https://doi.org/10.1039/C4RA13558J.

Shaikh, Abdul Aziz, Preetam Datta, Prithwish Dastidar, Arkadip Majumder, Maharghya Dyuti Das, Pratikrit Manna, and Subhasis Roy. 2024. "Biopolymer-Based Nanocomposites for Application in Biomedicine: A Review." *Journal of Polymer Engineering* 44 (2): 83–116. https://doi.org/10.1515/polyeng-2023-0166.

Shukla, Aparna, and Pralay Maiti. 2019. "Biodegradable Polymer-Based Nanohybrids for Controlled Drug Delivery and Implant Applications." In *Advances in Sustainable Polymers*, edited by Vimal Katiyar, Raghvendra Gupta, and Tabli Ghosh, 3–19. Materials Horizons: From Nature to Nanomaterials. Singapore: Springer Singapore. https://doi.org/10.1007/978-981-32-9804-0_1.

Song, Yilin, Huaqing Jing, Long Binh Vong, Jinping Wang, and Nan Li. 2022. "Recent Advances in Targeted Stimuli-Responsive Nano-Based Drug Delivery Systems Combating Atherosclerosis." *Chinese Chemical Letters* 33 (4): 1705–17. https://doi.org/10.1016/j.cclet.2021.10.055.

Stiller, Carl-Olav, and Paul Hjemdahl. 2022. "Lessons from 20 Years with COX-2 Inhibitors: Importance of Dose–Response Considerations and Fair Play in Comparative Trials." *Journal of Internal Medicine* 292 (4): 557–74. https://doi.org/10.1111/joim.13505.

Tanveer, Muhammad, Muhammad Imran, Shoomaila Latif, Nazim Hussain, and Muhammad Bilal. 2022. "Structural Design of Organic–Inorganic Nanohybrids." In *Hybrid Nanomaterials*, edited by Komal Rizwan, Muhammad Bilal, Tahir Rasheed, and Tuan Anh Nguyen, 29–36. Materials Horizons: From Nature to Nanomaterials. Singapore: Springer Nature Singapore. https://doi.org/10.1007/978-981-19-4538-0_2.

Tu, Zhaoxu, Yiling Zhong, Hanze Hu, Dan Shao, Rainer Haag, Michael Schirner, Jaewoo Lee, Bruce Sullenger, and Kam W. Leong. 2022. "Design of Therapeutic Biomaterials to Control Inflammation." *Nature Reviews Materials* 7 (7): 557–74. https://doi.org/10.1038/s41578-022-00426-z.

Van Noort, Johannes M., Malika Bsibsi, Peter J. Nacken, Wouter H. Gerritsen, Sandra Amor, Inge R. Holtman, Erik Boddeke, et al. 2013. "Activation of an Immune-Regulatory Macrophage Response and Inhibition of Lung Inflammation in a Mouse Model of COPD Using Heat-Shock Protein Alpha B-Crystallin-Loaded PLGA Microparticles." *Biomaterials* 34 (3): 831–40. https://doi.org/10.1016/j.biomaterials.2012.10.028.

Vargas-Bernal, Rafael. 2020. "Introductory Chapter: Hybrid Nanomaterials." In *Hybrid Nanomaterials – Flexible Electronics Materials*, edited by Rafael Vargas-Bernal, Peng He, and Shuye Zhang. IntechOpen. https://doi.org/10.5772/intechopen.92012.

Viana, Iara Maíra De Oliveira, Sabrina Roussel, Joan Defrêne, Eliana Martins Lima, Frédéric Barabé, and Nicolas Bertrand. 2021. "Innate and Adaptive Immune Responses toward Nanomedicines." *Acta Pharmaceutica Sinica B* 11 (4): 852–70. https://doi.org/10.1016/j.apsb.2021.02.022.

Vizuete, María, Myriam Barrejón, María José Gómez-Escalonilla, and Fernando Langa. 2012. "Endohedral and Exohedral Hybrids Involving Fullerenes and Carbon Nanotubes." *Nanoscale* 4 (15): 4370. https://doi.org/10.1039/c2nr30376k.

Wang, Qin, Liming He, Donghao Fan, Wenlang Liang, and Jiyu Fang. 2020. "Improving the Anti-Inflammatory Efficacy of Dexamethasone in the Treatment of Rheumatoid Arthritis with Polymerized Stealth Liposomes as a Delivery Vehicle." *Journal of Materials Chemistry B* 8 (9): 1841–51. https://doi.org/10.1039/C9TB02538C.

Wang, Qin, Xianyan Qin, Jiyu Fang, and Xun Sun. 2021. "Nanomedicines for the Treatment of Rheumatoid Arthritis: State of Art and Potential Therapeutic Strategies." *Acta Pharmaceutica Sinica B* 11 (5): 1158–74. https://doi.org/10.1016/j.apsb.2021.03.013.

Wu, Bohua, Yinjie Kuang, Xiaohua Zhang, and Jinhua Chen. 2011. "Noble Metal Nanoparticles/Carbon Nanotubes Nanohybrids: Synthesis and Applications." *Nano Today* 6 (1): 75–90. https://doi.org/10.1016/j.nantod.2010.12.008.

Wu, Jingjiao, Huiyi Liang, Yuanchao Li, Yi Shi, Massimo Bottini, Yongming Chen, and Lixin Liu. 2020. "Cationic Block Copolymer Nanoparticles with Tunable DNA Affinity for Treating Rheumatoid Arthritis." *Advanced Functional Materials* 30 (27): 2000391. https://doi.org/10.1002/adfm.202000391.

Xue, Hang, Zhenhe Zhang, Ze Lin, Jin Su, Adriana C. Panayi, Yuan Xiong, Liangcong Hu, et al. 2022. "Enhanced Tissue Regeneration through Immunomodulation of Angiogenesis and Osteogenesis with a Multifaceted Nanohybrid Modified Bioactive Scaffold." *Bioactive Materials* 18 (December): 552–68. https://doi.org/10.1016/j.bioactmat.2022.05.023.

Yu, Huanghe, Jialong Fan, Nuzhat Shehla, Yixing Qiu, Ye Lin, Zhou Wang, Liang Cao, et al. 2022. "Biomimetic Hybrid Membrane-Coated Xuetongsu Assisted with Laser Irradiation for Efficient Rheumatoid Arthritis Therapy." *ACS Nano* 16 (1): 502–21. https://doi.org/10.1021/acsnano.1c07556.

Yu, Seungjin, N. Sanoj Rejinold, Goeun Choi, and Jin-Ho Choy. 2025. "Revolutionizing Healthcare: Inorganic Medicinal Nanoarchitectonics for Advanced Theranostics." *Nanoscale Horizons*, 10.1039.D4NH00497C. https://doi.org/10.1039/D4NH00497C.

Zeb, Hassan, and Asim Riaz. 2022. "Introduction to Organic–Inorganic Nanohybrids." In *Hybrid Nanomaterials*, edited by Komal Rizwan, Muhammad Bilal, Tahir Rasheed, and Tuan Anh Nguyen, 1–27. Materials Horizons: From Nature to Nanomaterials. Singapore: Springer Nature Singapore. https://doi.org/10.1007/978-981-19-4538-0_1.

Zeng, Yujun, Zhiqian Li, Hongyan Zhu, Zhongwei Gu, Hu Zhang, and Kui Luo. 2020. "Recent Advances in Nanomedicines for Multiple Sclerosis Therapy." *ACS Applied Bio Materials* 3 (10): 6571–97. https://doi.org/10.1021/acsabm.0c00953.

Zhang, Songbai, Vega Lloveras, Daniel Pulido, Flonja Liko, Luiz F. Pinto, Fernando Albericio, Miriam Royo, and José Vidal-Gancedo. 2020. "Radical Dendrimers Based on Biocompatible Oligoethylene Glycol Dendrimers as Contrast Agents for MRI." *Pharmaceutics* 12 (8): 772. https://doi.org/10.3390/pharmaceutics12080772.

Zhao, Junkai, Xuan Chen, Kwun-Hei Ho, Chao Cai, Cheuk-Wing Li, Mo Yang, and Changqing Yi. 2021. "Nanotechnology for Diagnosis and Therapy of Rheumatoid Arthritis: Evolution towards Theranostic Approaches." *Chinese Chemical Letters* 32 (1): 66–86. https://doi.org/10.1016/j.cclet.2020.11.048.

Zhuo, Yue, Yong-Gang Zhao, and Yun Zhang. 2024. "Enhancing Drug Solubility, Bioavailability, and Targeted Therapeutic Applications through Magnetic Nanoparticles." *Molecules* 29 (20): 4854. https://doi.org/10.3390/molecules29204854.

6 Harnessing Multi-Enzymatic Activities of Single-Atom Nanozymes for Advanced Antimicrobial Applications

Suchika Burra and Firdoz Shaik

6.1 INTRODUCTION

The growing prevalence of multidrug-resistant (MDR) bacterial infections poses a serious global health challenge, driving the demand for innovative therapeutic solutions. Nanozymes the nanoscale artificial enzymes capable of replicating natural enzymatic activities have emerged as promising candidates for reactive oxygen species (ROS) based antibacterial therapy. By mimicking catalytic functions such as peroxidase (POD), oxidase (OXD), catalase (CAT), and superoxide dismutase (SOD), nanozymes provide versatile platforms for controlled ROS generation and microbial eradication (Wang et al., 2021).

Within this field, transition-metal single-atom nanozymes (SAZs), particularly those containing Pt, Fe, Cu, and Co, represent a transformative class of antimicrobial nanomaterials. Their defining feature is atomically dispersed active centers that ensure maximum atomic utilization, superior catalytic efficiency, and precise biochemical reactivity in complex microenvironments (Xu et al., 2021). For example, Hou et al. (2025) reported Fe–N–C SAZs synthesized via encapsulated pyrolysis, which displayed strong peroxidase-like activity by converting H_2O_2 into highly reactive •OH and $O_2•^-$ species. These nanozymes effectively killed both gram negative and gram positive bacteria, with antimicrobial potency further enhanced under near-infrared (NIR) irradiation through synergistic chemodynamic (CDT) and photothermal therapy (PTT).

Building on this, Xu et al. (2021) engineered Fe-doped polydiaminopyridine SAZs that were highly responsive to biofilm microenvironments characterized by low pH and elevated H_2O_2 . Under NIR exposure, these materials achieved efficient ROS generation and CDT/PTT synergy, with theoretical modeling confirming the

DOI: 10.1201/9781003563723-6

crucial role of Fe–N coordination geometry in enhancing catalytic output. Subsequent efforts by Liu et al. improved structural homogeneity and stability by uniformly dispersing Fe atoms on carbon frameworks, resulting in reproducible catalytic performance essential for clinical translation. Similarly, Feng et al. (2022) introduced mesoporous Fe–N–C SAZs with ~4 nm pore sizes, which enhanced mass transport, light absorption, and substrate accessibility. Innovations such as FeN_5–SA/CNF nanozymes demonstrated how tailored nitrogen coordination could amplify electron transfer and catalytic efficiency.

Recent studies further demonstrate the broad potential of SAZs. Huo et al. (2024) showed that Fe–N–C nanozymes with high density distributed active sites of Fe achieved superior antibacterial effects against *S. aureus* and *E. coli*, particularly under NIR activation. Feng et al. (2025) expanded this concept by designing Fe–SAZs with combined POD- and SOD-like activities, enabling balanced ROS regulation for both bacterial killing and wound healing. Parallel investigations have expanded single-atom nanozymes (SAZs) to transition metals such as Cu, Pt, and Co , highlighting their multifunctional behavior and tunable catalytic properties. These advances further emphasize their applicability in diverse biomedical contexts, including tissue repair (Qian et al., 2022).

Together, these advances highlight the progressive evolution of transition-metal SAZs, especially Fe–N–C systems, as multifunctional agents for combating MDR pathogens. Rational atomic-level design, photothermal integration, and optimized structural architectures not only enhance antibacterial performance but also support regenerative outcomes. This chapter systematically reviews their development, catalytic mechanisms, and translational prospects, with emphasis on ROS-driven antimicrobial therapy and clinical management of MDR infections and wound healing (Lan et al., 2024).

6.2 SYNTHESIS OF SINGLE METAL ATOM NANOZYMES BASED ON THERMAL ATOMIZATION

High-temperature thermal atomization has emerged as a robust strategy for synthesizing single-atom nanozymes (SAZs), enabling uniform dispersion of individual metal atoms on supportive matrices to optimize catalytic activity. In this process, metal nanoparticles undergo controlled thermal treatment, leading to their breakdown into isolated atoms that are subsequently stabilized on suitable supports – commonly nitrogen-doped carbon frameworks derived from metal-organic frameworks. For instance, Pt nanoparticles have been successfully atomized and anchored onto N-doped carbon matrices originating from zeolitic imidazolate frameworks (ZIF-8). This approach, often referred to as "reverse thermal sintering," which improved the availability and firmness of active sites by strengthening metal-binding interactions. It also improves catalytic efficacy by fine-tuning the electronic environment and maintaining the durability of single-atom centers (Zhang et al., 2024).

SAZs represent a breakthrough class of nanozymes in enzyme-mimetic catalysis, characterized by maximized atomic utilization, well-defined active centers, and high catalytic precision. Anchoring isolated metal atoms on heteroatom-doped carbon supports, particularly nitrogen, allows these materials to display versatile enzyme-like activities. Such features make SAZs highly attractive for biomedical applications, including antibacterial therapies and tissue repair (Wang et al., 2023).

6.2.1 Synthesis and Characterization of Fe-Based Single-Atom Nanozymes

Carbon supported nanomaterials are largely utilized in antibacterial and catalytic systems, largely because nitrogen atoms readily coordinate with metal ions to generate structurally stable metal–nitrogen ($M–N_x$) active sites. In fabricating Fe-based single-atom nanozymes (Fe-SAZs), urea serves as a nitrogen-rich precursor, polyvinylpyrrolidone (PVP) provides the carbon source, and $FeCl_3$ functions both as the iron precursor and as the catalytic center responsible for reactive oxygen species (ROS) generation to achieve antibacterial activity. The incorporation of a mesoporous structure ensures improved accessibility of Fe active sites, thereby enhancing peroxidase (POD)-like activity.

During synthesis, the mixture of urea, PVP, and $FeCI_3$ undergoes thermal decomposition at ~500 °C, releasing volatile byproducts such as ammonia $(NH\ )$, carbon dioxide (CO_2), and water vapor ($H_2\ O_2$). The release of these gases assists in forming a porous carbonaceous framework in which Fe atoms are doped into nitrogen-rich carbon and g-C_3N_4 matrices, producing a composite material denoted as NC@Fe/g-C_3N_4. A subsequent high-temperature calcination step, typically between 800 and 1000 °C, drives further carbonization of the organic matrix into activated carbon, enhancing porosity, refining morphology, and enabling uniform distribution of Fe single atoms within the carbon scaffold **(Figure 6.1 I.** This multi-step process results in highly active Fe-SAZs with optimized catalytic and structural features (Liu et al., 2024). Comparable high-temperature synthesis approaches for SAZs are summarized in **Table 6.1**

6.2.2 Synthesis and Characterization of Cu-Based Single-Atom Nanozyme

The synthesis of CuN_x-doped carbon nanosheets (CuN_x-CNS) is generally achieved through pyrolysis of copper–silk fibroin $(Cu-SF)$ complexes, where silk fibroin (SF) derived from *Bombyx mori* cocoons acts as a nitrogen-rich biopolymeric template. The coordination environment of $Cu(II)$ ions depends strongly on solution pH, producing either $Cu-2N_2O$ complexes at pH 5.0 or $Cu-4N$ complexes at pH 11.0. UV-Vis spectroscopy, showing a characteristic absorption peak at ~540 nm, confirmed the latter coordination mode, which ultimately evolves into CuN sites upon pyrolysis. Following freeze-drying and high-temperature treatment, the $Cu-SF$ precursors undergo carbonization to form two-dimensional carbon nanosheets decorated with atomically dispersed Cu centers. Acid etching of the resulting product effectively removes residual salts and metallic Cu particles, ensuring the uniform generation of CuN_x active sites within the carbon lattice. Microscopic characterization (TEM, AFM) reveals nanosheets with a layered morphology (~1.8 nm thick), mesoporous architecture induced by hypersaline-assisted pyrolysis, and well-dispersed Cu atoms as verified by HAADF-STEM. No Cu nanoparticles were detected, and elemental mapping (EDS)

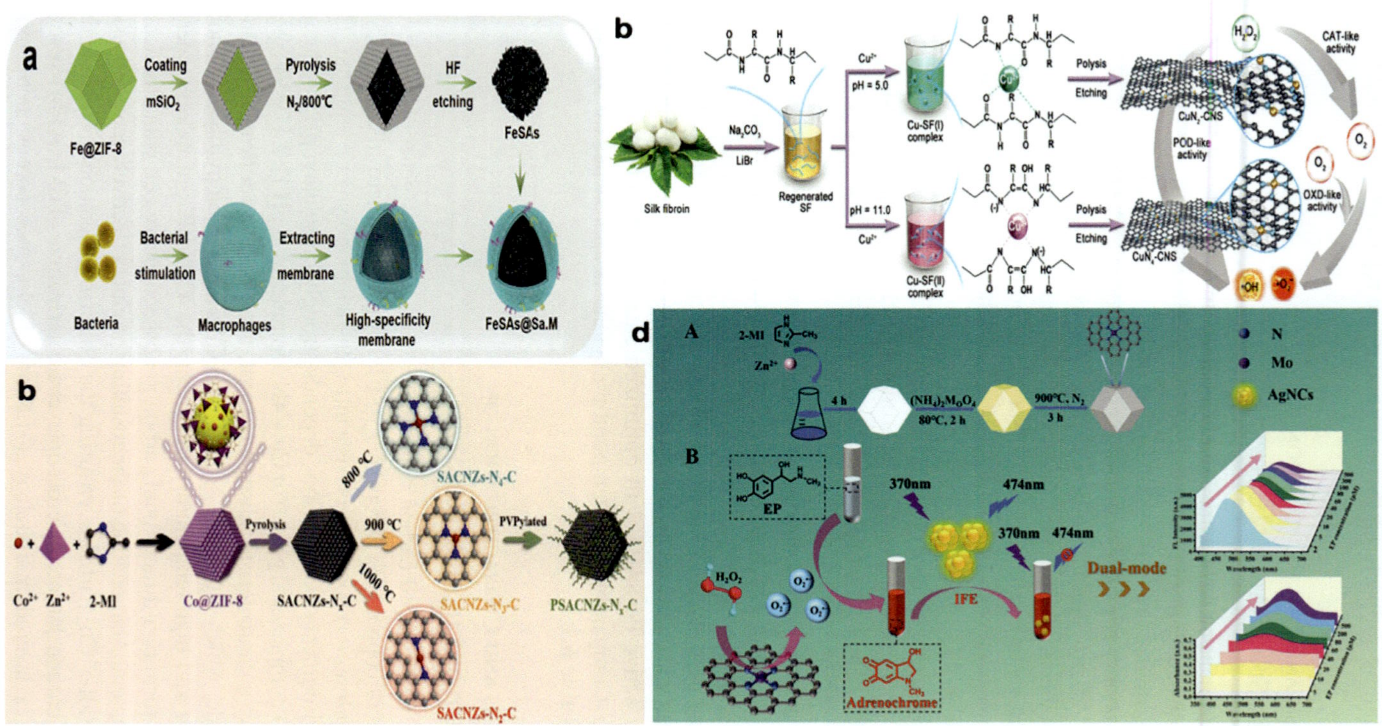

FIGURE 6.1 **(A)** A schematic illustration depicts the preparation process and properties of FeSAs@Sa.M (Liu et al., 2024). **(B)** The synthesis pathway and antibacterial therapy mechanism of CuN_x-CNS SAzyme are shown, highlighting its fabrication via pyrolysis of the Cu-SF complex. **(C)** The synthetic processes of SACNZs-N_x-C and PSACNZs-N_x-C are illustrated schematically. **(D)** (a) A diagram presents the synthesis of Mo/NC-SAN, while (b) illustrates its application in a dual-mode assay platform for EP detection.

TABLE 6.1
Synthesis Methods and Antibacterial Applications of SAZs

Synthesis Method	SAZs	Antibacterial Effect	Reference
Pyrolysis of (MOFs)	Fe-SAZS	Drug-resistant *S. pneumoniae*, Multidrug-resistant Tuberculosis, MRSA	(Liu et al., 2024)
Pyrolysis of (MOFs)	CO-SAZS	*S. aureus*	(Liu et al., 2023b)
	Cu-N-C	*P. aeruginosa*, *S. aureus*	(Zhu et al., 2022)
	Cu-N-CNS	MRSA, *E. coli*	(Bai et al., 2023)
	FeSAs@Sa.M	MRSA	(Liu et al., 2023a)
	FeN3P-SAzyme	*S. aureus, E. coli*	(Gao et al., 2024)
	Mn/HSAE@BCP-	*S. aureus, E. coli*	(Gao et al., 2024)
	scaffolds FeN5 SA/CNF	MRSA	(Li et al., 2023)
	Pt-Ti3C2	*S. aureus, P aeruginosa*	(Li et al., 2023)
	Au@CuBCat	MRSA, ESLP *E. coli*	(Fan et al., 2023)
	ENT	MRSA	(Fan et al., 2023)
	Co@SAHSS	*S. aureus, E. coli*	(Zhang et al., 2023)
	PtTS-SAzyme	*E. coli, P. aeruginosa, K. pueumoniae, S. enteritidis, S. aureus*	(Chen et al., 2021)
Wet Chemistry Synthesis (ALD)	Mo SA-N/C	*E. coli, S. aureus*	(Wang et al., 2022)
	CeO_2@Gox	*S. aureus, E. coli*	(Xu et al., 2024)(Xu et al., 2024)
	Pd-CeO_2@Gox	*S. aureus, E. coli*	
Surfactant-Assisted Synthesis	Pt/g-C3N4-K	*S. aureus, E. coli, B. cereus, Pseudomonas aeruginosa*	(Fan et al., 2022)
	RBC-HNTM-Pt@Au	MRSA	(Yu et al., 2021)

confirmed homogeneous distribution of Cu, N, and C . ICP-OES analysis indicated a Cu content of ~1.5 wt%. XRD patterns confirmed the presence of N-doped carbon nanosheets without crystalline Cu phases, while XPS identified both Cu(I) and Cu(II) states alongside multiple nitrogen species, including pyridinic, pyrrolic, graphitic, and Cu – N bonding environments. Raman spectra displayed a high D/G ratio, reflecting a defect-rich carbon framework, with slightly reduced disorder compared to N-CNS due to Cu incorporation **(Figure 6.1 iv)**; Bai et al., 2023).

6.2.3 Synthesis and Characterization of Platinum (Pt)-Based SAzymes

Single-atom nanozymes (SAZs) are commonly synthesized using high-temperature thermal atomization, a method that transforms metal nanoparticles into atomically dispersed species anchored onto porous supports. For instance, Pt-based SAZs have been produced by incorporating platinum atoms into graphitic carbon nitride (g-C N) nanorods, yielding materials with intrinsic peroxidase-like activity

(Wu et al., 2021). These Pt–SAZs effectively catalyze the decomposition of hydrogen peroxide (H O), generating reactive oxygen species (ROS) that disrupt bacterial membranes and intracellular structures, leading to strong antibacterial effects. Fan et al. (2022) reported the development of Pt/g-C_3N_4-K SAZs, where Pt atoms were immobilized on carbon nitride nanorods. The resulting material displayed multi-functional biomedical utility, including sensitive H O detection, antibiotic screening, and antibacterial therapy. Its peroxidase-like catalytic activity was confirmed through chromogenic assays using 3,3′,5,5′-tetramethylbenzidine (TMB), in which H O -driven TMB oxidation produced a blue signal with an absorbance peak at 652 nm. The catalytic behavior of these SAZs was both pH- and temperature-dependent, closely resembling that of natural horseradish peroxidase (HRP), with optimal activity observed between pH 4 and 8. Importantly, antibacterial tests demonstrated that SA-Pt/g-C N -K significantly inhibited *E. coli* biofilm formation, highlighting its therapeutic promise against persistent Gram-negative biofilm-related infections. Similarly, Chen et al. (2021) utilized high-temperature atomization of Pt nanoparticles on nitrogen-doped carbon frameworks derived from ZIF-8 to synthesize Pt–SAZs. This method improved the exposure of catalytic sites and further enhanced antibacterial performance. Comparable Pt–SAZ synthesis strategies are summarized in Table 6.1.

6.2.4 Synthesis and Characterization of Molybdenum (Mo) SA-N/C-Based Single-Atom Nanozymes

For the synthesis of molybdenum-based single-atom nanozymes (Mo-SAZs), Qiang et al. (2025) employed ZIF-8 as a structural precursor. ZIF-8 was first prepared by dissolving certain amounts of zinc nitrate hexahydrate $\left(Zn\left(NO_3\right)_2 \cdot 6H_2O\right)$ and 2-methylimidazole in 80 mL of methanol, followed by continuous stirring at room temperature for 4 hours. The resulting ZIF-8 crystals were isolated through centrifugation, washed thoroughly with methanol to eliminate the unused precursors, and subsequently dried at 40 °C.

For Mo incorporation, certain amount of dried ZIF-8 was dispersed in ethanol, to which an aqueous solution containing ammonium molybdate $\left(\left(NH_4\right)_2 MoO_4\right)$ was added. The mixture was subjected to reflux at 80 °C for 2 hours. The resulting Mo@ZIF-8 composite was separated using centrifugation, repeatedly washed with ethanol, and dried at 40 °C (Qiang et al., 2025). The dried Mo@ZIF-8 precursor was then subjected to pyrolysis at 900 °C for 3 hours under a nitrogen atmosphere resulting in carbonized material **(Figure 6.1 III).**

6.2.5 Synthesis and Characterization of Single-Atom Cobalt (Co) Nanozymes

Cobalt-based single-atom nanozymes (Co-SAZs) have attracted considerable interest owing to their oxidase- and peroxidase-like catalytic activities. Typically synthesized by pyrolyzing metal-organic frameworks (MOFs) such as Co@ZIF-8, these materials also exhibit strong photothermal antibacterial activity under near-infrared (NIR) light.

Their catalytic efficiency is closely linked to the local coordination environment of cobalt atoms; notably, a lower $Co-N$ coordination number enhances peroxidase-mimicking activity, as confirmed by kinetic studies and density functional theory (DFT) analyses.

Beyond MOF-derived routes, various Co-based SAZs (SAZs-Nn-C) have been fabricated through high-temperature pyrolysis of cobalt–ligand complexes anchored onto carbon skeletons. To further improve their stability and biocompatibility, polyvinylpyrrolidone (PVP) coating was applied, which enhanced dispersion and colloidal stability in aqueous media (**Figure 6.1 (II)**; Zhang et al., 2023).

6.3 ENZYMATIC ACTIVITY OF FE/CU/PT/CO/MO-BASED SAZS

6.3.1 Multi-Enzymatic Properties of Single-Metal-Atom Nanozymes

Single-atom nanozymes (SAZs) based on Fe, Cu, Pt, Co, and Mo exhibit remarkable multi-enzyme mimicking behavior, functioning simultaneously as superoxide dismutase (SOD), peroxidase, and oxidase analogs. This multifunctionality, often described as an "antioxidant enzyme cocktail" or "multi-enzyme system," enables precise modulation of reactive oxygen species (ROS), supporting both bactericidal action and antioxidant defense by maintaining redox homeostasis. Owing to their exceptional atomic utilization efficiency and strong catalytic activity, SAZs have emerged as a next-generation class of artificial enzymes. In particular, iron-based SAZs (Fe-SAZs) anchored onto carbon frameworks have displayed outstanding catalytic versatility, effectively replicating peroxidase, oxidase, and SOD activities. Their ability to promote ROS generation under physiological conditions makes them highly valuable for biomedical applications, including antibacterial therapy, biofilm disruption, and photothermal-assisted wound healing (Miao et al., 2024; Ajmal et al., 2024).

Single-atom nanozymes (SAZs) based on Fe, Cu, Pt, and Co demonstrate inherent peroxidase-like catalytic activity, closely resembling the enzymatic function of natural horseradish peroxidase (HRP). This ability highlights their potential as artificial peroxidases for diverse biochemical and biomedical applications. Incorporating these metals into nitrogen-doped graphitic carbon nitride $(g\text{-}C_3N_4)$ frameworks with atomically dispersed sites maximizes exposure of active centers, thereby enhancing catalytic efficiency.

Functioning as Fenton-like nanozymes, Fe/Cu/Pt/Co-SAZs catalyze the decomposition of H_2O_2 to generate hydroxyl radicals $(\bullet OH)$, which are highly reactive and capable of damaging bacterial cell membranes as well as essential biomolecules such as proteins, lipids, and nucleic acids. In addition, superoxide radicals $(O_2\bullet^-)$ are produced, which undergo superoxide dismutase (SOD)-like transformations into less reactive species including H_2O_2 and O_2 (Xi et al., 2019; Qu et al., 2024). Singlet oxygen $(^1O_2)$ is also generated, further intensifying bactericidal efficacy.

Their catalytic behavior can be synergistically enhanced through combination with antimicrobial agents (e.g., antibiotics or nanoparticles) or integration with photodynamic therapy (PDT). In colorimetric assays, the peroxidase-like function of these SAZs is validated by their ability to oxidize chromogenic substrates such as ABTS and TMB in the presence of H_2O_2, resulting in visible color changes.

Moreover, specific thermal treatments during synthesis – particularly high-temperature carbonization (800–1000 °C) – along with nitrogen doping, play a critical role in tailoring nanosheet morphologies, improving porosity, and optimizing the catalytic performance of Fe-based and other transition metal SAZs (Feng et al., 2023; Li et al., 2024).

6.4 ANTIBACTERIAL APPLICATIONS AND PROPERTIES OF SINGLE-METAL-ATOM NANOZYMES

The antibacterial activity of Fe/Cu/Pt/Co-based single-atom nanozymes (SAZs) was assessed under different conditions, including PBS (control), H_2O_2 alone, SAZs alone, and SAZs combined with H_2O_2 with or without near-infrared (NIR-I) irradiation. Results showed that the combination of SAZs with H_2O_2 and NIR-I produced the strongest bactericidal effect, effectively eliminating both Gram-positive and Gram-negative (MRSA) bacteria and (*E. coli*) respectively.

The atomically dispersed active sites of SAZs maximize catalytic efficiency compared to conventional nanoparticles. In the presence of H_2O_2, SAZs catalyze Fenton-like reactions to generate hydroxyl radicals, inducing oxidative damage to bacterial membranes, proteins, and nucleic acids, leading to cell death (Zhang et al., 2024). NIR-I irradiation further enhances ROS generation by promoting electron transfer through photoexcitation, thereby amplifying peroxidase-like activity (Sun et al., 2023).

This synergistic effect enables deeper tissue penetration, localized heating, and potent antibacterial performance, achieving > 95% bacterial inactivation in vitro. Importantly, SAZ dosage can be tailored according to infection severity to achieve complete eradication, including against multidrug-resistant pathogens (Hou et al., 2024).

(a) Temperature elevation curves demonstrated concentration-dependent photothermal effects of FeSAs@Sa.M under 808 nm laser irradiation (1 W cm^{-2}), **(b)** The percentage survival of extracellular MRSA varied significantly under different treatments, **(c)** Intracellular MRSA survival was markedly reduced following FeSAs@Sa.M exposure, **(d)** Colony formation assays confirmed the antibacterial efficacy against extracellular MRSA, while **(e–g)** Steady-state kinetic assays with H_2O_2 and TMB, along with UV-vis spectra, verified the peroxidase-like activity of FeSAs, FeSAs@M, FeSAs@Ec.M, and FeSAs@Sa.M in PBS buffer (10 mM, pH 4.0, 37 °C), **(h)** Statistical analyses indicated significant differences, and (i) bio-TEM imaging revealed the attachment of nanozymes to intracellular MRSA within infected macrophages of MRSA-infected RAW264.7.

6.4.1 Fe-Based Nanozymes

The antibacterial activity of Fe-SAZs was assessed in vitro and in vivo. When combined with H_2O_2, Fe-SAZs showed enhanced catalytic activity, and under NIR irradiation they effectively eliminated multidrug-resistant bacteria such as *E. coli* and MRSA, while also accelerating wound healing (Yan et al., 2023). NIR irradiation provides deeper tissue penetration, converting photon energy into localized heat that disrupts bacterial membranes and amplifies bactericidal efficiency.

Photothermal heating further promoted H_2O_2 decomposition into highly reactive •OH radicals, achieving ~95% MRSA inactivation in vitro **(Figure 6.2 b–d).** In vivo experiments confirmed accelerated wound healing in treated groups compared to controls. These findings demonstrate the multimodal antibacterial mechanism of Fe-SAZs, combining photothermal and catalytic effects for effective eradication of extracellular and intracellular pathogens (Liu et al., 2024).

Bio-TEM imaging **(Figure 6.2 i)** revealed that FeSAs@Sa.M specifically bound to MRSA-infected RAW264.7 macrophages, enabling direct association with intracellular MRSA, unlike FeSAs alone. This indicates that the Sa.M component mediates bacterial targeting and enhances phagocytosis, highlighting FeSAs@Sa.M as a promising targeted nanozyme system for treating resistant bacterial infections. A detailed study examined the synthesis, structure, and antibacterial performance of Fe-based single-atom nanozymes functionalized with Staphylococcus aureus

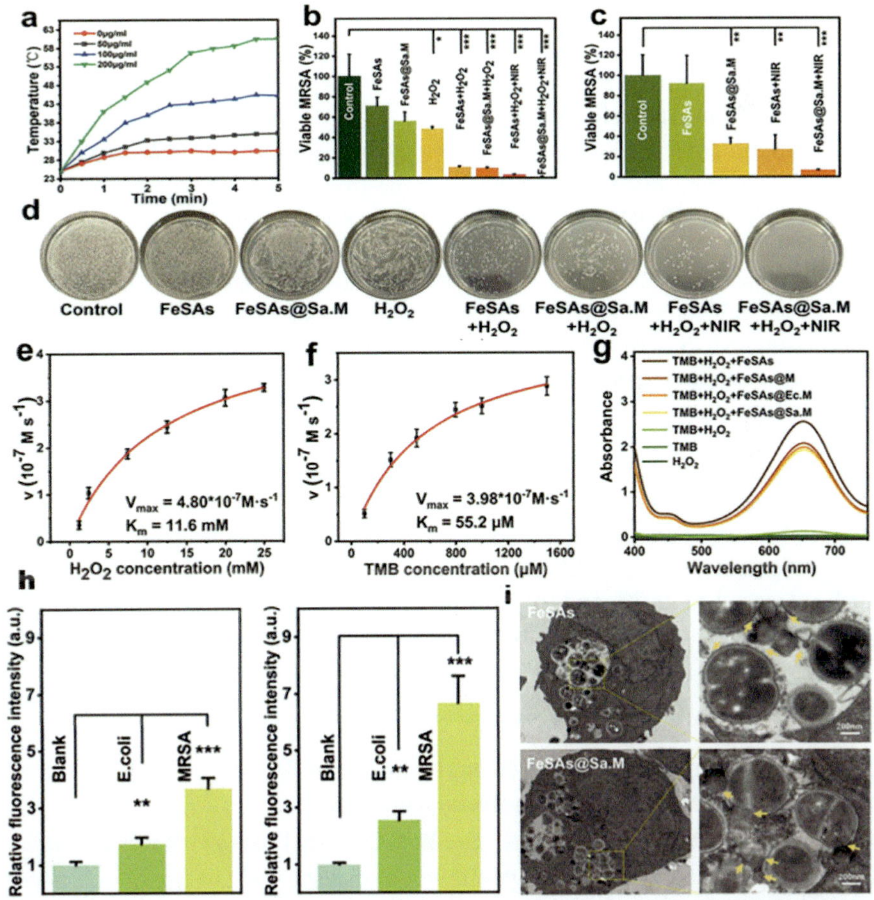

FIGURE 6.2 Focusing on the pathogen-targeting and catalytic performance of FeSAs @Sa.M.

membrane vesicles (FeSAs@Sa.M), designed to enhance catalytic, photothermal, and bactericidal effects against MRSA. Fe-SAZs in presence of H_2O_2, and NIR-I irradiation reduced the viability of *E. coli* to 0.2% and MRSA 1.5%, confirming the strong synergy of photothermal and catalytic mechanisms. NIR-I further amplified the activity of peroxidase-like Fe-SAZs, intensifying bacterial killing. Biofilm disruption was assessed by crystal violet staining, which showed that Fe-SAZs with H_2O_2 markedly suppressed MRSA biofilms, and with NIR-I irradiation, the disruption efficiency reached ~87.1% (Liu et al., 2024). The peroxidase-like activity of FeSAs, FeSAs@M, FeSAs@Ec.M, and FeSAs@Sa.M was evaluated using H_2O_2 and TMB as substrates in PBS buffer (10 mM, pH 4.0) at 37 °C, with UV-vis spectra confirming catalytic performance **(Figure 6.2 e–g).** Furthermore, the oxidase-like activity of FeSAs@Sa.M toward TMB was investigated through steady-state kinetic assays under identical buffer conditions. Immunofluorescence imaging confirmed the proper orientation of bacteria-pretreated macrophage membrane coating on FeSAs.

6.4.2 Cu-Based Nanozymes

6.4.2.1 Copper-Based Single-Atom Nanozymes (CuN_4-CNS) and Antibacterial Mechanism

Copper single-atom nanozymes (CuN_4-CNS), synthesized from $CuCl_2$ and 2-methylimidazole, display multiple enzyme-like activities, including oxidase (OXD), peroxidase (POD), and catalase (CAT) mimicking functions.

These activities promote the production of highly reactive oxygen species (ROS) such as superoxide ($O_2\bullet^-$) and hydroxyl (•OH)radicals (Figure 6.4E), which drive their strong antibacterial effect against a broad range of pathogens, including multi-drug-resistant MRSA. In combination with H_2O_2 and NIR irradiation, CuN_4-CNS effectively disrupted biofilms and reduced bacterial viability **(Figure 6.3 iv–v)**, demonstrating promise for infection control and wound healing applications (Bai et al., 2023).

Fluorescence and UV-vis analyses confirmed robust ROS generation, correlating with high bactericidal performance in vitro. While H_2O_2 alone had minimal effect, CuN_4-CNS catalyzed a Fenton-like reaction that amplified antibacterial activity. Against *E. coli* and MRSA, CuN_4-CNS achieved inhibition rates of 82.8%, which increased to 98.7% and 99.9% with H_2O_2, respectively. These results highlight their synergistic catalytic efficiency and therapeutic potential.

6.4.3 Pt-Based Nanozymes

6.4.3.1 Platinum-Based Single-Atom Nanozymes SA-Pt/g-C_3N_4-K and Antibacterial Mechanism

The single-atom Pt-doped g-C_3N_4-K (SA-Pt/g-C_3N_4-K) nanozyme was synthesized to improve catalytic efficiency by incorporating Pt atoms into the g-C_3N_4-K framework. This structural modification significantly enhanced its peroxidase-like activity compared with natural horseradish peroxidase (HRP) and pristine g-C_3N_4-K. To exploit this improvement, a colorimetric detection platform was constructed for sensitive H_2O_2 detection. The catalytic performance was systematically evaluated using Michaeli-Menten and Lineweaver-Burk analyses, which confirmed that SA-Pt/g-C_3N_4-K possessed the lowest Km values for both TMB and H_2O_2, reflecting superior substrate affinity. Mechanistic studies demonstrated that although both SA-Pt/g-C_3N_4-K and g-C_3N_4-K activate H_2O_2, the Pt-based system showed a reduced energy barrier in adsorption-desorption processes, facilitating efficient dissociation of H_2O_2 into reactive •OH radicals. Free energy calculations further indicated that OH* desorption from g-C_3N_4-K was energetically unfavorable (3.34 eV), while release from Pt–N_4 sites in SA-Pt/g-C_3N_4-K required substantially less energy (0.885 eV). This highlights the enhanced catalytic turnover rate enabled by Pt incorporation. UV-vis absorption spectra confirmed peroxidase-like behavior, where absorbance increased proportionally with rising H_2O_2 concentration. A strong linear correlation was observed between absorbance and H_2O_2 concentration over a range of 5–500 μM, with a low detection limit of 1 μM **(Figure 6.3 ii)**, demonstrating high sensitivity. Compared to conventional approaches, this platform provided broader applicability for reliable H_2O_2 sensing. The antibacterial properties were subsequently evaluated using confocal fluorescence imaging. Control groups displayed mainly live bacteria with dominant green fluorescence, while individual treatment with either SA-Pt/g-C_3N_4-K or H_2O_2 showed only limited bacterial death. In contrast, co-treatment with SA-Pt/g-C_3N_4-K and H_2O_2 led to a dramatic increase in bacterial mortality, evidenced by strong red fluorescence signals **(Figure 6.3 iii)**. These results were consistent with colony plate counting, confirming a synergistic antibacterial effect. Overall, SA-Pt/g-C_3N_4-K integrates efficient synthesis, superior catalytic activity, sensitive H_2O_2 detection, and potent antibacterial performance, establishing it as a promising nanozyme platform for biomedical applications, particularly in addressing gram-negative biofilm-associated infections.

6.4.4 Mo-Based Nanozymes

6.4.4.1 Molybdenum-Based Single-Atom Nanozymes for Antibacterial and Sensing Applications

Molybdenum-based single-atom nanozymes (Mo SA-N/C) showed the properties of haloperoxidase (HPO)-like activity which catalyzes the halide ion oxidation (e.g., Br^-, Cl^-, F^-) with H_2O_2, generating hypobromous acid (HOBr), a highly effective antimicrobial agent. Their antibacterial efficacy is further enhanced by visible light, where photothermal heating accelerates reaction kinetics and improves HOBr production, making Mo SA-N/C highly promising for biofilm disruption and marine antifouling.

A carbon-supported molybdenum nanozyme (Mo/NC-SAN) with nitrogen-doping was successfully synthesized with strong peroxidase-like activity **(Figure 6.3 III)**. In parallel, fluorescent silver nanoclusters (AgNCs) were prepared and integrated with Mo/NC-SAN to develop a dual-mode colorimetric and fluorescence sensor for epinephrine (EP). In this system, Mo/NC-SAN catalyzes EP oxidation to adrenochrome, producing a 485 nm absorption peak, while adrenochrome quenches AgNC fluorescence at 474 nm via the inner-filter effect, enabling sensitive EP detection.

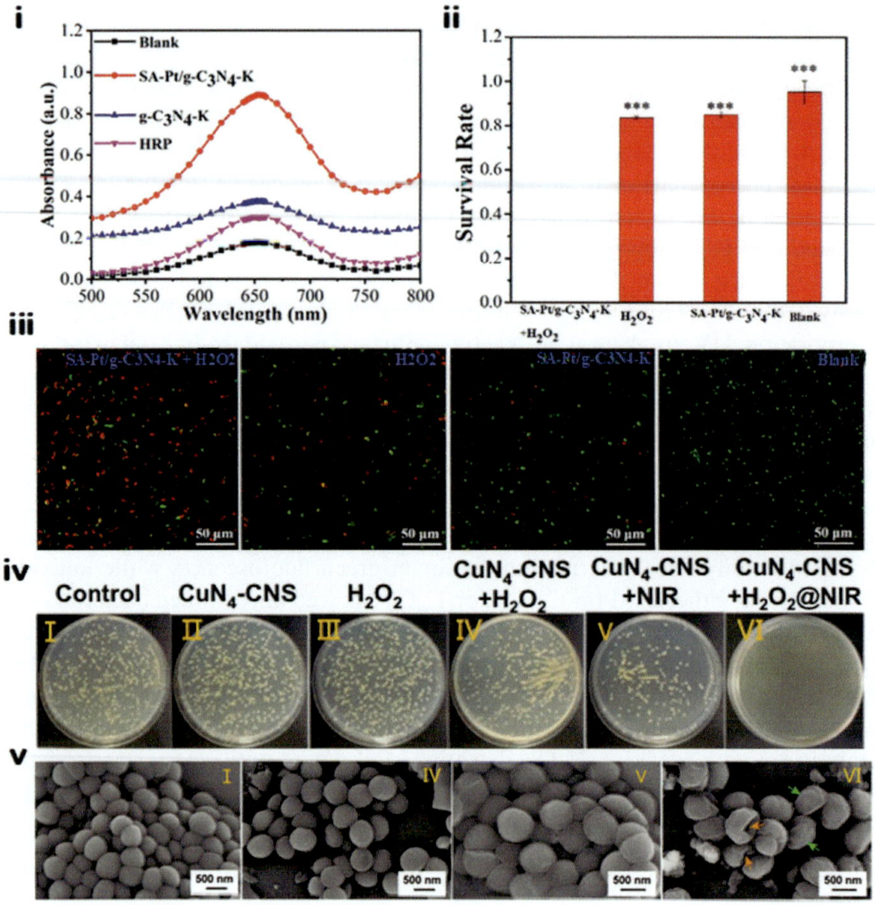

FIGURE 6.3 **(I)** UV-vis absorption spectra of SA-Pt/g-C_3N_4-K, g-C_3N_4-K, and HRP with 1 mM TMB and 1 mM H_2O_2 at pH 4 confirmed peroxidase-like activity. **(II)** The survival rate of ***E. coli*** cells (n = 3) showed significant reduction, with t-test analysis indicating ***p < 0.001 for combined SA-Pt/g-C_3N_4-K and H_2O_2 treatment. **(III)** Fluorescence imaging revealed green (live) and red (dead) signals in ***E. coli*** colonies, demonstrating enhanced bacterial killing under combined treatment compared to controls. **(IV)** The catalytic antibacterial and antibiofilm efficacy of CuN_4-CNS was validated through colony photographs and SYTOX/PI staining under different treatment conditions, including PBS, CuN_4-CNS, H_2O_2, and their combinations with NIR irradiation. **(V)** SEM images further confirmed morphological alterations in bacterial cells, supporting the observed antibacterial performance.

Density functional theory (DFT) studies confirmed Mo single atoms as efficient catalytic sites for bromide oxidation in the Mo SA-N/C + H_2O_2 + Br^- system. Antibacterial assays demonstrated broad-spectrum efficacy against *E. coli, P. aeruginosa, S. aureus, B. cereus, B. subtilis, V. alginolyticus,* and *V. vulnificus*, with visible light irradiation significantly amplifying bactericidal performance (Zhu et al., 2022; Qiang et al., 2025).

6.4.5 Co-Based Nanozymes

The microbicidal effect of the Co-based nanozymes (PSAZSNZs-N_x-C) nanoscale catalytic mimics was evaluated against Escherichia coli (ATCC 25922) as shown in **Figure 6.4(a-d)**. The results indicated that all three PSAZSNZs-N_x-C nanozymes exhibited significant reactive oxygen species (ROS) driven antibacterial activity, activated by H_2O_2, with PSAZSNZs-N_2-C demonstrating superior antibacterial efficacy. The observed enhancement in activity was ascribed to the optimization of its peroxidase-mimetic catalytic properties (Zhang et al., 2023).

Subsequent kinetic evaluations and density functional theory calculations (DFT) demonstrated a clear association between the catalytic behavior resembling peroxidase and the coordination structure of cobalt centers. Notably, a reduced coordination number of Co–N bonds correlated with improved catalytic performance. These observations indicate that precise modulation of Co–N ligand coordination during synthesis can strategically control the enzymatic activity of cobalt-based single-atom nanozymes (Liu et al, 2023b; Liang et al, 2022).

Biological wound healing investigations into in vivo catalytic therapy against bacteria of PSACNZs-N x -C and in vitro antimicrobial assays against E. coli, S. aureus confirmed the potent therapeutic effects of PSAZSNZs-N_2-C when combined in the form of PSACNZs-N 2 -C + H 2 O 2 + NaAc buffer compared to PSACNZs-N 3 -C, PSACNZs-N 4 – C as shown in **Figure 6.4(b-d)**. Upon 1064 nm laser irradiation, the Co-based SAzyme exhibited oxidase-like catalytic activity by converting molecular oxygen (O_2) to superoxide anion radicals (O_2^{-}•) and simultaneously increasing the local wound temperature to approximately 53 °C. The synergistic combination of photothermal therapy (PTT), chemo-dynamic therapy (CDT), and catalytic therapy (CT) enabled rapid bacterial eradication and accelerated wound healing. These results underscore the potential of cobalt-based single-atom nanozymes as versatile therapeutic agents with multifunctional capabilities for combating antibacterial activity while enhancing tissue repair and regeneration processes (Ren et al., 2023). A detailed antibacterial application of various single metal atom based nanozymes (SAZs) is summarized in **Table 6.2**.

6.5 IN VIVO AND CATALYTIC EVALUATIONS OF SINGLE-ATOM NANOZYMES

In vivo assessments of single-atom nanozymes rely on advanced structural and catalytic characterization. High-angle annular dark-field scanning transmission electron microscopy (HAADF-STEM) is used to visualize isolated single atoms as bright spots on the support, while X-ray absorption spectroscopy (XAS) reveals elemental distribution and oxidation states. Energy-dispersive X-ray spectroscopy (EDS) with elemental mapping further confirms uniform atomic dispersion.

Catalytic performance is evaluated using chromogenic substrates such as TMB and ABTS to probe peroxidase-like activity in the presence of H_2O_2. Reactive oxygen species (ROS) generation is monitored with fluorescent probes (DCFH-DA, HPF) to detect •OH and O_2•$^-$ radicals. Enzyme kinetics are analyzed through Michaelis-Menten modeling (Km, Vmax) to benchmark catalytic efficiency against natural

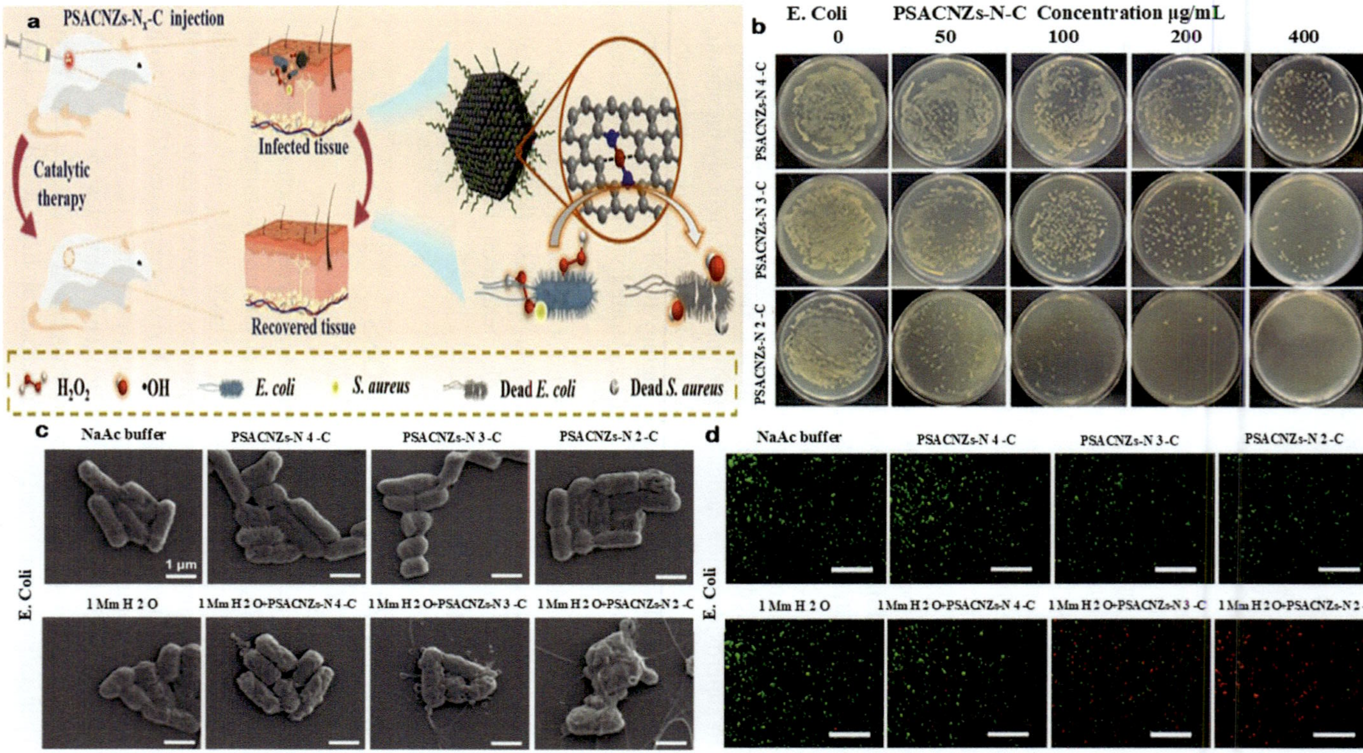

FIGURE 6.4 **(A)** In vivo antibacterial catalytic therapy of PSACNZs-N_x-C was evaluated under physiological conditions. **(B)** The survival of ***E. coli*** was assessed at varying concentrations of the material in the presence of 1 mM H_2O_2 . **(C)** SEM imaging revealed morphological changes in ***E. coli*** after different treatments compared with untreated controls. **(D)** ***E. coli*** was systematically tested across control (Group 1), individual treatments with PSACNZs-N_4-C (Group 2), PSACNZs-N_3-C (Group 3), PSACNZs-N_2-C (Group 4), and H_2O_2 (Group 5), as well as combined treatments with PSACNZs variants and H_2O_2 (Groups 6–8) in NaAc buffer (pH 4.5, 25 °C), all microscopy results confirmed enhanced antibacterial effects in co-treatment groups, with scale bars representing 50 μm (Fan et al., 2022; Zhang et al., 2023).

TABLE 6.2
Comparative Analysis of the Catalytic Functions and Therapeutic Potential of SAZs

SAZs	Catalytic Nodes	Support	Nanozyme Catalyze Behavior	Therapeutic Biomedical Applications	Reference
FeN5 SA/CNF	Fe-N5	Nitrogen-doped carbon	Cytochrome P450	Antibacterial	(Lan et al., 2024)
Fe-Art M	Fe2N6O	Nitrogen-doped carbon	POD and haloperoxidase	Antibacterial	(Long et al., 2021)
SA-Pt/g-C 3 N 4-K	Pt-N-C	pristine g-C3N4)	POD	Antibacterial	(Fan et al., 2022)
FeSAs@Sa.M	Fe–N4–O–Fe–N4	ZIF-8	POD	Antibacterial	(Liu et al., 2023a)
Mo SA-N/C	Mo	Nitrogen-doped carbon	HPO	Antibacterial	(Wang et al., 2022)
Co-SAC	Co	ZIF-8	OXD	Antibacterial	(Liu et al., 2023b)
Cu-N-C	Cu	CuCl2, KCl	POD, OXD	Antibacterial	(Zhu et al., 2022)
PSACNZs-N x -C	Co-N	Co@ZIF-8	POD	Antibacterial	(Zhang et al., 2023)
CuN_4-CNS	CuN	Silk fibroin	POD, OXD	Antibacterial	(Bai et al., 2023)
Cu SASs/NPC	Cu-N4	Nitrogen-doped carbon	POD and GPx	Antibacterial	(Jin et al., 2023)
PMCS	Zn-N4	Nitrogen-doped carbon	POD	Antibacterial	(Jin et al., 2023)
Co@SAHSs@IL-4@RCM	CoPc	SiO2@CN	POD, SOD, CAT	Antibacterial	(Zhang et al., 2023)
Mn/HSAE@BCP	Mn	ZIF-8 NCs	POD, SOD, CAT	Antibacterial	(Gao et al., 2024)
Au@CuBCat	Cu-Nx	CuBCats	POD	Antibacterial	(Fan et al., 2023)
Pt-Ti3C2	Pt	Ti3C2 lattice	POD	Antibacterial	(Li et al., 2023)
Pd–CeO 2 @ GOx	Pd	CeO2	POD, CAT	Antibacterial	(Xu et al., 2024)
PtTS-SAzyme	Pt	ZIF-8	POD	Antibacterial	(Chen et al., 2021)
(Dual) SAFe-NMCNs	Fe-N	F127/DA Micelle	CAT, POD	Anti-tumor	(Su et al., 2022a)
CrSA–CN	Cr-N4	Nitrogen-doped carbon	Haloperoxidase	Antibacterial against Biofouling in seawater	(Peng et al., 2024)
L-Arg@Cu–SAzymes	Cu	Cu–silk fibroin	POD, OXD, CAT	Antibacterial	(Lan et al., 2024)

enzymes. Electron spin resonance (ESR) spectroscopy is additionally employed to capture transient ROS intermediates, offering detailed mechanistic insights into catalytic pathways.

6.6 CONCLUSION

Iron-, copper-, platinum-, and cobalt-based single-atom nanozymes (Fe/Cu/Pt/Co SAZs) are a cutting-edge class of catalytic nanomaterials with potent antibacterial activity. Atomically dispersed metal centers, particularly Fe within nitrogen-doped carbon frameworks, enable enzyme-mimetic functions – including superoxide dismutase (SOD), peroxidase (POD), and oxidase (OXD) – while generating reactive oxygen species (ROS) to selectively inactivate bacteria. These nanozymes exhibit multimodal therapeutic potential, combining ROS-mediated killing with photothermal, chemodynamic, or antibiotic-assisted strategies, and can be integrated with diagnostic probes for real-time infection monitoring.

SAZs respond to pathogen-specific microenvironments, such as elevated H_2O_2 or acidic pH within biofilms, enhancing precision against multidrug-resistant (MDR) bacteria. Cu-, Pt-, and Co-based SAZs similarly show broad-spectrum antibacterial activity, with structural innovations like mesoporous architectures improving mass transport, surface exposure, and catalytic efficiency.

Key challenges remain, including long-term biocompatibility, in vivo safety, and scalable synthesis. Future efforts should optimize metal coordination, clarify catalytic mechanisms, and conduct rigorous preclinical validation. With interdisciplinary collaboration, SAZs hold significant promise as next-generation antimicrobial and wound-healing agents, offering an effective approach to combat antibiotic-resistant infections.

Funding Acknowledgment: Dr. Shaik Firdoz gratefully acknowledges the generous financial support provided by the Indian Council of Medical Research (ICMR) under the grant number EM/Dev/IG/17/1129/2023, which made the preparation of this book chapter possible.

REFERENCES

Ajmal, S., Zhao, Y., Yasin, G., Boakye, F. O., Tabish, M., Alam, M. M.,. . . Zhao, W. (2024). Transition metals based dual single-atom catalysts for oxygen electrocatalysis: Stunning advances and future prospects. *ChemCatChem*, 16(12), e202301392.

Bai, J., Feng, Y., Li, W., Cheng, Z., Rosenholm, J. M., Yang, H.,. . . Geng, D. (2023). Alternative copper-based single-atom nanozyme with superior multienzyme activities and NIR-II responsiveness to fight against deep tissue infections. *Research*, 6, 0031.

Chen, Y., Wang, P., Hao, H., Hong, J., Li, H., Ji, S.,. . . Li, Y. (2021). Thermal atomization of platinum nanoparticles into single atoms: An effective strategy for engineering high-performance nanozymes. *Journal of the American Chemical Society*, 143(44), 18643–18651.

Fan, X., Gao, Y., Yang, F., Low, J. L., Wang, L., Paulus, B.,. . . Haag, R. (2023). A copper single-atom cascade bionanocatalyst for treating multidrug-resistant bacterial diabetic ulcer. *Advanced Functional Materials*, 33(33), 2301986.

Fan, Y., Gan, X., Zhao, H., Zeng, Z., You, W., & Quan, X. (2022). Multiple application of SAzyme based on carbon nitride nanorod-supported Pt single-atom for H_2O_2 detection, antibiotic detection and antibacterial therapy. *Chemical Engineering Journal*, 427, 131572.

Feng, J., Kong, F., Yue, W. S., Yu, H., He, Z. L., Zhai, Y. N., & Dong, Y. B. (2023). Covalent organic framework-based nanozyme for cascade-amplified synergistic cancer therapy. *Science China Materials*, 66(10), 4079–4089.

Feng, H. X., Zhou, Z., Jiang, J., Hui, Y. F., Li, B. X., Li, S.,. . . Yan, L. P. (2025). A porphyrin-based metal–organic framework nanozyme with superior peroxidase-like activity for combating antibacterial infections and promoting wound healing. *Inorganic Chemistry*, 64(7), 3541–3552.

Feng, Y., Qin, J., Zhou, Y., Yue, Q., & Wei, J. (2022). Spherical mesoporous Fe-NC single-atom nanozyme for photothermal and catalytic synergistic antibacterial therapy. *Journal of Colloid and Interface Science*, 606, 826–836.

Gao, Z., Song, Z., Guo, R., Zhang, M., Wu, J., Pan, M.,. . . Zheng, J. (2024). Mn single-atom nanozyme functionalized 3D-printed bioceramic scaffolds for enhanced antibacterial activity and bone regeneration. *Advanced Healthcare Materials*, 2303182.

Hou, B., Li, B., Deng, W., Li, B., Ren, B., Hu, C.,. . . Xie, D. (2024). DHTPY-Cu@ ZOL-enhanced photodynamic therapy: A strategic platform for advanced treatment of drug-resistant bacterial wound infections. *International Journal of Nanomedicine*, 6319–6336.

Hou, X., Wang, H., Yao, X., Zhou, Q., & Niu, X. (2025). Pt-induced sublattice distortion facilitates enzyme cascade reactions for eradicating intracellularly methicillin-resistant Staphylococcus aureus and enhancing diabetic wound healing. *ACS Nano*, 19(18), 17709–17727.

Jin, C., Fan, S., Zhuang, Z., & Zhou, Y. (2023). Single-atom nanozymes: From bench to bedside. *Nano Research*, 16(2), 1992–2002.

Lan, X., Chen, M., He, X., Gao, S., & Zhao, X. (2024). Single atom nanozymes for bacterial infection therapy. *Biomaterials Science*, 12(1).

Li, Y., Ma, Q., Gong, H., Gu, J., Liu, T., & Wang, X. (2024). Superior oxidase-mimetic activity of FeCo-NC dual-atom nanozyme for smartphone-based visually colorimetric assay of organophosphorus pesticides. *Microchimica Acta*, 191(7).

Li, Z., Lu, X., Zhao, R., Ji, S., Zhang, M., Horton, J. H.,. . . Zhu, J. (2023). A heterogeneous single atom cobalt catalyst for highly efficient acceptorless dehydrogenative coupling reactions. *Small*, 19(18), 2207941.

Liang, X., Wang, D., Zhao, Z., Li, T., Gao, Y., & Hu, C. (2022). Coordination number dependent catalytic activity of single-atom cobalt catalysts for Fenton-like reaction. *Advanced Functional Materials*, 32(38), 2203001.

Liu, H., Liu, X., Wang, H., Ren, J., & Qu, X. (2023a). A homing missile-like nanotherapeutic with single-atom catalytic sites for in situ elimination of intracellular bacterial pathogens. *Small*, 19(37), 2207510.

Liu, Q., Liu, X., He, X., Wang, D., Zheng, C., Jin, L., & Shen, J. (2024). Iron-single-atom nanozyme with NIR enhanced catalytic activities for facilitating MRSA-infected wound therapy. *Advanced Science*, 11(15), 2308684.

Liu, X., Liu, Q., He, X., Yang, G., Chen, X., Meng, J.,. . . Zhang, X. (2023b). NIR-II-enhanced single-atom-nanozyme for sustainable accelerating bacteria-infected wound healing. *Applied Surface Science*, 612, 155866.

Long, Y., Li, L., Xu, T., Wu, X., Gao, Y., Huang, J.,. . . Zhao, C. (2021). Hedgehog artificial macrophage with atomic-catalytic centers to combat Drug-resistant bacteria. *Nature Communications*, 12(1), 6143.

Miao, J., Jiang, Y., Wang, X., Li, X., Zhu, Y., Shao, Z., & Long, M. (2024). Correlating active sites and oxidative species in single-atom catalyzed Fenton-like reactions. *Chemical Science*, 15(30), 11699–11718.

Peng, C., Pang, R., Li, J., & Wang, E. (2024). Current advances on the single-atom nanozyme and its bioapplications. *Advanced Materials*, 36(10), 2211724.

Qian, X., Shi, R., Chen, J., Wang, Y., Han, X., Sun, Y.,. . . Pan, Y. (2022). The single-atom iron nanozyme mimicking peroxidase remodels energy metabolism and tumor immune landscape for synergistic chemodynamic therapy and photothermal therapy of triple-negative breast cancer. *Frontiers in Bioengineering and Biotechnology*, 10, 1026761.

Qiang, J., He, J., Wang, B., Zhou, C., Liu, H., & Su, X. (2025). A novel nitrogen-doped carbon-based molybdenum single-atom nanozyme for the highly sensitive dual-mode detection of neurotransmitter epinephrine. *Microchemical Journal*, 212, 113565.

Qu, X., Yan, Y., Zhang, Z., Tian, B., Yin, S., Cheng, X.,. . . Sun, S. (2024). Regulation strategies for Fe–N–C and Co–N–C catalysts for the oxygen reduction reaction. *Chemistry–A European Journal*, e202304003.

Ren, X., Wang, X., Yang, J., Zhang, X., Du, B., Bai, P.,. . . Zhang, R. (2024). Multi-enzyme-based superabsorbent hydrogel for self-enhanced NIR-II photothermal-catalytic antibacterial therapy. *Advanced Healthcare Materials*, 13(12), 2303537.

Su, L., Qin, S., Xie, Z., Wang, L., Khan, K., Tareen, A. K.,. . . Zhang, H. (2022a). Multi-enzyme activity nanozymes for biosensing and disease treatment. *Coordination Chemistry Reviews*, 473, 214784.

Su, Y., Wu, F., Song, Q., Wu, M., Mohammadniaei, M., Zhang, T.,. . . Shen, J. (2022b). Dual enzyme-mimic nanozyme based on single-atom construction strategy for photothermal-augmented nanocatalytic therapy in the second near-infrared biowindow. *Biomaterials*, 281, 121325.

Sun, B., Wang, X., Ye, Z., Zhang, J., Chen, X., Zhou, N.,. . . Shen, J. (2023). Designing single-atom active sites on sp^2-carbon linked covalent organic frameworks to induce bacterial ferroptosis-like for robust anti-infection therapy. *Advanced Science*, 10(13), 2207507.

Wang, F., Wang, Y., Wang, H., Zhao, G., Li, J., & Wang, Y. (2023). Advances in the application of single-atom nanozymes for heavy metal ion detection, tumor therapy and antimicrobial therapy. *Microchemical Journal*, 191, 108817.

Wang, K., Wang, X., & Liang, X. (2021). Synthesis of high metal loading single atom catalysts and exploration of the active center structure. *ChemCatChem*, 13(1), 28–58.

Wang, W., Luo, Q., Li, J., Li, L., Li, Y., Huo, X.,. . . Wang, N. (2022). Photothermal-amplified single atom nanozyme for biofouling control in seawater. *Advanced Functional Materials*, 32(36), 2205461.

Wu, T., Sun, J., Lei, J., Fan, Q., Tang, X., Zhu, G.,. . . Shi, B. (2021). An efficient treatment of biofilm-induced periodontitis using Pt nanocluster catalysis. *Nanoscale*, 13(42), 17912–17919.

Xi, J., Wei, G., Wu, Q., Xu, Z., Liu, Y., Han, J.,. . . Gao, L. (2019). Light-enhanced sponge-like carbon nanozyme used for synergetic antibacterial therapy. *Biomaterials Science*, 7(10), 4131–4141.

Xu, Q., Hua, Y., Zhang, Y., Lv, M., Wang, H., Pi, Y.,. . . Yong, Y. (2021). A biofilm microenvironment-activated single-atom iron nanozyme with NIR-controllable nanocatalytic activities for synergetic bacteria-infected wound therapy. *Advanced Healthcare Materials*, 10(22), 2101374.

Xu, X., Zhang, J., Wang, X., Fang, H., Shi, S., Wu, F.,. . . Sun, B. (2024). Multifunctional Pd single-atom nanozyme for enhanced cascade chemodynamic therapy of chronic wounds. *ACS Applied Nano Materials*, 7(3), 3445–3457.

Yan, D., Huang, Y., Zhang, J., Wu, Q., Song, G., Ji, J.,. . . Tang, B. Z. (2023). Adding flying wings: Butterfly-shaped NIR-II AIEgens with multiple molecular rotors for photothermal combating of bacterial biofilms. *Journal of the American Chemical Society*, 145(47), 25705–25715.

Yu, Y., Tan, L., Li, Z., Liu, X., Zheng, Y., Feng, X.,. . . Wu, S. (2021). Single-atom catalysis for efficient sonodynamic therapy of methicillin-resistant *Staphylococcus aureus*-infected osteomyelitis. *ACS Nano*, 15(6), 10628–10639.

Zhang, S. L., Li, Y., Zhang, J., Wang, W., Tham, N. N., Li, B.,. . . Liu, Z. (2024). Anchoring metal–nitrogen sites on porous carbon polyhedra with highly accessible multi-channels for efficient oxygen reduction. *ACS Applied Materials & Interfaces*, 16(34), 44728–44736.

Zhang, Y., Hu, J., Zuo, W., He, P., Xue, Q., Feng, X.,. . . Maze, M. (2023). Longitudinal profiling of plasma cytokines and its association with postoperative delirium in elderly patients undergoing major lower limb surgery: A prospective observational study. *Anesthesia & Analgesia*, 136(1), 34–42.

Zhu, J., Li, Q., Li, X., Wu, X., Yuan, T., & Yang, Y. (2022). Simulated enzyme activity and efficient antibacterial activity of copper-doped single-atom nanozymes. *Langmuir*, 38(22), 6860–6870.

7 Smart Biosensors Based on Single-Atom Nanozymes for Biomedical Innovations

Manaswini Narapusetty, Akhila Karumuri, Weiqing Zhang, and Firdoz Shaik

7.1 INTRODUCTION

7.1.1 Background on Biosensors

A biological response can be transformed into a measurable and processable signal by analytical tools called biosensors (Naresh & Lee, 2021). These devices consist of a transducer, a signal processor, and a bioreceptor (such as enzymes, antibodies, or nucleic acids) (Liu, 2024). Due to their capacity to deliver quick, accurate, and economical analysis, biosensors have developed into essential instruments in the fields of clinical diagnostics, environmental monitoring, food safety, and biological research over the years (Haleem et al., 2021). The secret to their success is their capacity to identify even the smallest analyte concentrations in intricate biological matrices, which guarantees early disease detection and effective treatment intervention monitoring (Ahmad et al., 2023)

7.1.2 Importance of Biomarker Detection

The presence or advancement of a disease is frequently linked to biomarkers, which are quantifiable indicators of a biological condition or state (Ahmad et al., 2023). Nucleic acids, proteins, metabolites, or certain cells with diseases like cancer, heart disease, and infectious diseases are a few examples. For efficient illness management, early and precise biomarker detection is essential because it enables prompt intervention, therapy efficacy monitoring, and disease prognosis assessment (Jungblut et al., 1999). The need for highly precise, sensitive biomarker detection systems that can deliver results in real time has increased due to the increased focus on customized therapy.

DOI: 10.1201/9781003563723-7

7.1.3 Limitations of Conventional Biosensors

Conventional biosensors, although widely used, have several drawbacks: Traditional biorecognition elements such as enzymes and antibodies are often delicate and susceptible to denaturation under extreme pH or temperature conditions (Kulkarni et al., 2022) and can exhibit batch-to-batch variability; their high cost, limited stability, and relatively complex immobilization procedures further limit their practical applications; and the sensor's operational lifetime and robustness can be limited due to its reliance on natural enzymes, particularly in resource-constrained or point-of-care settings (Chakraborty, 2024).

7.1.4 Introduction to Nanozymes and Emergence of Single-Atom Nanozymes (SAzymes)

For biosensing applications, nanozymes – nanomaterials with catalytic capabilities similar to those of enzyme – have shown great promise as substitutes for natural enzymes (Wang et al., 2018). Since they were discovered in the early 2000s, nanozymes have demonstrated remarkable stability, easily adjustable surface modification, low production costs, and customizable catalytic activity. They are appealing candidates for incorporation into biosensor platforms because of their capacity to imitate a variety of enzyme activities, including oxidase, peroxidase, and catalase (Kucherenko et al., 2019). In addition to overcoming the inherent limitations of natural enzymes, nanozymes also pave the way for the development of reliable, sensitive, and compact diagnostic instruments. Their versatility and adaptability, which allow for the development of next-generation biosensors that can handle contemporary diagnostic difficulties, further emphasize their significance.

Single-atom nanozymes have recently attracted a lot of interest as the next generation of nanozymes because of their high surface-to-volume ratio, atomically distributed active sites, and catalytic specificity that is similar to that of enzymes. By providing improved control over active centers, customizable electronic architectures, and increased turnover frequency, these nanozymes combine the benefits of homogenous and heterogenous catalysts. SAzyme creation and integration in the biosensor platform for ultra-sensitive biomarker detection are the main topics of this chapter. The evolutionary path of the nanozymes and their advancements have been clearly depicted in Figure 7.1.

This figure presents a conceptual overview of the progression from natural enzymes to artificial enzymes and the development of nanozymes. It highlights key scientific discoveries, the introduction of various enzyme mimics, and the transition toward advanced nanozyme applications. The diagram emphasizes how nanomaterials have been engineered to replicate enzymatic functions, leading to innovations in biosensing, therapeutics, and catalysis (Das et al., 2021, https://doi.org/10.1007/s40820-021-00717-0).

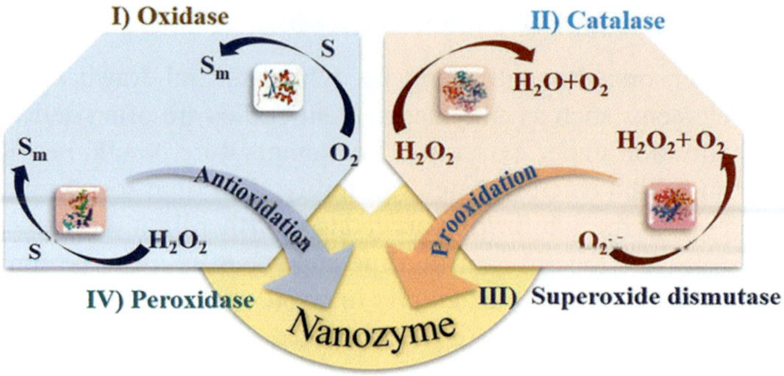

FIGURE 7.1 Evolution of enzyme mimics and advancements in nanozyme technology.

7.2 NANOZYMES: FUNDAMENTALS AND CLASSIFICATION

7.2.1 Definition and Historical Perspective

Catalytic activity akin to that of enzymes is inherent in nanozymes. The synthetic or designed inorganic nanostructures known as nanozymes are able to catalyze biochemical processes, in contrast to the biological macromolecules known as classical enzymes (Huang et al., 2019). In the early 2000s, when scientists found that certain nanomaterials, such as iron oxide nanoparticles, might imitate peroxidase activity, the name "nanozyme" was first used (Singh, S., 2019). This groundbreaking discovery sparked a new era in nano-biotechnology by encouraging a great deal of study into the creation of nanomaterials with specific catalytic properties.

Because of their exceptional catalytic efficiency and specificity, enzymes have long been vital biosensing instruments (Kucherenko et al., 2019). However, drawbacks including instability in challenging environments, expensive manufacturing, and short shelf life led scientists to look into reliable substitutes. By providing materials that not only mimic enzyme activity but also provide benefits like chemical stability, reusability, and simplicity of mass manufacturing, the discovery of nanozymes closed this gap (Abdel-Mageed, 2025).

7.2.2 Types of Nanozymes (Oxidase, Peroxidase, Catalase, etc.)

By mimicking a certain sort of enzyme activity, nanozymes may be categorized. The classes that are studied the most include:

Peroxidase-mimicking nanozymes: these catalyze the oxidation of substrates (such as TMB and ABTS) when hydrogen peroxide is present. Classic examples include cerium oxide and iron oxide nanoparticles (Mirra, 2025). The foundation of many biosensing technologies is their capacity to provide colorimetric signals. Without requiring H_2O_2 , oxidase-mimicking nanozymes use molecular oxygen to catalyze the oxidation of substrates. Typical examples are noble metal nanoparticles such as platinum and gold, and manganese oxide (Singh, S., 2019). Because their catalytic routes are independent of H_2O_2 , they can be used in safer biosensor designs. The nanozymes involved have been discussed in detail in Figure 7.2.

- Oxidase-Mimicking Nanozymes: These enzymes use molecular oxygen (O_2) to catalyze substrate oxidation without the need for H_2O_2. Manganese oxide and noble metal nanoparticles, such as gold and platinum, are frequent examples. They are appropriate for safer biosensor designs due to their catalytic pathways that are independent of H_2O_2 (Chong & Ge, 2022).
- Catalase-Mimicking Nanozymes: These nanozymes replicate the action of natural catalase enzymes by breaking down hydrogen peroxide into water and oxygen. They are frequently employed to modify the microenvironment in biosensors or to lessen oxidative stress in biological systems (Mishra et al., 2022).
- Superoxide Dismutase (SOD)-Like Nanozymes: By facilitating the conversion of superoxide radicals into oxygen and hydrogen peroxide, these substances resemble SOD enzymes. In this area, cerium-based nanozymes have demonstrated great potential (Singh, N. et al., 2023).
- Multifunctional Nanozymfbiosensorses: Certain nanozymes, like combination peroxidase and catalase activity, display multiple enzymatic activities based on the temperature or pH of the surrounding environment. Flexibility in sensor use and design is provided by this multifunctionality.

7.2.3 Introduction to Single-Atom Nanozymes (SAzymes)

The class of nanozymes known as single-atom nanozymes involves the dispersion of individual metal atoms, such as Fe, Co, and Pt, on substrates such as nitrogen-doped carbon. By simulating the active centers of natural metalloenzymes, this atomic dispersion optimizes the exposure of catalytic sites. In biosensing applications where ultrasensitive and low-background signal detection is necessary, SAzymes show great promise because of their remarkable activity, selectivity, and stability (Jiao et al., 2021; Xiao et al., 2023).

7.2.4 Comparison with Natural Enzymes

While natural enzymes are highly specific and efficient, they suffer from several drawbacks. As mentioned in Table 7.1, Nanozymes provide a synthetic alternative that addresses many of these limitations:

Although nanozymes currently cannot fully match the substrate specificity of natural enzymes, advances in surface engineering and hybrid material design are rapidly narrowing this gap.

7.2.5 Advantages and Challenges of SAzymes

Advantages:

- **Enhanced Stability**: Single-atom nanozymes are perfect for long-term usage and storage since they are resistant to denaturation and deterioration.
- **Cost-Effective Synthesis:** Scalable techniques may be used to create a large number of single-atom nanozymes from cheap precursors.

TABLE 7.1
Comparative Analysis of Natural Enzymes, Nanozymes, and Single-Atom Nanozymes (SAzymes)

Property	Natural Enzymes	Nanozymes	SAzymes (Single-Atom Nanozymes)
Stability	Sensitive to temperature, pH, and chemicals	Stable under harsh conditions	Extremely stable due to atomic dispersion
Cost	Expensive to produce and purify	Economical and scalable	Cost-effective with high atom utilization
Shelf life	Short, requires refrigeration	Long-term storage possible	Excellent stability with extended shelf life
Specificity	Highly specific	Moderate, tunable	Enhanced specificity due to uniform active sites
Reusability	Limited	Can be reused in many cases	High reusability with sustained activity
Biocompatibility	Generally biocompatible	Needs careful surface engineering	Good biocompatibility with proper functionalization

- **Tunable Activity:** Modulating their size, shape, composition, or surface chemistry influences the catalytic activity.
- **Multifunctionality:** Multiple types of reactions can be catalyzed by a single nanozyme, increasing versatility.
- **Integration-Friendly:** Single-atom nanozymes can be easily incorporated into various platforms such as paper strips, microfluidic devices, and wearable sensors (Wu, W. et al., 2020).

Challenges:

- **Lower Specificity:** Nanozymes often exhibit lower catalytic selectivity and a lower spectrum of substrates than natural enzymes.
- **Biocompatibility:** If not appropriately surface modified, certain metal-based nanozymes may be hazardous to biological systems.
- **Standardization:** Comparisons between research are hampered by the absence of common procedures for assessing nanozyme activity.
- **Understanding Mechanisms:** The logical design of many nanozymes is limited by the incomplete understanding of their catalytic processes.

7.3 SYNTHESIS AND CHARACTERIZATION OF NANOZYMES

Designing high-performance nanozymes begins with choosing a synthesis route that provides precise control over composition, size, shape, and surface chemistry – parameters that ultimately govern catalytic behavior in biosensing applications (Shen et al., 2020).

7.3.1 Synthetic Strategies

- **Chemical Routes**
    - Co-precipitation and sol-gel synthesis methods: extensively utilized for metal oxides, such as CeO_2 and FeO_4. Particle size and crystal phase are controlled by adjusting pH, temperature, and precursor ratios, resulting in gram-scale yields suitable for disposable biosensors.
    - Thermal Decomposition and Pyrolysis: Uniform noble metal or alloy nanozymes $\left(\text{Au, Pt, Pt-Ni}\right)$ are produced by the breakdown of organometallic precursors at high temperatures in inert or reducing atmospheres. Narrow size distributions are produced by precise heat control, which is necessary for repeatable catalytic kinetics.
    - Hydrothermal and Solvothermal Synthesis: Unusual morphologies (nanoflowers, hollow spheres) with a large number of active sites are made possible by autoclave-based processes, which enable high-pressure crystal formation. Defect density and oxidation states can be altered by customizing mineralizers and solvents (such as ethylene glycol and NaOH).
- **Green (Biogenic) Synthesis**
  Harsh chemicals are eliminated by using biomolecules or plant extracts as reducing and capping agents
    - Polysaccharide- or Protein-Mediated Reduction – For instance, metal-doped carbon dots made from starch produce luminous peroxidase mimics.
    - Microbial and Plant Extract-Assisted Routes – These routes facilitate downstream functionalization by reducing metal salts while forming biocompatible coatings through the use of live cells or phytochemicals (polyphenols).
    - In addition to improving environmental sustainability, green pathways frequently provide native bioligands that increase the colloidal stability of biological media.
- **Template-Directed and Confined Synthesis**
    - Hard templates such as mesoporous silica and anodic alumina produce size-confined nanozymes with ordered pores that promote substrate diffusion.
    - Anisotropic development is guided by soft templates and micelles, resulting in nanorods or nanosheets with facet-dependent catalytic performances.
    - The metal-organic framework-derived nanozymes, which are now the gold standard for sensitivity in paper-based biosensors, are created by pyrolyzing MOFs to create hollow, heteroatom-doped carbon shells that encase single-atom catalytic sites (Altaf et al., 2024).
    - SAzyme synthesis has found that carbon supports produced from metal-organic frameworks (MOFs) are the best templates. Through the pyrolysis of MOFs, metal can disperse atomically inside nitrogen-doped carbon matrices, creating M-N-C (such as Fe-N-C) single-atom sites that are stable and extremely catalytically active.

- **Microfluidic and Continuous-Flow Synthesis**

The exact residence time and mixing control made possible by microreactors provide batch-to-batch homogeneity, which is essential for commercial biosensor cartridge regulatory certification.

7.3.2 Structural and Functional Modifications

- Heteroatom Doping (N, S, P) lowers activation barriers for redox processes by modifying the electronic structure.
- By integrating synergistic activities like peroxidase + catalase, core-shell and alloy architectures (such as Au@Pt and Fe_3O_4@CeO_2) expand the operating pH windows.
- Surface Ligand Engineering – linkers with thiol, carboxyl, or amine groups give antibodies and aptamers places to attach while adjusting hydrophilicity.
- Support immobilization on hydrogels, graphene, or carbon nanotubes promotes electron transmission in electrochemical devices, improves surface area, and inhibits aggregation.

TABLE 7.2
Characterization Techniques and Their Relevance in Nanozyme-Based Biosensing Applications

Technique	Information Gained	Relevance to Biosensing
Transmission electron microscopy (TEM/HRTEM)	Particle size, lattice fringes, defect density	Correlates morphology with catalytic rate constants
Scanning electron microscopy (SEM)	Surface topography of assembled electrodes or paper strips	Quality control of sensor coatings
X-ray diffraction (XRD)	Crystal phase, grain size	Identifies active phases (e.g., spinel vs. wüstite FeOx)
UV-Vis and Raman spectroscopy	Valence-state transitions, plasmon bands	Monitors reaction intermediates during catalysis
Fourier-transform infrared spectroscopy (FTIR)	Surface functional groups, ligand attachment	Confirms biomolecule immobilization chemistry
X-ray Photoelectron spectroscopy (XPS)	Elemental composition, oxidation states	Quantifies heteroatom doping and active centers
Dynamic light scattering (DLS) and zeta potential	Hydrodynamic size, surface charge	Predicts colloidal stability in biological fluids
BET surface area analysis	Porosity, specific surface	Higher area often translates to enhanced sensitivity
Electrochemical Techniques (CV, EIS)	Electron-transfer kinetics, interfacial resistance	Directly ties nanozyme properties to sensor performance

- The coordination environment of SAzymes, such as Fe-N_4 and Co-N_4, can be engineered to improve their performance. These distinct active centers allow for precise tweaking of electronic structure and catalytic performance since they closely match genuine metalloenzymes (Song et al., 2022).

7.3.3 Characterization Techniques for SAzymes

Robust analytical verification, as detailed in Table 7.2, ensures the nanozyme's catalytic function aligns with biosensor design goals:

Collectively, these methods establish a feedback loop between synthesis parameters and catalytic outcomes, guiding rational optimization for high-sensitivity biomarker detection.

7.4 BIOSENSING MECHANISMS ENABLED BY SAZYMES

The basic idea behind nanozyme-based biosensors is that by using the catalytic activity of nanozymes, biochemical interactions may be transformed into quantifiable signals. The durability, tunability, and multifunctionality of nanozymes, in contrast to conventional enzyme-based systems, have greatly increased the sensitivity and range of biosensing platforms.

7.4.1 Signal Transduction Methods

The transduction mechanism used in a biosensor greatly influences the kind of signal that is produced. As adaptable catalysts, nanozymes facilitate a range of signal transduction techniques, such as:

- **Colorimetric Biosensors**
  Colorimetric detection is among the most popular and accessible techniques. When H_2O_2 is present or absent, nanozymes catalyze the oxidation of chromogenic substrates like 3, 3', 5, 5'-tetramethylbenzidine (TMB), o-phenylenediamine (OPD), or ABTS. This results in an apparent color shift that may be seen with the naked eye or with the use of a spectrophotometer (Aldewachi et al., 2018).
- Fe_3O_4 nanoparticles with peroxidase-like activity can accelerate the oxidation of TMB, producing a blue product. Analyte concentration and color intensity correspond, allowing for quantitative identification. These devices, especially when combined with paper-based sensors, are perfect for low-cost diagnostics. Biosensors based on electrochemical nanozymes are used in electrochemical biosensors to catalyze redox processes, producing electrical signals that may be detected as impedance, voltage, or current. Nanozymes increase signal-to-noise ratios, decrease overpotentials, and speed up electron transfer rates (Bilalis et al., 2022). Nanozymes made of cerium oxide, gold, and platinum are frequently employed in this configuration. Electrochemical detection in conjunction with nanozyme catalysis enables great sensitivity, compactness, and compatibility with portable readers.

- **Optical Biosensors**
  Surface plasmon resonance (SPR), chemiluminescence, or fluorescence signals are all impacted by nanozymes included in optical biosensors. For example, depending on the presence of target analytes, certain nanozymes either quench or increase fluorescence, while others catalyze luminol-based chemiluminescence to generate signals. Because spatial and temporal resolution are crucial for imaging biomarkers in biological samples, this modality is very helpful (Yang et al., 2024).
- **Photoelectrochemical (PEC) Biosensors**
  PEC sensors use nanozyme catalysis in conjunction with photoactive nanomaterials. Light causes the creation of electron-hole pairs, and the nanozyme catalyzes processes at the photoelectrode to improve the photoreaction. Excellent sensitivity is provided by these devices, which are appropriate for complicated materials such as serum or blood.

7.4.2 Role of SAzymes in Signal Amplification

The ability of nanozymes to amp up signals is one of the main benefits of utilizing them in biosensing; this ability is essential for identifying low-abundance biomarkers. In comparison to no-catalytic transducers, nanozymes may catalyze many substrate rotations per target-binding event, greatly increasing the signal that is produced.

Nanozymes attached to secondary antibodies, for instance, provide enhanced colorimetric or electrochemical signals in sandwich-type immunosensors when they interact with the target biomarker. To further amplify weak signals, one can also take advantage of the catalytic cascade that occurs between two or more enzymes or cofactors (Niu et al., 2020).

When a target is recognized, some sophisticated platforms use nanozyme-loaded nanocarriers, which release hundreds of catalytic units, increasing the reaction output and significantly reducing the detection limit.

Because of their large turnover rates and atomic-level homogeneity, SAzymes are especially effective in signal amplification techniques. Biosensors are essential for the detection of early-stage disease biomarkers because of their capacity to produce potent catalytic signals with little loading, enabling femtomolar or even attomolar sensitivity.

7.4.3 Catalytic Mechanisms in Biosensing (Peroxidase-Like, Oxidase-Like, etc.)

To maximize the efficacy of biosensors, it is essential to comprehend the catalytic mechanism of nanozymes (Yang et al., 2024). Among the important mechanisms are:

- **Peroxidase-Like Mechanism**
  As part of the peroxidase-like action, hydrogen peroxide breaks down into reactive oxygen species (ROS), notably hydroxyl radicals, which oxidize the chromogenic substrates. The activity of natural horseradish (HRP)

is mimicked by this. Fenton-like processes are frequently used by carbon-based materials and transition metal oxides.

- **Oxidase-Like Mechanism**
  To oxidize substrates, oxidase-mimicking nanozymes directly use dissolved oxygen, frequently producing H_2O_2 or other ROS in the process. This enhances biocompatibility and safety for biosensors that want to avoid external H_2O_2.
- **Catalase-Like Mechanism**
  Catalase-like nanozymes break down H_2O_2 into oxygen and water. In dual-enzyme systems, this activity can improve O_2-dependent sensing processes or control oxidative balance without directly generating a signal.
- **Electron Transfer Facilitation**
  Nanozymes lower the activation energy of redox reactions on electrochemical platforms by facilitating electron transport between the electrode surface and the bioreceptor. This improves responsiveness and decreases detection thresholds, particularly at low analyte concentrations.

7.5 FABRICATION OF SAZYME-BASED BIOSENSORS

The effectiveness of nanozymes' integration into sensor systems and their catalytic activity are both critical to their successful use in biosensing. In order to guarantee signal production, selectivity, and repeatability, fabrication entails assembling nanozymes with appropriate biorecognition components and transducers. Nanozymes may be immobilized and functionalized using a variety of engineering techniques, which enables the development of tiny and extremely sensitive biosensing devices.

7.5.1 Integration into Sensor Platforms

A variety of sensor designs, such as wearable platforms, screen-printed electrodes, paper-based devices, and microfluidic systems, can incorporate nanozymes. The target analyte, the kind of sample, and the detection technique (colorimetric, electrochemical, etc.) all influence the integration approach (Xia et al., 2024).

- **Paper-Based Sensors:** Nanozymes are infused into cellulose or nitrocellulose paper to create these inexpensive, disposable sensors. These are perfect for point-of-care diagnostics since the colorimetric reaction upon substrate oxidation may be readily detected.
- **Electrochemical Sensors:** Glassy carbon, gold, or carbon cloth are examples of conductive substrates on which nanozymes are commonly placed. Catalytic signal amplification and effective electron transfer are made possible by their high conductivity and surface area.
- **Microfluidic Devices:** These technologies allow for accurate fluid manipulation and regulated reagent mixing. Multiplexed analysis with little sample input is made possible by the immobilization of nanozymes in detection chambers, which catalyze reactions in small quantities.

- **Wearable and Flexible Sensors:** Nanozymes are being incorporated into flexible electronics, textiles, and tattoos to detect sweat or saliva biomarkers in response to the growing demand for real-time, on-body health monitoring.
- SAzymes can be uniformly adsorbed onto paper, flexible patches, or electrode surfaces because of their minuscule size and exceptional stability. This allows for efficient electron transmission and great signal repeatability. They are perfect for incorporating into wearable and portable biosensors due to their interoperability with smaller platforms (Zhang et al., 2025).

7.5.2 Surface Functionalization and Immobilization

In addition to preserving catalytic activity and for targeted target identification, surface functionalization guarantees that nanozymes are firmly attached to sensor substrates.

Typical Immobilization Techniques:

- **Physical Adsorption:** This type of binding is quick and easy, but it might eventually lead to instability or leaching.
- **Covalent Bonding:** Strong covalent bonds can be formed between functional groups $(-NH_2, -COOH, -SH)$ on nanozymes or substrates by coupling agents (e.g., EDC/NHS chemistry). This results in strong, sustained immobilization. This provides robust, long-term immobilization.
- **Affinity-Based Methods:** Systems of biotin and streptavidin are frequently employed to attach nanozymes conjugated to bioreceptors with great specificity.
- **Encapsulation/Entrapment:** Nanozymes can be encapsulated or entrapped in hydrogels, sol-gels, or polymer matrices to maintain their activity and provide regulated substrate and analyte diffusion.

Functionalization Strategies:

- **Polymer Coatings:** Conducting polymers such as polypyrrole or polyaniline enhance conductivity and biocompatibility in polymer coatings.
- **Biomolecule Conjugation:** For specific target binding, biomolecules such as enzymes, aptamers, or antibodies are coupled to the surface of the nanozyme.
- **Nanocomposite Formation:** Metal-organic frameworks (MOFs), graphene oxide, or carbon nanotubes can be combined with nanozymes to increase surface area and signal amplification.

7.5.3 Device Assembly and Miniaturization

For wearable diagnostics, field applications, and point-of-care testing, miniaturization is essential. Modern manufacturing processes allow for the creation of biosensors that are small, integrated, and easy to use.

Key Approaches:

- **Inkjet Printing and Screen Printing**: Nanozyme inks may be patterned or deposited onto substrates, including paper, plastic, or textiles, via inkjet printing and screen printing (Mostofian & McCutcheon, 2017; Lustig et al., 1998).
- **Laser Engraving and 3D Printing:** High precision microelectrode or microchannel fabrication is made possible by 3D printing, opening the door to intricate multiplexed sensing systems (Zhao et al., 2025).
- **Microfluidic Chip Fabrication:** The fabrication of microfluidic chips involves the use of photolithography and soft lithography to create microchannels in which nanozymes are implanted to provide automated fluid management and response control (Li et al., 2014).
- **Layer-by-Layer Assembly:** Featuring high loading capacity and structural integrity, thin films are created by building up alternating layers of functional polymers and nanozymes (Pavesi & Pavesi, 2016).
- **Smartphone Integration:** To provide portable and easily accessible data analysis, a large number of nanozyme-based biosensors are currently made to be compatible with smartphone cameras or readers (Wu et al., 2024; Sahare et al., 2024).

7.6 BIOMARKER DETECTION USING SAZYME-BASED BIOSENSORS

Biomarkers are important markers of physiological or pathological conditions, and the prompt and precise identification of these markers is essential for illness monitoring, diagnosis, and treatment management. The ability of nanozyme-based biosensors to identify a broad range of biomarkers in different disease domains has shown remarkable promise. Their durability, catalytic activity, and compatibility with various signal transduction systems make them perfect for quick and sensitive biosensing.

7.6.1 Cancer Biomarkers

One of the main causes of death worldwide is still cancer, and increasing survival rates require the early identification of cancer biomarkers. Biosensors based on nanozymes have been used to identify important indicators linked to cancer, including:

- **Alpha-fetoprotein (AFP):** It is a liver cancer biomarker. Sub-nanogram detection levels are now possible with colorimetric sensors that use Fe3O4 nanozymes conjugated with anti-AFP antibodies.
- **Carcinoembryonic antigen (CEA):** A crucial indicator for lung, breast, and colorectal malignancies. Au@Pt nanozymes have been used to create nanozyme-enhanced electrochemical immunosensors that can detect human serum with extreme sensitivity.

- **Prostate-specific antigen (PSA):** Both colorimetric and fluorescence-based PSA detection at picomolar levels is now possible thanks to peroxidase-mimicking nanozymes.
- **MicroRNA (miRNA):** Nanozyme-based hybrid sensors have been used to target miRNA-21 and other oncogenic miRNAs, combining catalytic amplification with DNA strand displacement for accurate quantification.
- For example, Fe-N-C SAzymes have been employed in electrochemical immunosensors to detect carcinoembryonic antigen (CEA) with high specificity and sub-picomolar LODs. Their high activity enables a robust signal even at trace analyte levels (Huang et al., 2024).

7.6.2 Infectious Disease Biomarkers

It is essential to diagnose infectious diseases quickly to manage and treat outbreaks. One benefit of using nanozyme-based biosensors in the field is their deployability:

- **HIV:** By using nanozymes (such as Pt-loaded MOFs) in paper-based lateral flow experiments, HIV antibodies or antigens can now be visually and quantitatively detected.
- **Tuberculosis:** Using colorimetric nanozyme-DNA hybrid biosensors to detect mycobacterium tuberculosis DNA has made it possible to diagnose the disease quickly and without the need for a label.
- **COVID-19 (SARS-CoV-2):** During the pandemic, nanozyme-enhanced biosensors were created to detect anti-SARS-CoV-2 antibodies, viral RNA, or spike proteins. For instance, lateral flow strips with peroxidase-mimicking nanozymes inserted into them increased sensitivity while keeping costs down.
- **Malaria and Dengue:** Even in isolated and resource-constrained areas, colorimetric nanozyme platforms have been utilized to identify parasite or viral antigens in blood.
- By enhancing lateral flow assays for COVID-19 antibody detection, Pt single-atom nanozymes have proven to be more stable and sensitive than traditional nanoparticle methods.

7.6.3 Metabolic and Cardiac Biomarkers

Certain biochemical markers must be accurately and continuously monitored in order to treat metabolic and cardiovascular diseases:

- **Glucose:** Glucose oxidase-mimicking nanozymes transformed glucose detection, one of the most researched targets. Because they can function in environments devoid of enzymes, they improve stability and do not require refrigeration.
- **Cholesterol:** High-sensitivity cholesterol detection has been achieved by the development of nanozyme-based devices that either integrate with peroxidase nanozymes or mimic cholesterol oxidase.

- **Lactate and Uric Acid:** Two metabolites that are essential in diseases like gout or metabolic acidosis can be detected simultaneously thanks to hybrid sensors that use nanozymes with oxidase or peroxidase activity.
- **Cardiac Troponin I (cTnI):** An important indicator of myocardial infarction. Clinical samples have shown quick and accurate measurement using nanozyme-functionalized immunosensors.

7.6.4 Environmental and Toxicological Biomarkers

In addition to clinical diagnoses, environmental exposure to toxins and pollutants is being tracked more frequently using nanozyme-based biosensors:

- **Heavy Metals (e.g., Hg^{2+}, Pb^{2+}):** The presence of certain metal ions can either increase or decrease catalytic activity, which can modify nanozyme activity and act as indirect markers of contamination.
- **Pesticides:** Water and agricultural goods can be colorimetrically tested for pesticide residues thanks to certain nanozymes that are sensitive.
- **Mycotoxins and Food Allergens:** Using immuno-recognition and catalytic amplification, biosensors with nanozymes can identify aflatoxins or food-borne allergens.
- **Endocrine Disruptors (e.g., BPA):** Assays based on nanozymes have been developed to detect endocrine disruptors, such as BPA, in plastic products or water.

7.7 SENSITIVITY, SELECTIVITY, AND PERFORMANCE EVALUATION

The analytical performance of any biosensor, which encompasses sensitivity, selectivity, reaction time, reproducibility, and robustness, is what essentially determines its efficiency. Nanozyme-based biosensors have demonstrated notable progress in these areas because of the distinct catalytic and structural characteristics of nanozymes. The evaluation and optimization of these performance characteristics are examined in detail in this section.

7.7.1 Limit of Detection (LOD), Dynamic Range, and Response Time

7.7.1.1 Limit of Detection (LOD)

The lowest concentration of a target analyte at which it can be consistently separated from the background signal is known as the LOD. Nanozymes greatly reduce the limit of detection (LOD) in biosensors by enhancing weak signals due to their potent catalytic properties. In electrochemical sensors, for instance, gold-platinum alloy nanozymes have reached femtomolar level detection for proteins and nucleic acids, while FeO_4 nanozyme-based colorimetric sensors have reported LODs as low as 0.1 ng/mL for protein biomarkers.

The LOD is usually calculated using the formula:

$$\text{LOD} = 3.3 \times \sigma/\text{slope of the calibration curve}$$

Where:

- σ\sigma is the standard deviation of the blank measurements.
- The slope corresponds to sensitivity.

7.7.1.2 Dynamic Range

The range of analyte concentrations across which a detectable and linear response is produced by the sensor is known as the dynamic range. Wide dynamic ranges, usually from picomolar to micromolar levels, are frequently displayed by nanozyme-based biosensors, contingent upon the analyte and sensing format.

- Using oxidase-like nanozymes, colorimetric glucose sensors can detect concentrations ranging from 0.1μM to 10mM.
- The range of PSA electrochemical nanozyme sensors, which include both diagnostic and prognostic thresholds, is 10pg/mL to 100ng/mL.

7.7.1.3 Response Time

The speed at which a biosensor achieves a steady signal following analyte exposure is known as response time. Because nanozymes catalyze reactions quickly, response times are usually less than 5 minutes and sometimes less than 60 seconds. This is essential for point-of-care and emergency diagnostic applications.

- SAzymes have better-defined catalytic sites and larger turnover numbers than traditional nanozymes, which results in much lower LODs. Fe-N-C and Pt-N-C enzymes have been used to attain femtomolar sensitivity in colorimetric and electrochemical sensors.

7.7.2 Selectivity and Interference Studies

The capacity of the sensor to differentiate the target analyte from other elements in the sample matrix is known as selectivity. High selectivity is attained by nanozyme-based biosensors using:

- **Bioreceptor Integration:** To give selectivity for certain biomarkers, nanozymes are coupled with antibodies, aptamers, or molecularly imprinted polymers.
- **Dual Catalytic Systems:** Selectivity is increased by employing two nanozymes that only work when a target and a co-factor are present.
- **Inhibition or Enhancement Modulation:** The presence of particular analytes may either boost or inhibit nanozyme activity, offering a method of selective detection.

Potentially interfering agents, including glucose, uric acid, ascorbic acid, or ions like Na^+, K^+, and Ca^{2+}, are added to the test system to perform interference investigations. It is crucial that the biosensor can continue to produce a consistent and targeted response when they are present.

7.7.3 Real Sample Analysis and Reproducibility

7.7.3.1 Real Sample Analysis

A nanozyme-based biosensor's clinical translation and commercial viability depend on its validation in actual biological or environmental samples, such as blood, serum, saliva, urine, or water. Important things to think about include:

- **Matrix Effects**: Proteins, salts, and other chemicals that interfere with sensor function can be found in complex matrices.
- **Recovery Studies:** To assess accuracy, known amounts of the target analyte are added to actual samples, and the percentage recovered is computed.
- **Comparison with Gold-Standard Methods:** The accuracy and dependability of nanozyme biosensors' results are frequently confirmed by comparison with gold-standard techniques, such as PCR or ELISA (Scarsi, 2024).

7.7.3.2 Reproducibility and Stability

With relative standard deviation (RSD) values usually less than 5%, nanozyme-based sensors show good repeatability across several batches and tests. Stability testing entails:

- **Storage Stability:** After being kept at ambient temperature or in a refrigerator for a few weeks to months, biosensors are frequently retested.
- **Operational Stability:** The performance of the sensor is tracked under continuous flow or after repeated use.
- Many Fe_3O_4 and Au-based nanozyme sensors, for example, maintain more than 90% of their original activity after 30 days of storage, demonstrating their suitability for commercial usage.

7.8 RECENT ADVANCES AND CASE STUDIES

Since proof-of-concept designs gave way to more reliable, sensitive, and even commercially viable diagnostic instruments, nanozyme-based biosensors have seen tremendous technological advancements in recent years. This section examines recent advancements and particular instances that demonstrate how nanozymes are revolutionizing the biosensing industry.

7.8.1 State-of-the-Art Examples of Nanozyme Biosensors

- **Single-Atom Nanozyme (SAzyme) Biosensors**
  One significant advancement in the field is represented by single-atom nanozymes. These nanozymes obtain enzyme-mimicking activity that is comparable to or even higher than that of natural enzymes in turnover frequency by atomically spreading catalytic metal atoms (e.g., Fe, Co, or Pt) onto substrates such as nitrogen-doped carbon.

For instance, a Fe–N–C single-atom nanozyme that demonstrated peroxidase-like activity was included in a paper-based sensor to detect glucose and H_2O_2 with femtomolar sensitivity (Liu et al., 2023).

- **Nanozyme-Aptamer Hybrid Sensors**
  Aptamers, being highly specific nucleic acid ligands, are often paired with nanozymes to enhance target specificity.
- Case: A colorimetric sensor with great selectivity for Aflatoxin B1 was developed utilizing CeO2 nanozymes and DNA aptamers. A visual signal was produced when the aptamer separated from the nanozyme surface after binding the toxin, restoring catalytic activity.
- Using CeO_2 nanozymes and DNA aptamers detected Aflatoxin B1 was detected with high selectivity. Upon binding the toxin, the aptamer detached from the nanozyme surface, restoring catalytic activity and generating a visible signal.
- **CRISPR-Nanozyme Integrated Systems**
  Ultra-precise nucleic acid detection is now possible with next-generation biosensors due to the recent integration of nanozymes with CRISPR-based systems.
- Application: A nanozyme (Pt-decorated MoS) was employed in a CRISPR-Cas12a-driven biosensor to catalyze the oxidation of TMB. Rapid COVID-19 detection was made possible by the activation of Cas12a by target DNA, which led to the formation of color by nanozymes.
- **Wearable Nanozyme Sensors**
  Flexible electronics and nanozyme integration have opened doors for non-invasive, real-time monitoring.
- Example: A wearable glucose sensor that wirelessly transmits data to smartphones uses Au–Pt nanozymes that resemble Gox and are implanted in a flexible patch to detect sweat glucose.

7.8.2 Comparison with Traditional Biosensors, as Shown in Table 7.3

Nanozyme biosensors are particularly well suited for field diagnostics, wearable forms, and resource-constrained environments since they beat conventional sensors in terms of operating stability and environmental resilience, even though they are still lagging behind in terms of molecular specificity.

7.8.3 Commercial Products and Prototypes

Some platforms are heading toward commercialization, even if nanozyme biosensors are still mostly in the academic and R&D stage:

- **Nanozyme-LFA (Lateral Flow Assay) Kits:** Commercial test strips with nanozyme labels (e.g., Pt nanoparticles) are undergoing pilot testing for the

TABLE 7.3
Comparative Features of Traditional Enzyme-Based and Nanozyme-Based Biosensors

Feature	Traditional Enzyme-Based Biosensors	Nanozyme-Based Biosensors
Stability	Poor (denatures easily)	High thermal, pH, and chemical stability
Cost	High (purification and storage)	Lower (scalable, robust synthesis)
Shelf life	Weeks (needs refrigeration)	Months (room temperature storage)
Specificity	Very high	Moderate to high (improving with aptamers)
Reusability	Limited	Often reusable and regenerable
Fabrication flexibility	Limited	Highly adaptable for integration

detection of infectious diseases and food safety. These kits are known as Nanozyme-LFA kits.

- **Point-of-Care Diagnostic Tools:** Hand-held devices that combine colorimetric nanozyme reactions with smartphone-based analysis for detecting blood glucose, cholesterol, and uric acid are being prototyped by startups and research laboratories.
- **Environmental Sensors:** Several environmental monitoring organizations are working on developing field-deployable instruments that use nanozymes to track pesticides and heavy metals in water sources.

Though they still need regulatory approval, extensive validation, and production standardization before they can be fully adopted in the market, these prototypes show promise in terms of cost, usability, and performance.

7.9 CHALLENGES AND FUTURE PERSPECTIVES

Despite remarkable advancements, a number of technological, biological, and regulatory obstacles still need to be overcome before clinical translation and commercialization of nanozyme-based biosensors can proceed. The nanozymes and their role in wearable biosensors and personalized healthcare has been incorporated in Figure 7.2. Meanwhile, fresh developments in biology, materials science, and nanotechnology keep creating new opportunities for creativity.

This figure demonstrates the interconnected roles of nanozymes in advancing biosensing, wearable biosensors, and personalized healthcare. Nanozymes serve as functional components enabling sensitive detection, real-time monitoring, and adaptive health management. The circular flow emphasizes its central role in bridging nanotechnology with smart, patient-centric medical innovations (Zhang et al., 2024, https://doi.org/10.1016/j.isci.2025.111763, Elsevier).

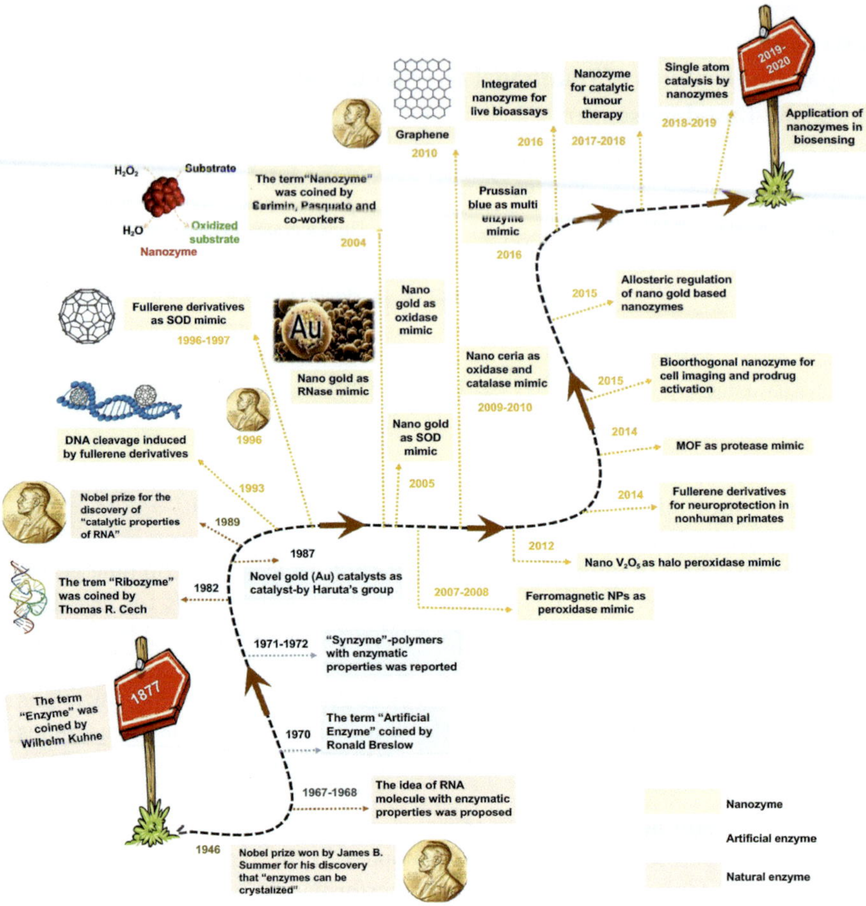

FIGURE 7.2 Nanozyme-driven integration in next-generation healthcare technologies.

7.9.1 Stability and Shelf Life of SAzymes

Current Advantage:

Compared to natural enzymes, nanozymes naturally have better thermal, chemical, and storage stability.

Challenges:

- Over time, oxidation, aggregation, or surface degradation may cause some nanozymes, particularly hybrid or doped systems, to lose their activity.
- Extended exposure to biological fluids, dampness, or UV light can affect catalytic activity.

Future Direction:

- Long-term performance can be improved by encapsulation within stable matrices like as silica shells, MOFs, or polymers
- Protective coatings and surface passivation methods (like PEGylation)

7.9.2 Biocompatibility and Toxicity Concerns

Concern:

Upon breakdown, many nanozymes, especially those made of metal oxides (e.g., Co_3O_4, CeO_2) or heavy metals (e.g., Pt, Pd), may produce reactive oxygen species (ROS) or release hazardous ions.

Future Direction

- Creating biodegradable or biosafe nanozymes via green synthesis techniques, carbon dots, or nanoparticles modified with amino acids.
- Developing tailored delivery methods to lessen off-target effects, such as functionalized coatings. Using human cell lines, rats, and zebrafish, a thorough in vivo toxicity profile was conducted.

7.9.3 Integration with IoT and Wearable Tech

Emerging Opportunity:

Intelligent, real-time biosensors that are coupled with wearable technology, smartphones, and cloud-based monitoring systems are being developed with great vigor.

Future Direction

- The creation of elastic and flexible substrates that are embedded with nanozyme inks.
- Real-time data interpretation and anomaly identification through the application of AI algorithms.
- Nanozyme-catalyzed sensors that run on biofuel or batteries (Wasilewski et al., 2024).

7.9.4 Challenges Specific to Single-Atom Nanozymes

Despite the great qualities of SAzymes, their manufacture frequently necessitates strict conditions to avoid aggregation into nanoparticles. Keeping single atoms stable over the long term, keeping them dispersed in biological media, and increasing production are all difficult tasks; furthermore, unless substituted with earth-abundant alternatives, the high cost of noble metal precursors (such as Pt and Au) may prevent their widespread usage.

7.10 CONCLUSION

The creation of biosensors based on nanozymes marks a major development in the field of diagnostics by overcoming the drawbacks of traditional enzyme-based devices. Nanozymes have transformed biosensing technology by providing improved stability, tunability, and cost-effectiveness while simulating enzyme activity. This has created new opportunities for the sensitive and targeted detection of a broad range of biomarkers.

The limitations of natural enzymes that sparked the development of nanozymes were highlighted in this chapter's introduction, which also provided an overview of biosensors and their crucial function in biomarker detection. We examined the basic ideas of nanozymes, including their synthesis, categorization, and characterization techniques, with a focus on how structural and compositional control directly affect their catalytic activity.

Next, we looked at the main biosensing platforms that nanozymes support, such as colorimetric, electrochemical, optical, and photoelectrochemical systems. Nanozymes are effective instruments for point-of-care, real-time detection because of their function in catalytic activity and signal amplification.

From surface functionalization and immobilization methods to device assembly and downsizing, fabrication methodologies for nanozyme-based biosensors were covered in depth. These methods make it possible to incorporate nanozymes into wearable, flexible, and even smartphone-compatible forms, increasing their use in a variety of contexts.

The use of nanozyme biosensors in the detection of environmental, metabolic, cardiac, infectious, and cancer biomarkers further shows their practical usefulness. These illustrations show the adaptability of nanozymes as well as their ability to operate with great precision and repeatability in intricate sample matrices.

Sensitivity, selectivity, LOD, response time, and real-sample analysis were among the performance assessment criteria that were examined, confirming the analytical superiority of nanozyme-based biosensors in several situations. Additionally, we examined current developments that are moving closer to commercialization, such as wearable diagnostic platforms, CRISPR-integrated systems, and single-atom nanozymes.

Nanozyme-based biosensors continue to encounter a number of obstacles in spite of their potential, from toxicity and biocompatibility issues to problems with regulatory approval, scalability, and integration with contemporary technology. However, these obstacles are being swiftly overcome by developments in synthetic biology, material science, and nanofabrication.

Biosensing has advanced significantly with the emergence of single-atom nanozymes. Together with their tunability and compliance with downsizing, their capacity to duplicate and even exceed natural enzyme activity makes them crucial parts of the next generation of biosensors for early and sensitive disease detection.

Emerging Trends

- Because of their high catalytic efficiency and adaptable selectivity, single-atom and multi-enzyme mimic nanozymes are probably going to dominate future designs.

- Remote health monitoring and tailored therapy will be made easier by NI-integrated biosensing technologies that combine data-driven diagnostics with nanozymes.
- As environmental issues gain priority and regulatory demands mount, sustainable and green synthesis methods will become crucial.
- Wearable technology, the Internet of Things (IoT), and nanozymes combined with smart diagnostics will allow for ongoing, on-body biomarker monitoring.

REFERENCES

Abdel-Mageed, H. M. (2025). Frontiers in nanoparticles redefining enzyme immobilization: A review addressing challenges, innovations, and unlocking sustainable future potentials. *Micro and Nano Systems Letters*, *13*(1), 7.

Ahmad, A., Imran, M., & Ahsan, H. (2023). Biomarkers as biomedical bioindicators: Approaches and techniques for the detection, analysis, and validation of novel biomarkers of diseases. *Pharmaceutics*, *15*(6), 1630.

Aldewachi, H., Chalati, T., Woodroofe, M. N., Bricklebank, N., Sharrack, B., & Gardiner, P. (2018). Gold nanoparticle-based colorimetric biosensors. *Nanoscale*, *10*(1), 18–33.

Altaf, A., Khan, I., Khan, A., Sadiq, S., Humayun, M., Khan, S., . . . & Bououdina, M. (2024). Metal/covalent organic framework encapsulated lead-free halide perovskite hybrid nanocatalysts: Multifunctional applications, design, recent trends, challenges, and prospects. *ACS Omega*, *9*(32), 34220–34242.

Bilalis, P., Karagouni, E., & Toubanaki, D. K. (2022). Peroxidase-like activity of Fe3O4 nanoparticles and Fe3O4-graphene oxide nanohybrids: Effect of the amino-and carboxyl-surface modifications on H2O2 sensing. *Applied Organometallic Chemistry*, *36*(9), e6803.

Chakraborty, S. (2024). Democratizing nucleic acid-based molecular diagnostic tests for infectious diseases at resource-limited settings–from point of care to extreme point of care. *Sensors & Diagnostics*, *3*(4), 536–561.

Chong, Y., & Ge, C. (2022). Oxidase-mimicking nanozymes: Recent development and biomedical applications. In *Nanozymes: Design, Synthesis, and Applications* (pp. 135–162). American Chemical Society.

Das, B., Franco, J. L., Logan, N., Balasubramanian, P., Kim, M. I., & Cao, C. (2021). Nanozymes in point-of-care diagnosis: An emerging futuristic approach for biosensing. *Nano-Micro Letters*, *13*, 193. https://doi.org/10.1007/s40820-021-00717-0.

Haleem, A., Javaid, M., Singh, R. P., Suman, R., & Rab, S. (2021). Biosensors applications in medical field: A brief review. *Sensors International*, *2*, 100100.

Huang, Y., Ren, J., & Qu, X. (2019). Nanozymes: Classification, catalytic mechanisms, activity regulation, and applications. *Chemical Reviews*, *119*(6), 4357–4412.

Huang, X., Deng, H., Deng, X., Li, L., Wu, M., Huang, C., . . . & Zhao, H. (2024). Single-atom iron boosts electrochemiluminescence for ultrasensitive carcinoembryonic antigen detectio. *Microchimica Acta*, *191*(2), 111.

Jiao, L., Xu, W., Wu, Y., Yan, H., Gu, W., Du, D.,. . . Zhu, C. (2021). Single-atom catalysts boost signal amplification for biosensing. *Chemical Society Reviews*, *50*(2), 750–765.

Jungblut, P. R., Zimny-Arndt, U., Zeindl-Eberhart, E., Stulik, J., Koupilova, K., Pleißner, K. P.,. . . Stöffler, G. (1999). Proteomics in human disease: Cancer, heart and infectious diseases. *ELECTROPHORESIS: An International Journal*, *20*(10), 2100–2110.

Kucherenko, I. S., Soldatkin, O. O., Kucherenko, D. Y., Soldatkina, O. V., & Dzyadevych, S. V. (2019). Advances in nanomaterial application in enzyme-based electrochemical biosensors: A review. *Nanoscale Advances*, *1*(12), 4560–4577.

Kulkarni, M. B., Ayachit, N. H., & Aminabhavi, T. M. (2022). Recent advancements in nanobiosensors: Current trends, challenges, applications, and future scope. *Biosensors*, *12*(10), 892.

Li, B., Li, L., Guan, A., Liu, H., & Du, H. (2014). A smartphone controlled handheld microfluidic liquid handling system. *arXiv preprint*. https://arxiv.org/abs/1405.5246

Liu, D. (2024). Biosensors. In *Handbook of Molecular Biotechnology* (pp. 473–482). CRC Press.

Liu, J., Pang, S., Wang, M., Yu, H., Ma, P., Dong, T., . . . & Liu, A. (2023). An ultrasensitive ELISA to assay femtomolar level SARS-CoV-2 antigen based on specific peptide and tyramine signal amplification. *Sensors and Actuators B: Chemical*, *387*, 133746.

Liu, Y., Zhang, Y., Wang, C., Wang, Y., Zhang, K., Yang, X., . . . & Gong, Y. (2024). Multiplexed optofluidic laser immunosensor for sensitive and rapid detection of biomarkers. *Sensors and Actuators B: Chemical*, *403*, 135198.

Lustig, D., Licari, J., & Enlow, D. (1998). Screen printing technology in disposable printed electrodes: Patterning of sensing materials and circuitry using conductive inks. *Sensor Review*, *18*(3), 208–212. https://doi.org/10.1108/02602289810219889

Mirra, G. (2025). *Comparing nanozymes catalytic activity and applications* (Doctoral thesis, Università degli Studi di Genova).

Mishra, P., Lee, J., Kumar, D., Louro, R. O., Costa, N., Pathania, D., Kumar, S., Lee, J., & Singh, L. (2022). Engineered nanoenzymes with multifunctional properties for next-generation biological and environmental applications. *Advanced Functional Materials*, *32*(8), 2108650. https://doi.org/10.1002/adfm.202108650

Scarsi, A. (2024). *Colorimetric nanodiagnostics of biomarkers in biological fluids* (Doctoral thesis, University of Genoa). https://hdl.handle.net/11567/1165055

Singh, L. (2022). Engineered nanoenzymes with multifunctional properties for next-generation biological and environmental applications. *Advanced Functional Materials*, *32*(8), 2108650.

Mostofian, B., & McCutcheon, J. R. (2017). Enzyme immobilization by inkjet printing on reagentless biosensors for electrochemical phosphate detection. *Biosensors*, *7*(4), 45. https://doi.org/10.3390/bios7040045

Naresh, V., & Lee, N. (2021). A review on biosensors and recent development of nanostructured materials-enabled biosensors. *Sensors*, *21*(4), 1109.

Niu, X., Cheng, N., Ruan, X., Du, D., & Lin, Y. (2020). Nanozyme-based immunosensors and immunoassays: Recent developments and future trends. *Journal of the Electrochemical Society*, *167*(3), 037508.

Pavesi, N. M., & Pavesi, J. (2016). Layer-by-layer assembled biofilms for biosensors: High loading and film integrity. *Journal of Materials Chemistry B*, *4*(21), 3839–3850. https://doi.org/10.1039/C6TB00157B

Sahare, T., Singh, N. N., & Sahoo, B. N. (2024). Smartphone-enhanced nanozyme sensors: Colorimetric and fluorescence sensing techniques. *Biosensors and Bioelectronics: X*, *42*, 100544. https://doi.org/10.1016/j.biosx.2024.100544

Shen, L., Ye, D., Zhao, H., & Zhang, J. (2020). Perspectives for single-atom nanozymes: Advanced synthesis, functional mechanisms, and biomedical applications. *Analytical Chemistry*, *93*(3), 1221–1231.

Singh, N., Sherin, G. R., & Mugesh, G. (2023). Antioxidant and prooxidant nanozymes: From cellular redox regulation to next-generation therapeutics. *Angewandte Chemie*, *135*(33), e202301232.

Singh, S. (2019). Nanomaterials exhibiting enzyme-like properties (nanozymes): Current advances and future perspectives. *Frontiers in Chemistry*, *7*, 46.

Song, H., Zhang, M., & Tong, W. (2022). Single-atom nanozymes: Fabrication, characterization, surface modification and applications of ROS scavenging and antibacterial. *Molecules*, *27*(17), 5426.

Wang, Q., Wei, H., Zhang, Z., Wang, E., & Dong, S. (2018). Nanozyme: An emerging alternative to natural enzyme for biosensing and immunoassay. *TrAC Trends in Analytical Chemistry*, *105*, 218–224.

Wasilewski, T., Kamysz, W., & Gębicki, J. (2024). AI-assisted detection of biomarkers by sensors and biosensors for early diagnosis and monitoring. *Biosensors*, *14*(7), 356.

Wu, T., Zhou, Q., & Chen, G. (2024). Rational integration of nanozyme probe and smartphone device for on-site analysis. *Analysis & Sensing*, *4*(3), e202300084. https://doi.org/10.1002/anse.202300084

Wu, W., Huang, L., Wang, E., & Dong, S. (2020). Atomic engineering of single-atom nanozymes for enzyme-like catalysis. *Chemical Science*, *11*(36), 9741–9756.

Xia, J., Li, Z., Ding, Y., Shah, L. A., Zhao, H., Ye, D., & Zhang, J. (2024). Construction and application of nanozyme sensor arrays. *Analytical Chemistry*, *96*(21), 8221–8233.

Xiao, X., Hu, X., Liu, Q., Zhang, Y., Zhang, G., & Chen, S. (2023). Single--atom nanozymes as promising catalysts for biosensing and biomedical applications-. *Inorganic Chemistry Frontiers*, *10*, 4289–4312. https://doi.org/10.1039/D3QI00430A

Yang, Z., Guo, J., Wang, L., Zhang, J., Ding, L., Liu, H., & Yu, X. (2024). Nanozyme-enhanced electrochemical biosensors: Mechanisms and applications. *Small*, *20*(14), 2307815.

Zhang, Y., Yang, Y., Yin, Z., Huang, L., & Wang, J. (2025, January 7). Nanozyme--based wearable biosensors for application in healthcare-. *iScience*, 28(2), 111763. https://doi.org/10.1016/j.isci.2025.111763. PMID: 39906563; PMCID: PMC11791255.

Zhao, Y., Chen, Y., Liu, X., Wang, Y., & Li, Z. (2025). Advancing transistor-based point-of-care (POC) biosensors: Additive manufacturing technologies and device integration strategies for real-life sensing. *Nanoscale*, Advance online publication. https://doi.org/10.1039/D4NR04441.

8 Carbon Dots and Dendrimer Nanohybrids for Biomedical Applications

Radhika Tippani, Sai Bhavani, and Mahendar Porika

8.1 INTRODUCTION

Carbon-based materials like fullerene, graphene, carbon nanotubes (CNT), and carbon nanofibers (CNF) have revolutionized material science and established a significant historical presence (Deshmukh et al., 2020a). Nanotechnology has enabled the development of carbon-based materials with precise nanoscale dimensional control and superior electrical characteristics, paving the way for new material technologies. Comprehending the improved properties and chemistry of carbon nanoparticles (NPs) is essential, as it facilitates a broad spectrum of applications and technologies for improved NPs (Deshmukh et al., 2020b; Jeon et al., 2020). Carbon nanoparticles are being utilized in cutting-edge research to broaden the boundaries of materials science and electrical engineering (Deshmukh et al., 2020a). Carbon nanomaterials are utilized in various customer and manufacturing application due to their adjustable nanoscale dimensions and potential influence from doping and charge transfer interactions (Kang et al., 2019).Carbon nanoparticles possess mechanical, optoelectronic, and physicochemical capabilities that may enhance existing technologies or facilitate next-generation applications, especially in sophisticated electronic technologies (You et al., 2020). In recent decades, transistors manufactured on silicon wafers contain enhanced the recital of consumer gadgets (Wang et al., 2018). A prominent research area focuses on the development of carbon nanomaterials that demonstrate markedly superior characteristics compared to conventional silicon-based materials, encompassing nanoscale physics and form-factor, cost-effectiveness, diminished electrical consumption, improved adaptability and longevity, along with large-area fabrication or roll-to-roll production capabilities (Kang et al., 2019). Scientists and engineers are increasingly interested in carbon nanohybrids due to their unique electrical, mechanical, chemical, and spectroscopic properties, as well as their high porosity (Yoon et al., 2019).

Hybrid nanomaterials have attracted considerable interest from the scientific community because of their capacity to utilize the unique features of their components.

 DOI: 10.1201/9781003563723-8

Exploiting this property allows hybrid nanomaterials to demonstrate unique behaviors and enhance performance, hence broadening their potential applications. Nanomaterials such as carbon dots (CDs) and dendrimers are extensively studied owing to their intriguing characteristics and prospective applications. CDs were identified in 2004 by Xu and Scrivens (Xu et al., 2004). The researchers identified minuscule particles as "fluorescent carbon" and later "carbon dots" due to quantum-size effects. The particles, measuring 30–50 nm, displayed reduced fluorescence compared to their smaller counterparts. CDs refer to a generic classification of certain carbon NPs that have distinctive physicochemical and photophysical characteristics. A novel categorization has been established to characterize the CDs, resulting in the emergence of four unique nanostructures: graphene quantum dots (GQDs), carbon quantum dots (CQDs), carbon nanodots (CNDs), and polymer dots (PDs) (Đorđević et al., 2022). Graphene quantum dots (CQDs) are composed of sp2 hybridized carbon atoms and have a honeycomb lattice structure, while CQDs have multiple π–π layered sp2/sp3 carbon sheet layers, surface-functionalized groups, and graphitic carbon topologies, with a spherical or quasi-spherical shape (1–10 nm), whereas GQDs have a disc-like morphology (< 20 nm).Nanodots (CNDs) are smaller than 10 nm with an amorphous carbon core, providing polymers with internal structures and surfaces. Synthesis conditions and methods affect CD design and production, affecting top-down (GQDs) or bottom-up (CQDs, CNDs, or PDs). The characteristics of the original precursor, including its type, temperature, and reaction length, might affect the degree of carbonization, hence impacting the synthesis of aromatic or polymeric compounds. Photoluminescence (PL) is an essential property shown by all types of carbon referenced. Although the origins and causes of PL remain unresolved, researchers have shown that the surface is a pivotal aspect affecting the PL characteristics of these materials (Wang and Lu, 2022). Additional attributes associated with CDs include their water solubility, surface functioning, and low cytotoxicity. Additional information on the nomenclature, structural elucidation, characteristics, design, and synthesis techniques of CDs is available in several recent studies (Đorđević et al., 2022; de Boëver et al., 2022). CDs, discovered recently, have various applications in biomedicine, detection of metal ions, biomolecules, drugs, explosive compounds, and energy conversion. They are suggested for drug and gene delivery and metal ion detection (Ge et al., 2021; Farshidfar and Fooladi, 2023).

Dendrimers are single-dispersed, branched polymeric nanoarchitectures, primarily grouped using George Newkome's names and terms (Newkome and Shreiner, 2010). Dendrimers' shape, stability, conformational flexibility, and viscosity are influenced by their chemical composition and architecture. They show a decrease in viscosity with successive generations due to their compact, globular shape. Dragon-tree-like structures, with minimal polydispersity, controlled molecular weight, aqueous solubility, surface functionality, and empty internal spaces, offer potential biological applications (Camacho et al., 2020, 2021; Mekuria et al., 2021).

Dendrimers have emerged as a potential category of materials in academic study, exhibiting considerable accomplishments throughout the years. Their distinctive characteristics and adaptable uses have made them a favored topic of research, facilitating several advancements. Large-scale synthesis, purification, and cytotoxicity challenges have limited their usefulness and delayed their clinical debut, as noted by Janaszewska et al. (2019). Despite being relatively novel parallel to different carbon-based nanomaterials, CDs exhibit specific limitations, including inadequate control over synthesis parameters, a lack of comprehensive understanding of the fluorescence mechanism, and poor synthesis yields (Mandal and Das, 2022). The combination of fluorescence, minimal cytotoxicity, loading capacities, and surface functions of carbon dots and other nanomaterials could potentially create efficient nanohybrid (NH) systems. This chapter explores the production and utilization of nanohybrid materials made from carbon dots and dendrimers, extending beyond biological applications, focusing on synthesis strategies and techniques for NPs and nanofilms. It is also highlights their potential use in biomedicine and concludes with a summary of key findings and projections for the future of this field.

8.2 SYNTHESIS

This section outlines the synthesis processes for NHs, categorized into covalent, non-covalent, casting, and sandwich techniques (**Table 8.1**). It also discusses various dendrimer types used, including peptides, PAMAM, silicone, and triazine dendrimers, for nanohybrid creation.

8.2.1 Covalent Approach

The covalent technique is commonly used for synthesizing NHs like carbon dots and dendrimers, enhancing their affinities, stability, and size distribution. Amide coupling chemistry uses carbodiimide agents like EDC/NHS and DCC to activate the surface of carbon dots and facilitate the covalent attachment of dendrimers, resulting in a covalent nanohybrid. In 2013, the first scientific paper described the synthesis of Au-PAMAM-carbon dot NHs via amide coupling. 3-mercaptopropionic acid (MPA) was used to functionalize Au colloids before conjugating them to PAMAM dendrimers. CDs were included in the next reaction phase and reacted for 24 hours at room temperature to create the necessary Au-PAMAM-CDs NHs (Zong et al., 2013). In a separate investigation, carbon nanodots, synthesized from the dehydration of starch NPs using sulfuric acid, were activated with EDC/NHS to interact with both G0 and G1 PAMAM-NH2 dendrimers. Covalent bonding was accomplished either at ambient temperature for 6 hours or by microwave irradiation at 60 W for 15 minutes at 75°C (Ngu-Schwemlein et al., 2016). Bhatnagar et al. (2017) developed a NH for cardiac biomarker detection using commercial graphene quantum dots conjugated to G3 PAMAM-NH2 dendrimers via EDC/NHS.

Feng and colleagues (2019) similarly used the same generation of PAMAM dendrimers to synthesize a NH including red-fluorescent carbon dots. Citric acid and formamide were mixed in a hydrothermal reactor to create carbon dots, which were then dispersed in methanol and covalently attached to G3 PAMAM-NH2. A separate research created peptide dendritic carbon dots for antitumor purposes. CDs were synthesized by only glucose and microwaved at 800 W for 3 minutes. The surface was functionalized with sulfhydryl groups (CDs-SH) to facilitate the attachment of G3 peptide dendrimers via a disulfide exchange process, resulting in the formation of CD-S-S-peptide dendrimer covalent NHs (Ma et al., 2018). Covalent-type

TABLE 8.1
Overview of Nanohybrids Produced by Various Methods and Applications

S.No.	Carbon dots	Dendrimer	Nanohybrid Size (nm)	Application	Reference
Covalent					
1	CNDs	G0 and G1 PAMAM-NH2	30–60	Antimicrobial activity	Ngu-Schwemlein et al., 2016
2	CQDs	G3 PAMAM-NH2	27	DOX drug delivery	Feng et al., 2019
3	CQDs	G1, G2, and G3 PAMAM-NH2	2–27	Sensing and gene therapy	Ghosh et al., 2019
4	CDs	G3 Triazine	400	DOX drug delivery	Karimi and Namazi, 2021
5	GQDs	G3 PAMAM-NH2	55	DOX drug delivery	Pooresmaeil et al., 2020
6	GQDs	G3 Triazine	111–112	DOX drug delivery	Karimi and Namazi, 2020
Non-covalent					
7	**CDs**	G4-G6 PAMAM-NH2	20–40	Bioimaging and gene delivery	Martins et al., 2021
8	**CDs**	G5 PAMAM-NH2	131.8 ± 29.4	DOX drug delivery	Li et al., 2019
9	**CDs**	G5 PAMAM-NH2	101.8	DOX drug delivery	Li et al., 2021
10	**GQDs**	G5 Guanidyl-PAMAM	342	Heparin and chondroitin sensing	Li et al., 2015
11	**CQDs**	G4 PAMAM-NH2	65 ± 5.3	Sensing of nitroaromatic Explosives	Campos et al., 2016b
12	**CQDs**	G5 PAMAM-NH2	6.9 ± 0.77	EPI drug delivery	Matai et al., 2015
Biorecognition					
13*	**Si-CDs**	Silicone dendrimer	NA	Solar cells	Wu et al., 2021
14*	**GQDs**	G2 PAMAM-NH2	NA	Fluorescence enhancement	Lin et al., 2016
15#	**CDs**	G4 PAMAM-NH2	NA	Immunosensing	Hamd-Ghadareh et al., 2017
16#	**CDs**	G4 PAMAM-NH2	NA	Immunosensing	Mohammadi et al., 2018

***Casting; # Sandwich**

nanohybrids were synthesized using low-generation PAMAM dendrimers (G1, G2, and G3) and carboxylated cyclodextrins. The CDs were first synthesized from delicious lemon peel by hydrothermal carbonization. The conjugation of CDs with G1-G3 PAMAM dendrimers was facilitated by EDC/NHS, resulting in the formation of three distinct NHs, designated as CDP1, CDP2, and CDP3 (Ghosh et al., 2019; **Figure 8.1**). Employing an alternative methodology, Pooresmaeil and colleagues (2020) used GQDs that had been functionalized with (3-aminopropyl)triethoxysilane (APTES), resulting in GQDs-NH2, to facilitate the growth of PAMAM-NH2 dendrimer on the altered surface. Karimi and Namazi (2020) synthesized G3 triazine dendrimers on magnetic iron oxide NPs and conjugated them with graphene quantum dots using DCC, forming nanoplatform core-shell structured Fe3O4@C@TDGQDs microspheres. Recently, the same team of researchers functionalized

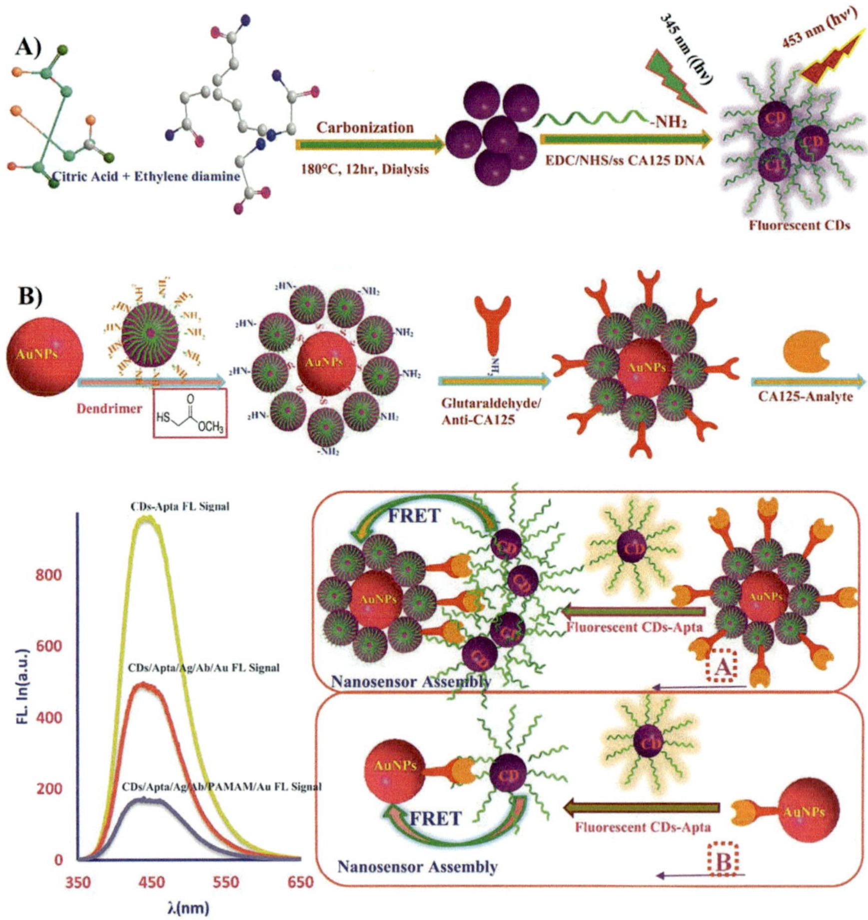

FIGURE 8.1 Schematically representation of CD and CDPs and theratostics of TNBC. Replicated with permission (Ghosh et al., 2019).

magnetic Fe_3O_4 NPs using triazine dendrimers and folic acid-derived carbon dots (Karimi and Namazi, 2021).

The CDs were first synthesized from folic acid as the precursor by the hydrothermal technique, resulting in N-doped CDs. A magnetic nanoplatform was created by covalently binding triazine magnetic dendrimers to carbon dots using DCC coupling chemistry for 24 hours at room temperature. The nanoplatform, Fe_3O_4@ SiO_2-G2.5–CDs, was used for targeted administration of doxorubicin. Covalent NHs were primarily synthesized using low-generation dendrimers (G0-G4), which have reduced steric effects and may enhance carbon dots' photoluminescence. However, the covalent technique requires more time for refinement and purification. The specificity of terminal functional groups in carbon dots and dendrimers is crucial for preserving the nanomaterials' integrity and properties.

8.2.2 Non-Covalent Approach

Non-covalent nanohybrids were created by linking CDs and dendrimers through non-covalent interactions, primarily through the attraction of opposing surface charges. This technique simplifies experimentation and setup, maintains photoluminescent properties of carbon dots, and creates NHs with enhanced loading capacities, simplifying the use of higher-generation dendrimers. Anionic surface-presenting CDs were engaged with cationic dendrimers. Li et al. (2015) studied the self-assembly of G5 PAMAM-Gu+ with graphene quantum dots, using non-covalently coupled graphene quantum dots and functionalized with univalent guanosine radical (Li et al., 2015). Researchers from different group used the same generation of PAMAM dendrimer to create nanohybrids containing CQDs, synthesized using chitosan and PEG-4000 hydrothermally. The G5 PAMAM dendrimer was acetylated with acetic anhydride, encapsulating anticancer anthracyclineepirubicin (EPI). CQDs@EPI⊂G5-Ac85 fluorescent NHs were created by combining them with cationic EPI⊂G5-Ac85 dendrimer complexes (Matai et al., 2015). A study by Campos et al. (2016a) found that carbon quantum dots (CQDs) can be enhanced for explosive chemical detection by conjugating with G4 PAMAM dendrimers. The fabrication of nanohybrids for cancer theranostics uses non-covalent interactions, using RGD as a targeted ligand and TPGS as a drug efflux inhibitor. The study by Li et al. (2019) utilized sodium citrate and ammonium bicarbonate to create CDs, which were then formed using hydrogen bonding and electrostatically attached to G5 PAMAM-RGD-TPGS. They also demonstrated the creation of G5-TPGS@y-CDs-DOX complexes through non-covalent interactions for chemotherapy applications. Acetylsalicylic acid and chemical method were used to create yellow-fluorescent carbon dots, which connect with G5 PAMAM-TPGS via electrostatic interactions, creating a y-CD/dendrimer NH for delivering TPGS and DOX to immune cancers (Li et al., 2021). Martins et al. (2021) synthesized carbon dot/dendrimer nanohybrids for bioimaging and gene transfer using hydrothermal synthesis of anionic carbon dots and cationic PAMAM dendrimers. The carbon dots were synthesized using ascorbic acid, and G4-G6 PAMAM-NH_2 dendrimers were electrostatically attached to the carbon dots, resulting in G4-G6 CDs@PAMAM NHs. The non-covalent technique of nanohybrids has drawbacks such as uneven shape and significant size fluctuations, as it relies on generational advancement and cationic concentrations, while the globular shape strengthens with successive generations.

8.2.3 Biorecognition Approach

The combination of CDs and dendrimers was achieved through modifying biorecognition methods for casting and sandwich fabrication processes. Lin et al. (2016) used a simple and effective process to combine GQDs with low-generation PAMAM dendrimers (G2). GQDs were created using laser ablation, followed by spin-coating a silicon substrate with PAMAM dendrimers. The GQDs were then drop-cast onto the dendrimers' surface, demonstrating the effectiveness and simplicity of this method. A group developed Si-CDs/Si-dendrimer composites for solar cell applications, using citric acid, dicyandiamide, and APTES. These nanofilms, which cured for 48 hours, effectively concentrate brilliant solar cells (Wu et al., 2021). The sandwich approach was used to combine CDs and PAMAM dendrimers for immunosensing applications. Hydrothermal treatment created CDs, which were surface functionalized with the ssCA125DNA aptamer, resulting in the formation of sandwich-type NH (Hamd-Ghadareh et al., 2017; **Figure 8.2**). A nanohybrid FRET immunosensor was developed by combining carbon dots and gold-polyamidoamine dendrimers, functionalized with the CA 15–3 antibody, and enhanced detection by forming an interaction with AuNPs-PAMAM-aptamer (Mohammadi et al., 2018).

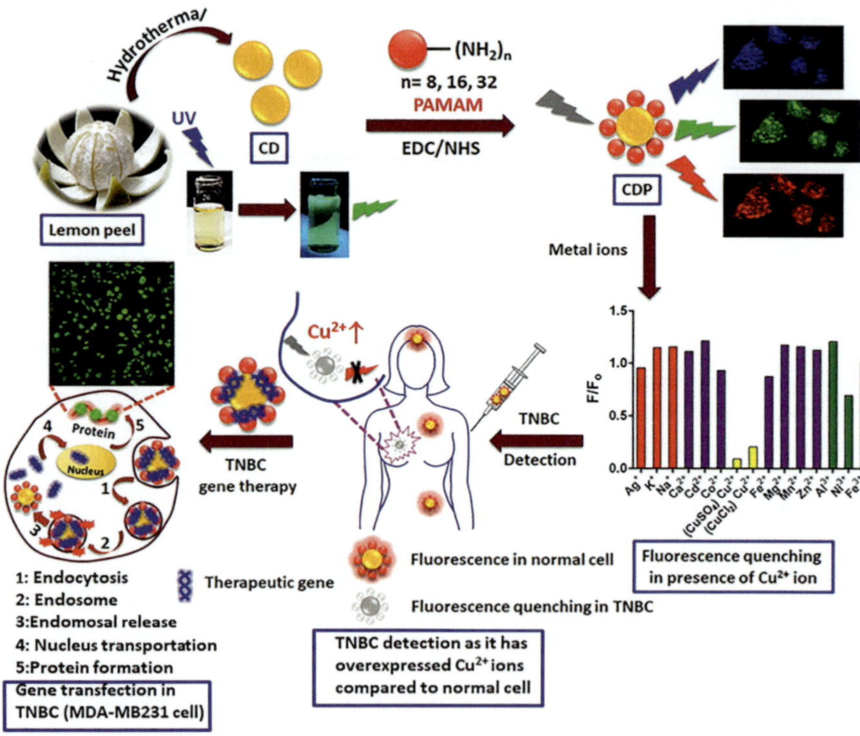

FIGURE 8.2 The FRET-based detection method involves conjugating fluorescent carbon dots to DNA, quenching the reaction with gold nanoparticles (AuNPs), and then using PAMAM-Ab via FRET in the presence of CA125 analyte. Replicated with permission (Hamd-Ghadareh et al., 2017).

8.3 BIOMEDICAL APPLICATIONS

NHs composed of carbon dots and dendrimers may possess prospective uses in biomedicine. The literature clearly indicates that a substantial number of these nanohybrids was specifically designed for medication and gene delivery, bioimaging, and antibacterial applications. The following sections provide and discuss the main findings and conclusions from those investigations.

8.3.1 Bioimaging and Drug Delivery

Bioimaging is perhaps the predominant use of carbon dots owing to their photoluminescence, photostability, and low cytotoxicity. The excitation-dependent behavior of some CDs produced multi-color emissions that illuminated cells. The NH, when combined with dendrimers, offers protection against environmental quenching and the ability to acquire target ligands, improving cellular uptake. The fluorescence of CDs can be preserved or enhanced, preserving their imaging use (Martins et al., 2021). Researchers found that CQDs are primarily internalized within the cell cytoplasm, making it the primary target for free CQDs. CQDs@EPI⊂G5-Ac85 NHs were identified in the cytoplasm, indicating colocalization of green and red fluorescence, suggesting CQDs could serve as fluorescent tracers for intracellular transport of therapeutic agents (Matai et al., 2015). A study used blue fluorescence emitted by CDs to track (CDs/DOX)@G5 PAMAM–RGD–TPGS complexes inside A549 cells (Li et al., 2019). After six hours of incubation, cells showed blue and red fluorescence signals, resulting in purple fluorescence in bright-field photos. These complexes were located in the cytoplasm, enabling monitoring of CDs and DOX. Li et al. (2021) studied the uptake of G5-TPGS@y-CDs-DOX complexes in multidrug-resistant neoplastic cells. After a 6-hour treatment, MCF-7/ADR cells showed yellow-green and red fluorescence, with composite pictures showing orange fluorescence due to colocalization. Martins et al.'s 2021 study explored the use of G4-G6 CDs@PAMAM NHs for bioimaging. They used flow cytometry to monitor cellular internalization in HEK 293T cells for 24 hours. The results showed nanohybrids were present in cells when exposed to green and red light, and the amount of PAMAM dendrimers could be adjusted to alter fluorescence intensity. A study modified CDs-PAMAM G3 conjugates with RGDs to improve cellular absorption in MDA-MB-231 cancer cells. Confocal imaging showed consistent distribution of CDs-PAMAM G3-RGDS conjugates inside the cell cytoplasm. When excited at 405, 473, and 559 nm, the conjugates produced green, blue, and red fluorescence, indicating their potential as an imaging agent for TNBC cells (Ghosh et al., 2019).

Drug delivery nanosystems provide significant promise for cancer therapy, offering targeted therapeutic benefits while minimizing harm to healthy tissues. Consequently, much research on NHs has concentrated on their prospective anticancer uses. CDs, with their multifunctionality, imaging capabilities, surface modifications, and stimuli responsiveness, show promise for intelligent transport, tracking, and delivery in cancer theranostics, enabling drug encapsulation and targeted ligand binding. Matai et al. (2015) developed CQDs@EPI⊂G5-Ac85 NHs by encapsulating

EPI-epirubicin in G5 PAMAM-Ac dendrimers and coupling them with CQDs. The NHs showed significant anticancer effects on MCF-7 cells, eliminating 70% of cancer cells at a 5 μM EPI dose. The NHs increased the sub G0/G1 phase and decreased the S phase, causing cell death through apoptosis. Ma et al. (2018) developed a nanoplatform for oncological treatment using carbon dots, peptide dendrimers, and pCBMA. The technique allows for future bioimaging CDs carrying DOX. In vivo studies showed 75.4% tumor inhibition in BALB/c mice with subcutaneous mammary carcinoma compared to 42.3% with DOX.HCl. Feng et al. (2019) synthesized carbon quantum dots and G3 PAMAM dendrimers, assessing drug release at pH 5.5 and 7.0 using a DOX model. Results showed 70% and 48% drug release after 70 hours, suggesting potential oncological applications. Li and colleagues (2019) synthesized CDs/DOX compounds using hydrogen bonding and conjugated them with G5 PAMAM-RGD-TPGS to form complexes. The NH s showed anticancer efficacy and target specificity in A549 cells, with 9% cell viability and inhibition of cancer cell growth at a concentration of 35 μg/mL. The integration of RGD in the NH s allowed for precise delivery of CDs/DOX@G5-RGD-TPGS complexes to A549 cells. Pooresmaeil et al. (2020) developed a NH with GQDs and PAMAM dendrimers to deliver DOX into MDA-MB 231 cells, modifying the GQDs-PAMAM NH with cyclodextrin for biocompatibility. The dendrimer structure held 62% DOX, demonstrating pH-sensitive drug release. Karimi and Namazi's (2020) study tested new triazine dendrimer-conjugated GQDs attached to Fe3O4@C@NH2 core-shell microspheres as a possible DOX carrier. The Fe3O4@C@TDGQDs microspheres loaded 63.1% of drugs and released 65.1% and 28.5% after 72 hours at pH 5.0 and 7.4, respectively. However, Fe3O4@C@TDGQDs-DOX reduced A549 cells' viability across a concentration range of 2–32 μg/mL, leading to higher cell death rates against A549 cancer cells.

Karimi and Namazi's 2021 study developed a new method for sending drugs to specific locations using iron oxide NPs, triazine dendrimers, and carbon dots. They modified Fe_3O_4 NPs with TEOS and used G2.5 triazine dendrimers on the surface. The researchers created $Fe_3O_4@SiO2-G2.5-CD-DOX$ complexes, which were effective at enclosing DOX and showed pH-dependent release. However, the combination was more harmful to A549 cells after 48 hours. This method demonstrates improved drug delivery systems using cyclodextrins and triazine-type dendrimers. Li et al. (2021) developed a nanoplatform using carbon dots and polyamidoamine dendrimers, called (G5-TPGS@y-CDs)-DOX complexes, to treat cancer resistant to multiple drugs. By altering the surface of G5 PAMAM with D-α-tocopheryl polyethylene glycol 1000 succinate (TPGS), the killing effect was enhanced in MCF-7 and MCF-7/ADR-adriamycin resistant cells. The anticancer and treatment effects were enhanced by ultrasound-targeted microbubble destruction technology.

8.3.2 Gene Delivery

Few groups have studied NHs made of carbon dots and dendrimers as gene transporters, which facilitate the creation of stable complexes that act as nucleic acid carriers and prevent enzymes from breaking down DNA. Ghosh et al. (2019) performed a research using CDs-PAMAM G3-RGDS conjugates to bind and complex pDNA encoding GFP in human Caucasian breast cancer cells, MDA-MB-231(**Figure 8.3**). The CDs-PAMAM G3-RGDS/pDNA complexes exhibited effective DNA condensation characteristics and emitted green light after 4 hours of treatment. The research indicated that CDs-PAMAM G3 conjugates may attach to DNA and inhibit enzymatic degradation, demonstrating safety at concentrations up to 500 μg/mL. Furthermore, they enhanced gene transfer, indicating their potential use as gene delivery vehicles for gene therapy in triple-negative breast cancer (TNBC). Martins et al. (2021) synthesized G4-G6 CDs@PAMAM nanohybrids via non-covalent interactions

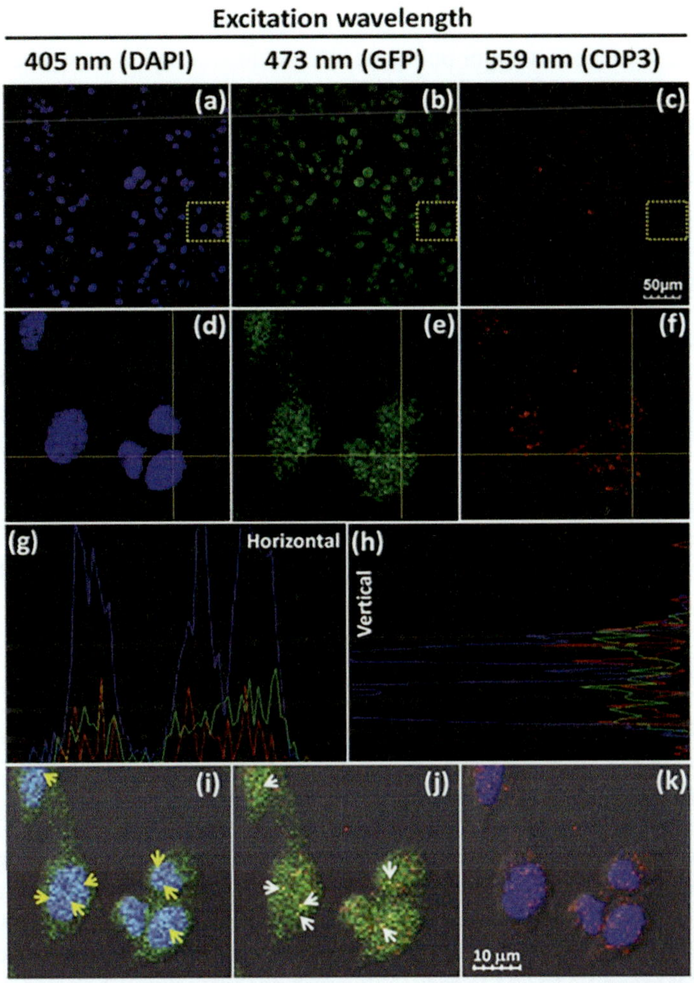

FIGURE 8.3 The study involved in vitro transfection of CDP3-RGD in MDA-MB-231 cells, accompanied by confocal fluorescence microscopy images at a wavelength of 405 nm. Replicated with permission (Ghosh et al., 2019).

and assessed their efficacy in DNA condensation and transport. The PicoGreen® experiment demonstrated that the NHs could condense pDNA more effectively than unmodified dendrimers. The research further validated their elevated transfection efficiency using HEK 293T cells, GFP, and fluorescence microscopy. The G5 NHs exhibited superior efficacy as delivery agents relative to earlier dendrimer generations. Wei et al. (2023) developed a nanocarrier using carbon NPs and G3 PAMAM dendrimers, which demonstrated long-wavelength emissive properties and the ability to encapsulate and deliver small interfering RNA for gene silencing in neuronal PC-12 cells.

8.3.3 Antimicrobial Activity

Antibiotic resistance is a major public health and healthcare system threat, and it is producing a broad variety of ailments. To tackle this, corporations and institutions must constantly study and create new solutions. Potentially effective against bacteria either alone or in tandem with antibiotics, carbon dot-dendrimer NH should the key to this mystery. To improve the antibacterial efficacy of low-generation PAMAM dendrimers, Ngu-Schwemlein et al. (2016) used CDs as a molecular scaffold. The antibacterial activity of the surface polyaminated CNDs scaffold was shown against a variety of bacteria, including those that are resistant to antibiotics as well as those that are not. Both CNDPAM1 and CNDPAM2, which are NHs combining CDs with dendrimers from PAMAM's first and zero generations, exhibited comparable selectivity and antibacterial activity. This suggests that CDs might help modulate the cationic densities of tiny polycationic amines so that they interact optimally with the anionic surfaces of bacterial membranes, hence increasing their antibacterial effectiveness. Because the NHs are able to penetrate bacterial membranes, the antibiotics (tetracycline and colistin) may be absorbed more quickly, leading to a faster reduction of bacterial growth. In addition, the NH system may be able to perform imaging and diagnostics thanks to the CNDs' intrinsic and enhanced fluorescence.

8.3.4 Sensors

The advancement of rapid and accurate detection instruments for particular analysis is a prominent scientific issue (Fan et al., 2023). A substantial portion of the research on nanohybrids including carbon dots and dendrimers concentrated on their prospective uses in sensing, namely for biological and chemical detection. NHs, sensitive, persistent, and precise, were created by combining dendrimer's surface activity with CDs' intrinsic fluorescence, reduced by FRET. These NHs regulate and target important analytes, such as anticoagulant heparin and chondroitin sulphate (CS), in cancer, myocardial infarction, and postoperative care. This technique uses dendrimer NHs of GQDs and PAMAM to reduce fluorescence intensity. When Hep and CS are added, they are strongly attached to PAMAM-Gu+, allowing them to be isolated from GQDs and restoring their intrinsic fluorescence. This fluorescence method offers a sensitive and rapid detection option for Hep or CS in pharmaceutical solutions (Li et al., 2015). A GQD-PAMAM nanohybrid modified gold screen-printed electrode was developed for the electrochemical detection of cardiac troponin I antibody (cTnI). The electrode was functionalized with 4-ATP and immobilized with GQDs and G3 PAMAM dendrimers. The antigen (cTnI) was captured by applying an anti-troponin I antibody. Bipolar and cyclic voltammetry were used to evaluate the changes. The Au/GQDs/PAMAM NHs connected to the biosensor could detect a minimum of 20 fg/mL of cardiac troponin I within 10 minutes, aiding in the risk assessment of myocardial infarction (Bhatnagar et al., 2017).

Hamd-Ghadareh et al. (2017) evaluated the immunosensing properties of CDs-AuNPs-PAMAM-antibody NHs for detecting the CA125 cancer marker. After modification with ssCA125DNA, the CA125 antibody was used to conjugate AuNP-PAMAM. The lowest detection limit was 0.5 fg/mL, and the immunosensor showed high sensitivity and specificity in ovarian cancer cell identification, indicating potential clinical use. Mohammedi et al.'s 2018 study developed an immunosensor to detect the CA 15–3 tumor antigen, using fluorescence resonance energy transfer (FRET). The C-dots and AuNPs were functionalized with the antigen, and the immunoassay was tested on blood samples and CA 15–3 extracts from breast MDA-MB-231 cancer cells, showing promising results. Campos et al. (2016b) developed chemical sensors for detecting chloroplatinate ions in platinum nanoparticle solutions using CQDs@ PAMAM dendrimer NH devices. The sensors enhanced green fluorescence and quenched chloroplatinate ions by 91.5%. The sensor had a sensitivity of 77.9 nM and a limit of detection (LOD) of 657.4 mM and a limit of quantification (LOQ) of 2.2 mM. A new sensor developed by Campos et al. (2016b) uses nanohybrids made from carbon quantum dots and G4 PAMAM dendrimers to detect nitroaromatic explosives. The target analyte is 4-chloro-2,6-dinitroaniline, a potent explosive initiator. The fluorescence quenching of CQDs@PAMAM conjugates enables the identification of this hazardous analyte, with detection limits and sensitivity measured at 2.6 and 111.6 mM, respectively.

8.4 CHALLENGES AND PERSPECTIVES

NHs made of carbon dots and dendrimers are challenging to prepare due to their complex synthesis and lack of repeatability. Despite increased research, issues remain, including the repeatability of carbon dots. A systematic methodology involving parameter changes like reaction time, temperature, and precursor concentration is proposed to improve control over carbon dot production and understand mechanistic features, with purification being a crucial component. The authors advocate for a definitive agreement on the nomenclature and categorization of carbon dots, and emphasize the importance of simplifying structures for large-scale synthesis and imaging capabilities. Big data and machine learning methodologies can enhance the properties of CDs and their NHs with dendrimers, improving their chemical, optical, and biological properties. This can optimize reaction conditions and expedite the synthesis process, thereby facilitating scale-up. The rapid development of NH materials requires increased investment in physical and human resources, as well as enhanced cooperation between academics and industry. By cultivating robust relationships, we can expedite the development of these materials and uncover novel and intriguing applications.

8.5 CONCLUSIONS

This book chapter explains the development of nanohybrid materials derived from carbon dots and dendrimers. Notwithstanding its promise, the domain remains little investigated. Diverse synthesis strategies are being investigated, including non-covalent methods, covalent techniques, casting, and biorecognition processes, to amalgamate both species. The characteristics of the NHs, whether as NPs or films, are influenced by both the synthesis process and the origin and preparation method of the original CDs, as well as the generation and type of dendrimers employed. Notably, the photoluminescent capabilities imparted by the carbon dots to the NH materials may be adjusted based on the synthetic method used and the creation of the dendrimer utilized. Enhanced efforts are required in characterization approaches to validate the NH nature of these novel materials and comprehend the interactions present within them. These endeavors will be essential for the applications examined for these materials, which show potential to enter the market and enhance people's lives.

REFERENCES

Bhatnagar, Deepika, Inderpreet Kaur, and Ashok Kumar. "Ultrasensitive cardiac troponin I antibody based nanohybrid sensor for rapid detection of human heart attack." *International Journal of Biological Macromolecules* 95 (2017): 505–510.

Campos, Bruno B., Rafael Contreras-Cáceres, Teresa J. Bandosz, José Jiménez-Jiménez, Enrique Rodríguez-Castellón, Joaquim C.G. Esteves da Silva, and Manuel Algarra. "Carbon dots as fluorescent sensor for detection of explosive nitrocompounds." *Carbon* 106 (2016a): 171–178.

Campos, Bruno B., María Moreno Oliva, Rafael Contreras-Cáceres, Enrique Rodriguez-Castellón, José Jiménez-Jiménez, Joaquim C.G. Esteves da Silva, and Manuel Algarra. "Carbon dots on based folic acid coated with PAMAM dendrimer as platform for Pt (IV) detection." *Journal of Colloid and Interface Science* 465 (2016b): 165–173.

Camacho, Cláudia S., Helena Tomás, and João Rodrigues. "Use of half-generation PAMAM dendrimers (G0. 5–G3. 5) with carboxylate end-groups to improve the DACHPtCl2 and 5-FU efficacy as anticancer drugs." *Molecules* 26, no. 10 (2021): 2924.

Camacho, Cláudia S., Marta Urgellés, Helena Tomás, Fernando Lahoz, and João Rodrigues. "New insights into the blue intrinsic fluorescence of oxidized PAMAM dendrimers considering their use as bionanomaterials." *Journal of Materials Chemistry B* 8, no. 45 (2020): 10314–10326.

de Boëver, Raphaël, Jason R. Town, Xu Li, and Jerome P. Claverie. "Carbon dots for carbon dummies: The quantum and the molecular questions among some others." *Chemistry–A European Journal* 28, no. 47 (2022): e202200748.

Deshmukh, Megha A., Sang-Joon Park, Byeong-Cheol Kang, and Tae-Jun Ha. "Carbon nanohybrids for advanced electronic applications." *Physica Status Solidi (A)* 217, no. 17 (2020a): 2000199.

Deshmukh, Megha A., Byeong-Cheol Kang, and Tae-Jun Ha. "Non-enzymatic electrochemical glucose sensors based on polyaniline/reduced-graphene-oxide nanocomposites functionalized with silver nanoparticles." *Journal of Materials Chemistry C* 8, no. 15 (2020b): 5112–5123.

Đorđević, Luka, Francesca Arcudi, Michele Cacioppo, and Maurizio Prato. "A multifunctional chemical toolbox to engineer carbon dots for biomedical and energy applications." *Nature Nanotechnology* 17, no. 2 (2022): 112–130.

Fan, Jiang, Lei Kang, Di Liu, and Sufeng Zhang. "Modification of carbon dots for metal-ions detection." *Chemistry Select* 8, no. 19 (2023): e202300062.

Farshidfar, Nima, Saba Fooladi, Mohammad Hadi Nematollahi, and Siavash Iravani. "Carbon dots with tissue engineering and regenerative medicine applications." *RSC Advances* 13, no. 21 (2023): 14517–14529.

Feng, Hao-Hui, Long Pang, Hai-Lin Cong, You-Qing Shen, and Bing Yu. "Preparation and application of fluorescence dendritic macromolecular nanoparticles." *Integrated Ferroelectrics* 197, no. 1 (2019): 99–110.

Ge, Guili, Lin Li, Dan Wang, Mingjian Chen, Zhaoyang Zeng, Wei Xiong, Xu Wu, and Can Guo. "Carbon dots: Synthesis, properties and biomedical applications." *Journal of Materials Chemistry B* 9, no. 33 (2021): 6553–6575.

Ghosh, Santanu, Krishanu Ghosal, S.K. Arif Mohammad, and Kishor Sarkar. "Dendrimer functionalized carbon quantum dot for selective detection of breast cancer and gene therapy." *Chemical Engineering Journal* 373 (2019): 468–484.

Hamd-Ghadareh, Somayeh, Abdollah Salimi, Fardin Fathi, and Saman Bahrami. "An amplified comparative fluorescence resonance energy transfer immunosensing of CA125 tumor marker and ovarian cancer cells using green and economic carbon dots for bio-applications in labeling, imaging and sensing." *Biosensors and Bioelectronics* 96 (2017): 308–316.

Janaszewska, Anna, Joanna Lazniewska, Przemysław Trzepiński, Monika Marcinkowska, and Barbara Klajnert-Maculewicz. "Cytotoxicity of dendrimers." *Biomolecules* 9, no. 8 (2019): 330.

Jeon, Jun-Young, Byeong-Cheol Kang, and Tae-Jun Ha. "Flexible pH sensors based on printed nanocomposites of single-wall carbon nanotubes and Nafion." *Applied Surface Science* 514 (2020): 145956.

Kang, Byeong-Cheol, Ban-Suk Park, and Tae-Jun Ha. "Highly sensitive wearable glucose sensor systems based on functionalized single-wall carbon nanotubes with glucose oxidase-nafion composites." *Applied Surface Science* 470 (2019): 13–18.

Karimi, Soheyla, and Hassan Namazi. "A photoluminescent folic acid-derived carbon dot functionalized magnetic dendrimer as a pH-responsive carrier for targeted doxorubicin delivery." *New Journal of Chemistry* 45, no. 14 (2021): 6397–6405.

Karimi, Soheyla, and Hassan Namazi. "Simple preparation of maltose-functionalized dendrimer/graphene quantum dots as a pH-sensitive biocompatible carrier for targeted delivery of doxorubicin." *International Journal of Biological Macromolecules* 156 (2020): 648–659.

Li, Dan, Yu Fan, Mingwu Shen, István Bányai, and Xiangyang Shi. "Design of dual drug-loaded dendrimer/carbon dot nanohybrids for fluorescence imaging and enhanced chemotherapy of cancer cells." *Journal of Materials Chemistry B* 7, no. 2 (2019): 277–285.

Li, Dan, Lizhou Lin, Yu Fan, Long Liu, Mingwu Shen, Rong Wu, Lianfang Du, and Xiangyang Shi. "Ultrasound-enhanced fluorescence imaging and chemotherapy of multidrug-resistant tumors using multifunctional dendrimer/carbon dot nanohybrids." *Bioactive Materials* 6, no. 3 (2021): 729–739.

Li, Yan, Hongcheng Sun, Fanping Shi, Nan Cai, Lehui Lu, and Xingguang Su. "Multi-positively charged dendrimeric nanoparticles induced fluorescence quenching of graphene quantum dots for heparin and chondroitin sulfate detection." *Biosensors and Bioelectronics* 74 (2015): 284–290.

Lin, T.N., M.R. Inciong, S.R. Santiago, C.W. Kao, G.W. Shu, C.T. Yuan, J.L. Shen, J.M. Yeh, and Y.W. Chen-Yang. "Electron injection from graphene quantum dots to poly (amido amine) dendrimers." *Applied Physics Letters* 108, no. 16 (2016).

Ma, Jin, Ke Kang, Yujia Zhang, Qiang Ying Yi, and Zhongwei Gu. "Detachable polyzwitterion-coated ternary nanoparticles based on peptide dendritic carbon dots for efficient drug delivery in cancer therapy." *ACS Applied Materials & Interfaces* 10, no. 50 (2018): 43923–43935.

Mandal, Saptarshi, and Prolay Das. "Are carbon dots worth the tremendous attention it is getting: Challenges and opportunities." *Applied Materials Today* 26 (2022): 101331.

Martins, Ivo, Helena Tomás, Fernando Lahoz, and João Rodrigues. "Engineered fluorescent carbon dots and G4-G6 PAMAM dendrimer nanohybrids for bioimaging and gene delivery." *Biomacromolecules* 22, no. 6 (2021): 2436–2450.

Matai, Ishita, Abhay Sachdev, and Packirisamy Gopinath. "Self-assembled hybrids of fluorescent carbon dots and PAMAM dendrimers for epirubicin delivery and intracellular imaging." *ACS Applied Materials & Interfaces* 7, no. 21 (2015): 11423–11435.

Mekuria, Shewaye Lakew, Zhijun Ouyang, Cong Song, João Rodrigues, Mingwu Shen, and Xiangyang Shi. "Dendrimer-based nanogels for cancer nanomedicine applications." *Bioconjugate Chemistry* 33, no. 1 (2021): 87–96.

Mohammadi, Somayeh, Abdollah Salimi, Somayeh Hamd-Ghadareh, Fardin Fathi, and Farzad Soleimani. "A FRET immunosensor for sensitive detection of CA 15-3 tumor marker in human serum sample and breast cancer cells using antibody functionalized luminescent carbon-dots and AuNPs-dendrimer aptamer as donor-acceptor pair." *Analytical Biochemistry* 557 (2018): 18–26.

Newkome, George R., and Carol Shreiner. "Dendrimers derived from 1→ 3 branching motifs." *Chemical Reviews* 110, no. 10 (2010): 6338–6442.

Ngu-Schwemlein, Maria, Suk Fun Chin, Ryan Hileman, Chris Drozdowski, Clint Upchurch, and April Hargrove. "Carbon nanodots as molecular scaffolds for development of antimicrobial agents." *Bioorganic & Medicinal Chemistry Letters* 26, no. 7 (2016): 1745–1749.

Pooresmaeil, Malihe, Hassan Namazi, and Roya Salehi. "Synthesis of photoluminescent glycodendrimer with terminal β-cyclodextrin molecules as a biocompatible pH-sensitive carrier for doxorubicin delivery." *Carbohydrate Polymers* 246 (2020): 116658.

Wang, Boyang, and Siyu Lu. "The light of carbon dots: From mechanism to applications." *Matter* 5, no. 1 (2022): 110–149.

Wang, Sihong, Jie Xu, Weichen Wang, Ging-Ji Nathan Wang, Reza Rastak, Francisco Molina-Lopez, Jong Won Chung et al. "Skin electronics from scalable fabrication of an intrinsically stretchable transistor array." *Nature* 555, no. 7694 (2018): 83–88.

Wei, Fangdi, Yuan Yao, Qiutong Chen, Jiamei Song, Zhen Xie, Li Ai, Guanhong Xu et al. "Dendrimer-modified carbon nanoparticles with excitation-independent long wavelength emission for siRNA delivery." *ACS Applied Nano Materials* 6, no. 2 (2023): 1083–1092.

Wu, Jun, Wei Xin, Yuhan Wu, Yuan Zhan, Jinhua Li, Jianying Wang, Shiqiang Huang, and Xianbao Wang. "Solid-state photoluminescent silicone-carbon dots/dendrimer composites for highly efficient luminescent solar concentrators." *Chemical Engineering Journal* 422 (2021): 130158.

Xu, Xiaoyou, Robert Ray, Yunlong Gu, Harry J. Ploehn, Latha Gearheart, Kyle Raker, and Walter A. Scrivens. "Electrophoretic analysis and purification of fluorescent single-walled carbon nanotube fragments." *Journal of the American Chemical Society* 126, no. 40 (2004): 12736–12737.

Yoon, Saemon, Su Ryong Ha, Taeho Moon, Sang Mun Jeong, Tae-Jun Ha, Hyosung Choi, and Dong-Won Kang. "Carbon nanotubes embedded poly (3, 4-ethylenedioxythiophene): Poly (styrenesulfonate) hybrid hole collector for inverted planar perovskite solar cells." *Journal of Power Sources* 435 (2019): 226765.

You, Rui, Yu-Qing Liu, Yi-Long Hao, Dong-Dong Han, Yong-Lai Zhang, and Zheng You. "Laser fabrication of graphene-based flexible electronics." *Advanced Materials* 32, no. 15 (2020): 1901981.

Zong, Jie, Xiaoling Yang, Adrian Trinchi, Simon Hardin, Ivan Cole, Yihua Zhu, Chunzhong Li, Tim Muster, and Gang Wei. "Photoluminescence enhancement of carbon dots by gold nanoparticles conjugated via PAMAM dendrimers." *Nanoscale* 5, no. 22 (2013): 11200–11206.

9 Semiconductor-Based Nanohybrids for Biomedical Applications

Taniya Sribhashyam

9.1 INTRODUCTION

Nanotechnology refers to a field of science and engineering that focuses on the design, creation, and use of materials, structures, devices, and systems by controlling processes at the nanoscale level (a billionth of a meter). It involves understanding and using phenomena that occur at this tiny scale for various practical applications. The concept of nanotechnology was first introduced in 1959 by physicist Richard Feynman, who gave a talk about building things at the atomic and molecular level (Roco, 2003). It is now considered one of the most promising technologies of the 21st century, and researchers are exploring it as a new approach in medical research. It is expected to bring a new era of growth and progress, as shown by the significant increase in public funding for its research and development over the past decade (Gonzalez et al., 2013).

Nanomedicine involves many areas of science and technology that work together to improve healthcare. It includes the diagnosis and treatment of diseases, ways to prevent illnesses, pain relief methods, improving overall health, using nanoscale techniques to treat injuries, and providing new treatment options for different medical conditions (Vaishampayan et al., 2023).

Today, nanomedicine is one of the most important applications of nanotechnology. It focuses on developing tiny medical tools at the nanoscale to improve healthcare systems. This approach helps us better understand how the human body works and supports the fight against serious diseases like cancer and heart conditions. Nanomedicine is especially important in areas like medical imaging, disease diagnosis, tissue repair, and creating safer, more effective, and affordable drug delivery systems. These systems are designed to target specific areas in the body, which helps improve treatment results and reduce side effects and toxicity (Dobrovolskaia, 2015).

In nanomedicine, nanohybrids are advanced materials made by combining organic and inorganic components at the nanoscale. This combination gives them multiple useful functions for medical applications. Their special physical and chemical properties – such as a large surface area compared to their volume, adjustable optical features, and ability to respond to different conditions – make them useful for advanced drug delivery, medical imaging, and combined treatment methods (Cheng et al., 2023).

DOI: 10.1201/9781003563723-9

In recent years, combining semiconductor nanomaterials with other functional components has led to the creation of semiconductor-based nanohybrids, opening new possibilities in biomedical research and treatments (Y. Chen et al., 2020). Semiconductor-based nanohybrids are materials made by combining semiconductor nanoparticles with other useful components like metals, metal oxides, or organic molecules (Ratner, 2019). These nanohybrids have adjustable electronic, optical, and surface properties, making them highly useful in healthcare. Researchers are increasingly exploring their potential in various areas, such as disease diagnosis, targeted drug delivery, bioimaging, photothermal therapy, and biosensing. Their ability to perform multiple functions and interact safely with the human body makes them ideal for advanced medical applications (Y. Chen et al., 2020).

9.1.1 Core Innovations in Biomedical Fields

Targeted drug delivery systems use nanohybrids to carry medicines and release them directly at the site of the disease. For example, mesoporous silica nanoparticles modified with ligands help control the release of cancer drugs like doxorubicin, reducing side effects on healthy tissues. Similarly, plasmonic platinum nanoclusters improve targeted drug delivery in breast cancer treatment, making the therapy more effective and lowering overall toxicity in the body. Theranostic systems combine diagnosis and treatment in one approach. For example, gadolinium-doped silica hybrids enable real-time MRI monitoring while delivering drugs to treat bone metastasis. Also, nanozymes made from noble metals act like enzymes and carry therapeutic agents, helping to effectively treat heart diseases (Malik et al., 2023).

Advanced treatments include photothermal therapy (PTT), which uses tungsten disulfide–iron oxide hybrids to destroy tumors when exposed to near-infrared light. Carbon nanohybrids, such as modified graphene oxide, help repair tissues by mimicking the structure of the natural extracellular matrix. They are especially useful in bone and nerve tissue engineering (Singh, 2024).

9.1.2 Types of Nanohybrids and Their Customization

Recent progress in microfluidic techniques and surface modification has made it possible to design nanohybrids with more control and precision. These methods help scientists create materials that work better inside the human body.

There are different types of nanohybrids based on how they are made and what they are made of. They are:

9.1.2.1 Metal–Organic Frameworks (MOFs)

Metal-organic frameworks (MOFs) are crystal-like materials with tiny pores, formed by the self-assembly of metal ions or clusters and organic molecules connected through special bonds. Their unique structure makes them very useful in medicine, especially when combined with nanoparticles to form MOF-based nanohybrids. These hybrids make use of MOFs' key features – such as large surface area, adjustable pore size, and strong chemical stability – along with the added benefits of nanoparticles for improved medical use (S. Wang et al., 2017).

These hybrid materials offer many advantages. They have a very large surface area (over 7,000 m^2/g), which helps them carry large amounts of drugs or genes. MOFs can also break down safely in the body because of their weak metal-ligand bonds, making them biodegradable. Another key benefit is their dual functionality – they can be specially designed for specific medical uses, like releasing insulin in response to glucose levels (Wu and Yang, 2017).

MOF-based nanohybrids show great promise in medical applications. For example, gadolinium-doped Zr-MOFs can be used both as MRI contrast agents and drug carriers, delivering doxorubicin and reducing tumors by up to 92% in mice. Some combination therapies use hybrids like Fe_3O_4@MIL-100(Fe), which combine chemotherapy with sound-based treatment by creating reactive oxygen species when exposed to ultrasound. MOF-based nanohybrids are also useful against infections – for instance, silver-based MOFs loaded with vancomycin have been very effective in destroying MRSA biofilms (Wu and Yang, 2017).

To make MOF nanohybrids work better, their surfaces are often changed. For example, PEGylation helps them stay in the blood longer – from 2 to 18 hours – by avoiding the immune system. This makes treatments more effective. Adding aptamers, which are targeting molecules, helps the nanohybrids reach tumors more accurately, improving drug delivery. In the future, AI may help design better metal-ligand combinations, while safer biodegradable materials can reduce side effects. Also, new systems may combine both imaging and therapy in one platform. These improvements make MOF nanohybrids powerful tools for accurate and effective treatment in modern medicine (S. Wang et al., 2017).

9.1.2.2 Semiconductor-Based Nanohybrids

Quantum dots (QDs) and metal oxides are becoming important tools in medical imaging and treatment because of their unique optical and electronic properties. For example, quantum dots like CdSe/ZnS core-shell particles linked with folic acid have shown high accuracy in detecting early-stage ovarian cancer using near-infrared (NIR-II) imaging, showing their value in advanced diagnostics. Metal oxide-based hybrids, such as TiO_2–graphene composites, are improving photodynamic therapy for melanoma. These hybrids produce much more reactive oxygen species (ROS) under UV light than TiO_2 alone, which makes the treatment more effective.

New techniques are expanding the use of semiconductor nanohybrids in medicine. For example, WO_3–C_3N_4 nanosheets use 660 nm light to create hole-electron pairs that damage the DNA of drug-resistant bacteria, offering a new way to fight infections. Electroresponsive systems, like polyaniline-coated ZnO nanowires, release drugs when triggered by electricity, making them useful for targeted treatment of brain diseases like Parkinson's. Another example is silicon–gold nanorods (Si–AuNRs), which combine strong heat generation (42% efficiency) with siRNA delivery. They reduce EGFR expression in brain cancer (glioblastoma) by 78% and also support real-time tracking through photoacoustic imaging.

These semiconductor nanohybrids combine advanced material properties with medical applications, helping to improve precision medicine. They support better imaging, targeted treatments, and multi-purpose therapy systems. Their flexibility and strong performance show great promise for solving complex health problems in the future.

9.1.2.3 Plasmonic Metal-Based Nanohybrids

These advanced materials use localized surface plasmon resonance (LSPR) for applications in photothermal therapy (PTT) and diagnostics through surface enhanced Raman scattering (SERS). They are designed to make use of the unique optical properties of metals like gold and silver in medicine. A key feature is photothermal conversion, where gold nanoshells can raise temperatures by up to 55°C when exposed to an 808 nm laser, making them effective for tumor treatment. Additionally, SERS uses the enhanced electromagnetic field around plasmonic nanostructures to detect biomolecules at extremely low concentrations, enabling highly sensitive diagnostics (Malhotra and Ali, 2018).

Advanced systems show how flexible plasmonic nanohybrids can be. For example, Pt–protein nanoclusters with HER2 antibodies effectively shrink tumors in HER2-positive breast cancer using NIR-II photothermal treatment. Similarly, Au–MOF composites, like Au@ZIF-8 core-shell structures, contain immunoadjuvants that increase dendritic cell activation by 12 times, boosting the effectiveness of cancer vaccines. Their potential for multiple uses is also clear – Ag–Fe_3O_4 "nanorattles" can detect circulating tumor cells with high precision using SERS, while Au–Cu_2O Janus particles kill 99.9% of *Pseudomonas aeruginosa* under 650 nm light by generating reactive oxygen species and releasing Cu^+ ions (Aldosari et al., 2023).

These plasmonic nanohybrids combine both diagnostic and therapeutic abilities, making them key to precision medicine. Their ability to mix photothermal treatment, molecular sensing, and immune system modulation shows their important role in solving complex medical problems (Malhotra and Ali, 2018).

9.2 SYNTHESIS OF NANOHYBRIDS

The synthesis of semiconductor-based nanohybrids is an important part of nanotechnology, allowing for advanced uses in electronics, energy, and medicine. These nanohybrids can be made in two main ways: the bottom-up approach, where structures are built step by step from atoms or molecules, and the top-down approach, where larger materials are broken down into nanoscale structures with specific functions.

9.2.1 Bottom-Up Approach

Bottom-up approaches can be divided into different methods like colloidal synthesis, the sol-gel method, and hydrothermal/solvothermal synthesis.

9.2.1.1 Collodial Synthesis

Colloidal synthesis is a powerful and flexible method used to create semiconductor nanohybrids, allowing precise control over their size, shape, and composition. The hot-injection method is commonly used to make CdSe/ZnS core/shell quantum dots (QDs). This technique produces uniform nanoparticles with adjustable optical properties, sharp emission peaks, and high photoluminescence efficiency (PLQY), making them ideal for use in bioimaging, sensing, and optoelectronics (Liu et al., 2019). Recently, lead halide perovskite nanocrystals (NCs), like $CsPbBr_3$, have attracted a lot of interest because of their excellent optoelectronic properties, such as very high PLQYs, wide color tunability, and strong resistance to defects. Improvements in surface ligand design and protective coatings have also made these nanocrystals more stable in water and body-like environments, increasing their potential use in biomedical imaging, combined therapy, and diagnostics and LEDs (Tsai et al., 2021).

9.2.1.2 Sol-Gel Synthesis

The sol-gel method is a flexible and widely used chemical technique for making oxide-based nanohybrids. It allows control over features like porosity, surface area, and surface chemistry. This bottom-up process involves turning a liquid mixture (sol) into a gel-like structure (gel), which is then carefully dried and heated to form solid materials. For instance, TiO_2@SiO_2 core-shell nanostructures, where the outer silica (SiO_2) layer improves biocompatibility and provides many silanol (Si-OH) groups. These groups are useful for attaching drugs and enabling their controlled release (Liu et al., 2020). The sol-gel method is especially useful for creating mesoporous structures, which have high surface areas and interconnected pores that improve drug-loading capacity (Hu et al., 2017).

9.2.1.3 Hydrothermal/Solvothermal Synthesis

Hydrothermal and solvothermal synthesis are powerful and flexible methods used to create highly crystalline nanohybrids. These techniques involve chemical reactions carried out at high temperatures and pressures inside a sealed container called an autoclave. By adjusting factors like the type of solvent (water for hydrothermal, non-water-based for solvothermal), temperature, pressure, and chemical ingredients, researchers can control the shape, structure, and composition of the resulting nanomaterials. A good example is ZnO-Au nanohybrids, where gold nanoparticles (Au NPs) are combined with zinc oxide (ZnO) structures. These hybrids use the special light-absorbing ability of gold, known as localized surface plasmon resonance (LSPR), to boost light absorption and produce reactive oxygen species (ROS). This makes them highly useful in cancer treatment, antibacterial therapies, and biosensing applications (Y. Zhang et al., 2012).

9.2.2 Top-Down Approach

Top-down approaches can be divided into different methods like mechanical exfoliation and the thermal decomposition method

9.2.2.1 Mechanical Exfoliation

Mechanical exfoliation is a useful top-down method for producing high-quality two-dimensional (2D) materials with special optoelectronic and biomedical properties. For example, Liu et al. (2020) showed that using sound waves (sonication) to help exfoliate MoS_2-WS_2 heterostructures creates very thin nanosheets with improved ability to convert light into heat. This makes them promising for use in cancer treatment (Liu et al., 2020). Black phosphorus (BP) nanosheets emerged as a promising material for cancer treatment because they are biocompatible, biodegradable, and can effectively convert near-infrared (NIR) light into heat. Recent research has shown that BP nanosheets can be modified with targeting molecules, chemotherapy drugs, or light-activated agents to enable multiple types of cancer therapy. These BP-based systems can turn NIR light into heat for photothermal therapy (PTT), while also delivering drugs or producing reactive oxygen species (ROS) for combined treatments like chemo-photothermal therapy or photodynamic therapy (PDT) (Tao et al., 2020).

9.2.2.2 Thermal Decomposition Method

Thermal decomposition is a new and effective method for synthesizing stable, uniform (monodispersed) metal nanoparticles. It is considered one of the most practical techniques for producing these types of nanoparticles. This method has emerged as a powerful technique for synthesizing high-quality semiconductor nanohybrids for biomedical applications. Wang et al. (2024) developed a thermal decomposition method to synthesize bimetallic Au-Pd nanohybrids with adjustable metal ratios. Their study shows that this simple technique allows precise control over the composition of the nanostructures, leading to improved catalytic performance. The enhanced efficiency in catalytic reactions is due to the combined electronic and structural (geometric) effects between the gold (Au) and palladium (Pd) atoms.

9.3 OTHER SYNTHESIS METHODS

9.3.1 Green Synthesis

Green synthesis, also known as biosynthesis, has become a popular eco-friendly method for making semiconductor nanohybrids. It uses natural plant extracts, microorganisms, or biomolecules instead of harmful chemicals. This approach reduces energy use, avoids toxic substances, and often improves the biocompatibility of the materials. Because of these benefits, green synthesis is especially useful for biomedical and environmental applications. El Golli A and his co-workers (2024) explored the green synthesis of zinc oxide (ZnO) nanohybrids using Moringa oleifera leaf extract as a reducing and stabilizing agent, demonstrating their enhanced photocatalytic activity in degrading methylene blue (MB) under sunlight irradiation. The biosynthesized ZnO nanohybrids exhibited superior degradation efficiency compared to conventional ZnO nanoparticles, attributed to their reduced particle size, increased surface area, and improved charge separation facilitated by phytochemicals from Moringa oleifera. The research highlights the potential of plant-mediated synthesis in producing eco-friendly and cost-effective photocatalysts for wastewater treatment (El Golli et al., 2023).

9.3.2 Biomineralization

Biomineralization, inspired by natural processes, uses living organisms like bacteria, diatoms, and proteins to form inorganic semiconductor nanostructures under gentle conditions. It offers special benefits for creating bio-integrated hybrid materials and supports the development of eco-friendly nanotechnology. The study by Y.

Zhang et al. (2024) introduces a new method for creating Fe_3O_4/ZnO nanohybrids using magnetotactic bacteria (MTB), which naturally produce magnetite (Fe_3O_4) nanoparticles inside their cells. The researchers grew these bacteria in an iron-rich environment, allowing them to form uniform Fe_3O_4 crystals with specific sizes and magnetic properties. These naturally made magnetite particles were then combined with ZnO using a gentle chemical process to create a heterostructured nanohybrid. The resulting (Fe_3O_4)/ZnO nanocomposites showed strong photocatalytic activity under visible light, effectively breaking down pollutants like methylene blue and tetracycline in water (Y. Zhang et al., 2024).

9.4 CHARACTERISTICS OF SEMICONDUCTOR NANOHYBRIDS

9.4.1 Size of Semiconductor Nanohybrids

Particle size is one of the most important factors when studying semiconductor nanohybrids. It helps determine how big the particles are, how they are spread out, and whether they fall under the micro or nanoscale range. To measure particle size and distribution, scientists often use electron microscopy. Images from scanning electron microscopes (SEM) or transmission electron microscopes (TEM) are commonly used to analyze the size of individual particles and their clusters. For solid bulk samples, laser diffraction techniques are used. In the case of liquid samples, methods like photon correlation spectroscopy and centrifugation are applied to measure particle size. However, for particles in the gas phase, it is usually difficult or not practical to use imaging techniques. Instead, a scanning mobility particle sizer (SMPS) is preferred because it provides fast and accurate results (Marsalek, 2014).

9.4.2 Surface Area of Semiconductor Nanohybrids

Surface area is an important factor to consider when studying semiconductor nanohybrids. The ratio of surface area to volume plays a key role in determining their properties and performance. One of the most common methods used to measure surface area is BET analysis (Hwang and Barron, 2021). In the liquid phase, surface area can be measured using a simple titration method, but this process is slow and time consuming. Therefore, nuclear magnetic resonance (NMR) spectroscopy is often used instead. To measure the surface area of semiconductor nanohybrids in the gas phase, instruments like the differential mobility analyzer (DMA) and a modified scanning mobility particle sizer (SMPS) are used.

9.4.3 Composition of Semiconductor Nanohybrids

The purity and performance of semiconductor nanohybrids are closely linked to their chemical or elemental composition. If there are too many unwanted or secondary elements present, it can lower the efficiency of the nanohybrids and may also cause side reactions or contamination during processing. To check the composition, a common method used is X-ray photoelectron spectroscopy (XPS) (Greczynski and Hultman, 2021). In some cases, the nanohybrids are first chemically digested and then analyzed using wet chemical methods such as mass spectrometry, atomic emission spectroscopy, or ion chromatography. For nanohybrids in the gas phase, the particles can be collected using filters or electrostatic methods, and then examined using either spectrometric or wet chemical techniques (Thangadurai and Islam, 2022).

9.4.4 Optical Characteristics

In semiconductor nanohybrids, optical properties – especially bandgap tuning and exciton lifetime – are very important as they directly affect how these materials behave under light. These properties determine how efficiently nanohybrids can absorb and emit light, making them valuable for applications in optoelectronics, photocatalysis, and solar energy conversion (photovoltaics) (Tang et al., 2018).

Bandgap tuning involves adjusting the energy gap between a material's valence and conduction bands to control its light absorption properties. Techniques such as UV-Vis diffuse reflectance spectroscopy (DRS) and photoluminescence (PL) spectroscopy help analyze these optical features by revealing details about the material's electronic structure. By modifying the composition, particle size, or surface chemistry of nanohybrids – like quantum dots, metal-semiconductor systems, or perovskite-based materials – the bandgap can be precisely tailored. This enables improved performance in applications such as solar cells, LEDs, and photocatalysts by enhancing light absorption or emission in targeted wavelength ranges (Edelstein and Cammarata, 1996).

Exciton lifetime is another important optical property and is usually studied using time-resolved fluorescence spectroscopy. It helps us understand how long charge carriers (electrons and holes) exist before they recombine. This gives valuable information about the efficiency and behavior of nanomaterials under light. In semiconductor nanohybrids, exciton lifetime can be affected by various factors such as the presence of interfaces, structural defects, or added materials like gold (Au) or silver (Ag) nanoparticles. These components can create new pathways for energy to be released, such as through energy transfer, charge separation, or non-radiative decay (Edelstein and Cammarata, 1996).

9.5 PROPERTIES OF SEMICONDUCTOR NANOHYBRIDS

Semiconductor nanohybrids have different properties that can be categorized into physical and chemical properties.

9.5.1 Physical Properties

Semiconductor nanohybrids have special properties that allow them to control light absorption, glow when exposed to light, and enhance light interactions. These features are important for technologies like solar panels, LEDs, and optoelectronics. They also have mechanical properties like flexibility, strength, and stretchability, making them useful for flexible electronics. Additionally, their interaction with water, stability in suspension, and sedimentation affect their use in coatings, sensors, and biomedical systems. With excellent electrical and magnetic properties, they are perfect for transistors, energy storage, spintronics, and heat management in modern electronics.

9.5.2 Chemical Properties

The chemical stability, reactivity, and surface characteristics of semiconductor nanohybrids determine how well they perform in different conditions. They must be carefully managed to prevent damage from moisture, temperature, light, or oxidation, especially for uses in photocatalysis, chemical sensors, and environmental cleanup. It can be designed to have antibacterial, antifungal, and photocatalytic properties, making them useful for medical devices, water purification, and antimicrobial coatings. Their resistance to fire, corrosion, and their ability to undergo chemical reactions also make them suitable for use in energy storage devices like batteries and supercapacitors, as well as in protective coatings.

9.6 BIOMEDICAL APPLICATIONS

Semiconductor nanohybrids are tiny particles that combine metals and organic material that help medicine by delivering drugs precisely, finding diseases early, scanning the body clearly, fighting germs, and treating cancer safely as shown in Figure 9.1. They work better with fewer side effects than regular treatments.

The diagram highlights five key applications. First, they are used in drug delivery, acting as tiny carriers to transport drugs directly to a targeted site in the body, which

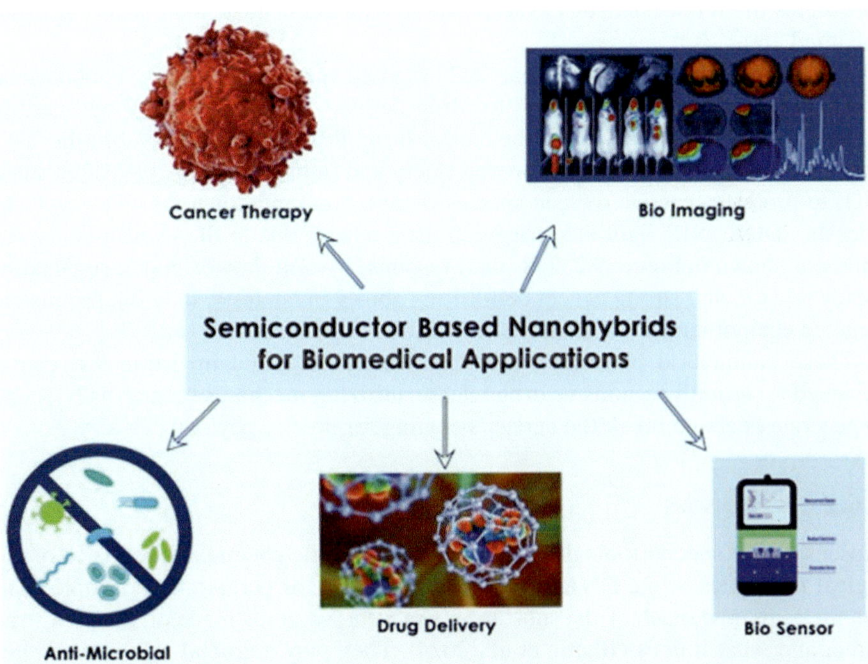

FIGURE 9.1 This image provides a summary of the various biomedical applications of semiconductor-based nanohybrids. These are advanced materials that combine the properties of semiconductors with other materials on a tiny, nanometer scale.

can increase effectiveness and reduce side effects. Second, their unique optical and electronic properties make them useful for bio-imaging, allowing scientists and doctors to visualize biological processes, tissues, and diseases with high resolution. They can also function as biosensors, detecting specific biological molecules like proteins or DNA to diagnose diseases or monitor health. Third, they are used in cancer therapy, often for targeted treatment that can destroy cancer cells with minimal harm to healthy tissue. Lastly, their ability to produce reactive species makes them effective as antimicrobials.

9.6.1 Drug Delivery System

In recent years, semiconductor nanohybrids – such as quantum dots, metal oxide hybrids, and carbon-semiconductor composites – have become important in medicine. They have special optical, electronic, and catalytic properties that help improve how well drugs work in the body. These nanohybrids make it easier for drugs to reach the right place, stay in the body longer, and be released in a controlled way. By combining semiconductors with organic or inorganic materials (which can be natural, synthetic, or similar to biological materials), they make treatments more effective. They also allow doctors to track the treatment in real time using fluorescent or photoacoustic imaging (Lu et al., 2019). These can be designed to react to external signals like light, magnetic fields, or changes in pH. This helps them release drugs exactly where they are needed, such as in tumors or inflamed areas.

Zhang and his team in the year 2023 created mesoporous TiO_2 nanoparticles coated with polydopamine (PDA) for drug delivery triggered by UV and near-infrared (NIR) light. They loaded the cancer drug doxorubicin (DOX) into the TiO_2 pores, while the PDA coating improved safety and light absorption. UV light caused TiO_2 to produce reactive oxygen species (ROS), breaking down the PDA shell and releasing DOX. NIR light also triggered drug release due to PDA's heat-generating ability as shown in Figure 9.2. This dual-response system showed good drug loading, steady release, and strong cancer cell-killing ability in lab tests, showing promise for targeted chemotherapy (X. Zhang et al., 2023).

These nanohybrid platforms, many of which are listed in **Table 9.1**, can be designed for stimuli-responsive drug release, utilizing mechanisms such as NIR light to generate heat and break the carrier's coating for precise payload delivery.

9.6.2 Biosensors

Biosensors are special tools designed to detect specific chemical substances or biological molecules – like DNA, proteins, genes, cells, or germs – in a sample. They can measure how much of the substance is present, what it's made of, how it's structured, and what it does (Bhatia et al., 2024). They play a crucial role in accurately detecting and analyzing these target molecules, making them essential in fields such as medical diagnostics, environmental monitoring, food safety, and biotechnology. These systems combine biological detection components, such as antibodies or enzymes, with transducers that translate biological interactions into quantifiable

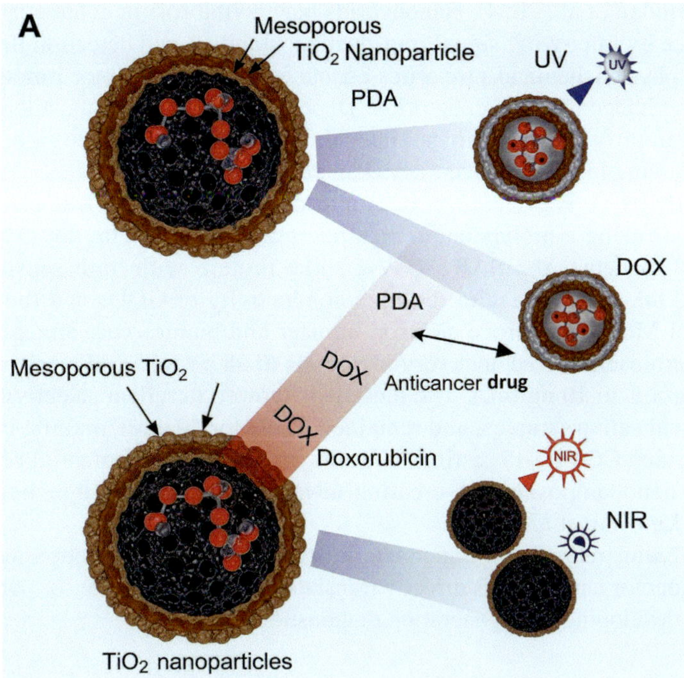

FIGURE 9.2 This image illustrates a method for delivering a drug called doxorubicin using mesoporous titanium dioxide (TiO_2) nanoparticles. These nanoparticles have a porous structure, which allows them to be loaded with the doxorubicin, a common anticancer drug. The process involves coating the drug-loaded nanoparticles with a material called polydopamine (PDA). This coating acts as a protective shell, preventing the drug from being released prematurely. The final step shows the drug being released from the nanoparticles. This can be triggered by external stimuli, such as ultraviolet (UV) light or near-infrared (NIR) light. When exposed to either UV or NIR light, the PDA coating breaks down, releasing the doxorubicin to target cancer cells. This method offers a targeted approach to drug delivery, potentially reducing the side effects of chemotherapy.

TABLE 9.1
Includes Various Nanohybrid Materials, the Drugs they Carry, and Their Specific Target Applications

S. No	Nanohybrid Material	Drug Loaded	Target Application
1.	Quantum Dot-Polymer	Doxorubicin, siRNA	Cancer Therapy, Imaging
2.	Metal Oxide-Graphene	Curcumin, Paclitaxel	Anti-inflammatory, Tumor Targeting
3.	Carbon Dot-Mesoporous Silica	Insulin, Antivirals	Diabetes, Infectious Diseases
5.	Perovskite-Lipid	Gene Therapeutics	Gene Delivery, Photodynamic Therapy
6.	MoS_2-PEG Nanosheets	Cisplatin, Antibiotics	Chemotherapy, Bacterial Infections

signals (Hemdan et al., 2024). Nanohybrids play a vital role in enhancing biosensor performance by improving signal transduction, stability, and detection limits. Their distinctive physicochemical properties enable efficient bioreceptor immobilization, leading to enhanced target recognition. Depending on their composition, nanomaterials can amplify electrochemical, optical, thermal, and magnetic signals, significantly improving biosensing accuracy (Pan et al., 2020).

The study by L. Wang et al. (2024) introduced a new label-free electrochemical biosensor using a molybdenum disulfide-graphene quantum dot (MoS_2-GQD) nanohybrid to detect the SARS-CoV-2 spike protein with high sensitivity. The nanohybrid takes advantage of the high conductivity of GQDs and the large surface area of MoS_2 to improve electron transfer and biomolecule attachment. This allowed the biosensor to detect very low levels (0.38 pg/mL) and work over a wide range (1 pg/mL to 10 ng/mL). The biosensor showed excellent selectivity, worked well with real saliva samples, and remained stable for 30 days, making it a promising tool for fast COVID-19 testing. The study highlights the potential of 2D material-based nanocomposites for creating advanced sensors for infectious disease detection (L. Wang et al., 2024).

Table 9.2 illustrates that unique material composition and detection mechanisms of semiconductor nanohybrids directly translate to enhanced biosensor performance, crucial for developing next-generation diagnostic tools.

TABLE 9.2
Compares Key Properties of Semiconductor Nanohybrids and Their Applications in Biosensors

S. No	Property	Semiconductor Nanohybrids	Biosensor Applications
1.	Material Composition	Combination of semiconductors (e.g., CdS, TiO_2, ZnO) with metals, carbon, or polymers.	Enhanced sensitivity due to high surface area and tunable electronic properties.
2.	Detection Mechanism	Optical (fluorescence, plasmonics), electrochemical, or field-effect sensing.	Used for detecting biomolecules (DNA, proteins, glucose, pathogens) via signal amplification.
3.	Sensitivity	Ultra-high sensitivity due to quantum confinement and plasmonic effects.	Enables detection at low concentrations (e.g., fM levels for biomarkers).
5.	Response Time	Fast electron transfer and signal transduction.	Real-time monitoring in medical diagnostics and environmental sensing.
6.	Selectivity	Functionalized with biorecognition elements (antibodies, aptamers, enzymes).	Specific detection of target analytes with minimal cross-reactivity.
7.	Stability and Durability	Improved stability via hybrid structures (e.g., graphene-semiconductor hybrids).	Long-term usage in implantable or wearable biosensors.

9.6.3 Cancer Therapy

Semiconductor nanohybrids are bringing big changes to cancer treatment by combining imaging and therapy in one powerful system. These nanohybrids are usually made of semiconductor nanoparticles (like quantum dots, silicon, or metal oxides) mixed with organic or metallic materials. They help deliver cancer treatment more accurately and effectively using methods such as photodynamic therapy (PDT), photothermal therapy (PTT), and smart drug delivery that respond to specific triggers (Bogdan et al., 2017). For example, nanohybrids made with materials like TiO_2 or ZnO can produce harmful reactive oxygen species (ROS) when exposed to light, which can kill cancer cells during PDT. On the other hand, nanohybrids that include gold, graphene, or carbon nanotubes can absorb NIR light and turn it into heat. This heat can destroy tumors through PTT while causing less harm to healthy tissue as shown in Figure 9.3 (Bisht and Rayamajhi, 2016). In 2023, Jundong Shao and his team developed an easy top-down method to create titanium nitride quantum dots (Ti_2N QDs), a new type of nitride-based MXene with great potential for cancer treatment. These very small quantum dots (about 5 nanometers in size) showed excellent ability to convert light into heat in both the first (NIR-I, 808 nm; 48.62%) and second (NIR-II, 1064 nm; 45.51%) near-infrared light ranges. This makes them perfect for photothermal therapy (PTT) using two different wavelengths (Shao et al., 2020). Lab tests and animal studies showed that the Ti_2N QDs are safe for the body (biocompatible), give strong photoacoustic imaging signals, and work well at killing tumors through PTT. The quantum dots quickly gathered in tumors within 4 hours after injection, allowing for precise imaging and treatment using both NIR-I and NIR-II

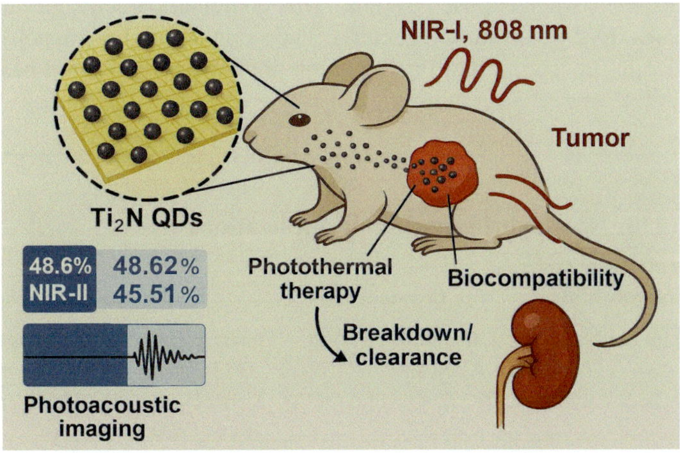

FIGURE 9.3 This diagram illustrates the use of titanium nitride quantum dots (Ti_2N QDs) for cancer therapy in a mouse model. The Ti_2N QDs are administered to the mouse, where they accumulate in the tumor tissue. A key feature of these quantum dots is their ability to generate heat when exposed to near-infrared light (NIR-I, specifically at a wavelength of 808 nm). This process is known as photothermal therapy (PTT). The heat generated by the QDs selectively destroys the tumor cells while minimizing damage to surrounding healthy tissue.

light. Importantly, the QDs also broke down safely in the body and were cleared through the kidneys, reducing the risk of long-term side effects while keeping the treatment stable and effective (Shao et al., 2023).

The diagram also shows the use of photoacoustic imaging, which uses sound waves created by light to visualize the quantum dots and monitor their distribution within the body. The results show high absorption percentages at both NIR-I and NIR-II wavelengths, indicating the QDs are effective. Finally, the diagram highlights that these nanoparticles are biocompatible and can be broken down and cleared from the body, showing a promising and safe application for cancer treatment.

Table 9.3 shows that combining semiconductors with other materials like metals or polymers results in versatile nanohybrids. These combinations can be used for many different cancer treatments, including hyperthermia and making tumors more responsive to radiation or immunotherapy.

9.6.4 Antimicrobial

Semiconductor nanohybrids have shown great potential in fighting harmful microbes. These materials can generate reactive oxygen species (ROS) when exposed to light, which helps in killing bacteria and viruses. Their high surface area and unique properties make them effective against a wide range of pathogens. They are being explored for use in wound dressings, water purification, and coating surfaces in hospitals to reduce infections (Yan et al., 2023).

A 2020 study focused on using graphene-based semiconductor nanohybrids – graphene-TiO_2 and graphene-ZnO – for medical use. These materials combine graphene's large surface area and fast charge transfer with the antibacterial effects of TiO_2 and ZnO when exposed to light. This combination helps produce reactive oxygen species (ROS) that can kill bacteria. The study found these nanohybrids were very effective in preventing biofilm formation and promoting wound healing. They

TABLE 9.3
Semiconductor Nanohybrids and Their Applications

S. No	Semiconductor Nanohybrid	Components	Cancer Therapy Application
1.	Quantum Dot-Metal NPs	CdSe/ZnS QDs + Au/Ag NPs	Imaging-guided photothermal therapy (PTT), photosensitizer delivery
2.	Metal Oxide-Polymer	TiO_2/ZnO + PLGA/PEG	Light-activated drug delivery, oxidative stress-induced apoptosis
3.	Carbon-Based Hybrids	Graphene QDs + MoS_2	Photothermal ablation, chemo-phototherapy (e.g., doxorubicin loading)
5.	Perovskite Nanocrystals	$CsPbBr_3$ + Lipid Coating	Tumor microenvironment sensing, radiation sensitization
6.	Silicon-Based Hybrids	Porous Si + Fe_3O_4 NPs	Magnetic hyperthermia, chemo-immunotherapy (e.g., siRNA co-delivery)

TABLE 9.4
Overview of Different Semiconductor Nanohybrids, Their Nanostructure Types and Their Antimicrobial Activities

S. No	Semiconductor Nanohybrid	Nanostructure Type	Antimicrobial Activity
1.	ZnO-TiO_2 nanocomposite	Core-shell nanoparticles	Antibacterial (*E. coli*, *S. aureus*)
2.	Ag/Ag_2S-QDs on graphene oxide	Quantum dots-decorated graphene oxide sheets	Broad-spectrum antibacterial and antifungal
3.	Cu_2O-MoS_2 nanosheets	Heterostructured 2D nanocomposite	Antibacterial (*P. aeruginosa*, MRSA)
4.	CdSe/ZnS QDs with chitosan	Polymer-coated quantum dots	Photodynamic antimicrobial therapy
5.	Fe_3O_4-SiO_2-Ag nanohybrid	Silica-coated magnetic nanoparticles with Ag	Antibacterial (*E. coli*, *B. subtilis*)
6.	Black phosphorus-Au nanohybrid	2D nanosheets with gold nanoparticles	NIR-responsive antibacterial and biofilm disruption

work by damaging bacterial membranes and supporting tissue repair. This research shows that graphene-based nanohybrids could be a strong new solution to fight antibiotic-resistant infections and improve wound treatment in healthcare (Hassen et al., 2024).

Micochova P and the coworkers studied how titanium dioxide (TiO_2) coatings on tiles can help stop the spread of SARS-CoV-2, the virus that causes COVID-19. They tested TiO_2 and TiO_2 with silver coatings, using both a harmless version and the real virus. After exposing the coated tiles to light, virus levels dropped sharply – by 10,000 times in one hour. For the real virus, most of it was killed within 20 minutes, and none remained after 5 hours. In comparison, the virus stayed active on uncoated tiles. The study shows TiO_2 coatings can reduce surface infection risk under indoor lighting (Micochova et al., 2021).

The potent and versatile antimicrobial capabilities of various semiconductor nanohybrids are showcased in Table 9.4. The table links specific nanostructure types – from core-shell nanoparticles to 2D heterostructures – to their activity against a range of challenging pathogens, including drug-resistant bacteria (MRSA) and fungal species, through mechanisms like photodynamic therapy and biofilm disruption.

9.7 IONIC BASIC NANOHYBRIDS

Ionic liquids are a type of salt that remain in liquid form at temperatures below 100°C (Kondrat et al., 2023). Ionic liquids (ILs) have been successfully used for a long time in many areas, especially in biomedicine. When turned into polymers at the nanoscale, polymeric ILs (PILs) bring together the useful features of ionic liquids with the benefits of solid polymers and tiny particles (Shiflett, 2020). Structures made with ILs and nanomaterials in different shapes have been created to stop breakdown, increase the concentration of active substances, and improve the movement, distribution, and release of drugs. For example, polymeric nanoparticles covered with IL coatings last longer in the body after being injected into the bloodstream and can be directed to specific organs for targeted delivery (Hamadani et al., 2023). Surface-active ILs are especially useful in drug formulation and delivery because they work as eco-friendly surfactants, offering better performance than traditional surfactants (Moshikur et al., 2021).

The diverse therapeutic potential of ionic liquids is highlighted in **Table 9.5**, which connects specific chemical structures to their engineered nanostructures – such as grafted copolymers and responsive micelles – and their resulting biological activities.

Jahed et al. proposed a new IL design that includes carboxylic and vinylic functional groups in a 1,2,3-benzotriazole cation. This IL was inserted into the layers of montmorillonite and then copolymerized with either just the IL monomer or with methacrylic acid to create pH-sensitive nanocomposite carriers (Jahed et al., 2019). The goal of a study by Júlio and her team was to create PIL-nanocarrier hybrids using choline-based ILs and PLGA to deliver drugs that are poorly soluble. However, the expected loading efficiency for the drug model, rutin, was not supported by drug release tests (Júlio et al., 2020). Bielas et al. developed a variety of PIL-grafted polymeric nanostructures to deliver biologically active salicylates. They added choline-supported PILs into the polymer matrix as side chains, where salicylates are attached ionically. These grafted copolymers then self-assembled into spherical nanoparticles. The release of salicylates in PBS was possible because phosphate ions can replace salicylate ions. The proposed nanocarriers showed low toxicity to human

TABLE 9.5
Diverse Therapeutic Potential of Ionic Liquids

Ionic Liquid	Nanostructure type	Biological activity	Reference
2-(Methacryloyloxy)ethyl]-trimethylammonium chlor	Grafted methacrylate-methyl methacrylate copolymeride	Normal human cells (NHDF and BEAS-2B), pro-inflammatory interleukins (IL-6 and IL-8), *E. coli* bacteria	(Bielas et al., 2019).
1-Vinyl-3-hexylimidazolium bromide bis(trifluromethane) sulfonamide	Hyaluronic acid-grafted block polymer micelle (based on polyethylene glycol methyl ether)	MCF-7 and CT26 cancer cells	(Lu et al., 2019).
1-Vinyl-3-hexylimidazolium bis(trifluromethane) sulfonamide	Light and pH-responsive polymer blocks copolymerized on the PIL	Different cancer cells/ animal model (mice)	(Lu et al., 2020).
Tetra-*n*-butylphosphonium styrenesulfonate	Silica-coated $CuCo_2S_4$ core	MCF-7 cell line/animal model (mice) assisted by photoacoustic imaging	(Fan et al., 2020)

cells, anti-inflammatory effects when tested with pro-inflammatory interleukins, and antibacterial activity against *Escherichia coli* (Bielas et al., 2019).

Recent research in environmental cleanup has shown that ionic liquid-functionalized nanohybrids can efficiently remove heavy metals from wastewater. L. Wang et al. (2024) created new nanohybrid materials modified with ionic liquids, which have a strong ability to adsorb and selectively bind toxic metals like lead, cadmium, and mercury. These nanohybrids take advantage of the unique properties of ionic liquids, such as high thermal stability, low volatility, and adjustable chemistry, to improve their ability to bind metals and be reused effectively. This method holds great potential for tackling industrial pollution and ensuring water safety in polluted ecosystems (L. Wang et al., 2024). H. Chen et al. (2023) studied ionic liquid (IL)-modified nanocatalysts for converting CO_2 into useful chemicals, showing their potential in eco-friendly chemistry. The study found that IL-functionalized nanocatalysts improved reaction efficiency and selectivity under mild conditions. By adjusting the properties of the ILs, they boosted catalytic performance. The research highlights how surface modification helps in CO_2 activation and conversion, offering valuable ideas for designing better catalysts to reduce greenhouse gas emissions (H. Chen et al., 2023).

9.8 CONCLUSION AND FUTURE PERSPECTIVES

Semiconductor-based nanohybrids have emerged as a transformative class of materials in biomedical applications due to their unique optical, electronic, and catalytic properties. By integrating semiconductors with other nanomaterials (such as metals, polymers, or carbon-based structures), these hybrids exhibit enhanced functionalities, including improved biocompatibility, targeted drug delivery, real-time imaging, and efficient photothermal/photodynamic therapy (S. Wang et al., 2017). Their tunable bandgap and surface chemistry allow for precise control over interactions with biological systems, making them ideal for biosensing, theranostics, and regenerative medicine (Zhang et al., 2024). Recent advances in semiconductor nanohybrids, such as quantum dots (QDs), metal-oxide-semiconductor composites, and perovskite-based nanostructures, have demonstrated significant potential in cancer therapy, neural interfacing, and infection control (H. Chen et al., 2023). However, challenges remain in ensuring long-term stability, minimizing toxicity, and achieving scalable synthesis (Yan et al., 2023). Future research should focus on optimizing these nanomaterials for clinical translation while addressing regulatory and safety concerns. Over the next few years, semiconductor-based nanohybrids (tiny engineered particles combining nanomaterials and electronics) will transform medicine in incredible ways. These ultra-small devices will act like smart doctors inside the body – detecting diseases early, delivering drugs exactly where needed, and even repairing damaged cells. Imagine nanorobots that swim through blood vessels to clear blockages, or tiny sensors that monitor your health 24/7 and alert you before an illness gets serious. Advanced materials like quantum dots and graphene will make medical imaging sharper than ever, helping doctors spot tumors or infections at the smallest stage. AI-powered nanohybrids could learn your body's patterns and adjust treatments in real time, offering personalized medicine for diseases like cancer,

Alzheimer's, or diabetes. In the future, these technologies might connect with wearable devices or brain-computer interfaces, blurring the line between biology and machines. While challenges like safety and cost remain, the potential is enormous – leading to longer, healthier lives where diseases are stopped before they even cause harm. By 2040, nanohybrids could make today's medicine look like science fiction, bringing sci-fi dreams of microscopic healers into reality.

REFERENCES

Aldosari, B. N., Abd El-Aal, M., Abo Zeid, E. F., Faris, T. M., Aboelela, A., Abdellatif, A. A. H., & Tawfeek, H. M. (2023). Synthesis and characterization of magnetic Ag-Fe3O4@ polymer hybrid nanocomposite systems with promising antibacterial application. *Drug Development and Industrial Pharmacy*, *49*(12), 723–733.

Bhatia, D., Paul, S., Acharjee, T., & Ramachairy, S. S. (2024). Biosensors and their widespread impact on human health. *Sensors International*, *5*, Article 100257.

Bielas, R., Mielanczyk, A., Skonieczna, M., Mielanczyk, L., & Neugebauer, D. (2019). Choline supported poly(ionic liquid) graft copolymers as novel delivery systems of anionic pharmaceuticals for anti-inflammatory and anti-coagulant therapy. *Scientific Reports*, *9*, 14410.

Bisht, G., & Rayamajhi, S. (2016). ZnO nanoparticles: A promising anticancer agent. *Nanobiomedicine*, *3*, 9.

Bogdan, J., Pławińska-Czarnak, J., & Zarzyńska, J. (2017). Nanoparticles of titanium and zinc oxides as novel agents in tumor treatment: A review. *Nanoscale Research Letters*, *12*, 225.

Chen, H. et al. (2023). Perovskite nanocrystals in bioimaging and photodynamic therapy. *Nature Nanotechnology*, *18*(3), 234–245.

Chen, Y., Wang, H., Zhao, R., & Zhang, X. (2020). Functionalized semiconductor-based nanohybrids for biomedical imaging and cancer therapy. *ACS Nano*, *14*(3), 3195–3210.

Cheng, X., Xie, Q., & Sun, Y. (2023). Advances in nanomaterial-based targeted drug delivery systems. *Frontiers in Bioengineering and Biotechnology*, *11*, 1177151. https://doi.org/10.3389/fbioe.2023.1177151

Dobrovolskaia, M. A. (2015). Pre-clinical immunotoxicity studies of nanotechnology formulated drugs: Challenges, considerations and strategy. *Journal of Controlled Release*, *220*(Pt B), 571–583.

Edelstein, A. S., & Cammarata, R. C. (1996). *Nanomaterials: Synthesis, properties and applications*. Bristol: Institute of Physics.

El Golli, A., Contreras, S., & Dridi, C. (2023). Bio-synthesized ZnO nanoparticles and sunlight-driven photocatalysis for environmentally-friendly and sustainable route of synthetic petroleum refinery wastewater treatment. *Scientific Reports*, *13*, 20809.

Fan, S.-Y., Hao, Y.-N., Zhang, W.-X., Kapasi, A., Shu, Y., Wang, J.-H., & Chen, W. (2020). Poly (ionic liquid)-gated CuCo2S4 for pH-/thermo-triggered drug release and photoacoustic imaging. *ACS Applied Materials & Interfaces*, *12*, 9000–9007.

Gonzalez, L. et al. (2013). Nanotechnology in corneal neovascularization therapy – a review. *Journal of Ocular Pharmacology and Therapeutics*, *29*(2), 124–134.

Greczynski, G., & Hultman, L. (2021). The same chemical state of carbon gives rise to two peaks in X-ray photoelectron spectroscopy. *Scientific Reports*, *11*, 11195.

Hamadani, C. M., Dasanayake, G. S., Gorniak, M. E., Pride, M. C., Monroe, W., Chism, C. M., Heintz, R., Jarrett, E., Singh, G., Edgecomb, S. X., & Tanner, E. E. (2023). Development of ionic liquid-coated PLGA nanoparticles for applications in intravenous drug delivery. *Nature Protocols*, *18*, 2509–2557.

Hassen, A., Moawed, E. A., Bahy, R., El Basaty, A. B., El-Sayed, S., Ali, A. I., & Tayel, A. (2024, October 3). Synergistic effects of thermally reduced graphene oxide/zinc oxide composite material on microbial infection for wound healing applications. *Scientific Reports*, *14*(1), 22942.

Hemdan, M., Ali, M. A., Doghish, A. S., Mageed, S. S. A., Elazab, I. M., Khalil, M. M., Mabrouk, M., Das, D. B., & Amin, A. S. (2024). Innovations in biosensor technologies for healthcare diagnostics and therapeutic drug monitoring: Applications, recent progress, and future research challenges. *Sensors*, *24*.

Hu, M., Cao, Y., Li, Z., Yang, S., & Xing, Z. (2017). Ti 3+ self-doped mesoporous black TiO2/SiO2 nanocomposite as remarkable visible light photocatalyst. *Applied Surface Science*, *426*, 734–744.

Hwang, N., & Barron, A. R. (2021). *BET surface area analysis of nanoparticles*. Houston, TX: Rice University.

Jahed, F. S., Galehassadi, M., & Davaran, S. (2019). A novel 1,2,3-benzotriazolium based ionic liquid monomer for preparation of MMT/POLYIONIC liquid (PIL) pH-sensitive positive charge nanocomposites. *Journal of Chemical Sciences*, *131*, 1–9.

Júlio, S. A., Lima, S. A. C., Reis, S., de Almeida, T. S., & Fonte, P. (2020). Development of ionic liquid-polymer nanoparticle hybrid systems for delivery of poorly soluble drugs. *Journal of Drug Delivery Science and Technology*, *56*, Article 100915.

Kondrat, S., Feng, G., Bresme, F., Urbakh, M., & Kornyshev, A. A. (2023). Theory and simulations of ionic liquids in nanoconfinement. *Chemical Reviews*, *123*, 6668–6715.

Liu, Y. et al. (2019). Aqueous synthesis of core/shell/shell CdSe/CdS/ZnS quantum dots for photocatalytic hydrogen generation. *The Journal of Materials Science*, *54*, 8571–8580.

Liu, Y., Bhattarai, P., Dai, Z., & Chen, X. (2020). Photothermal therapy and photoacoustic imaging via nanotheranostics in fighting cancer. *Chemical Society Reviews*, *49*(4), 1253–1321.

Lu, B., Li, Y., Wang, Z., Wang, B., Pan, X., Zhao, W., Ma, X., & Zhang, J. (2019). A dual responsive hyaluronic acid graft poly (ionic liquid) block copolymer micelle for an efficient CD44-targeted antitumor drug delivery. *New Journal of Chemistry*, *43*, 12275–12282.

Lu, B., Zhou, G., Xiao, F., He, Q., & Zhang, J. (2020). Stimuli-responsive poly(ionic liquid) nanoparticles for controlled drug delivery. *The Journal of Materials Chemistry B*, *8*, 7994–8001.

Malhotra, B., & Ali, M. (2018). Plasmonic nanostructures. *Nanomaterials for Biosensors*, 161–181.

Malik, **S.,** Muhammad, **K.,** & Waheed, **Y.** (2023**). Emerging potential of nano-based techniques in targeted drug delivery and diagnosis: A comprehensive review.** *Biotech*, *13*(6)**, 198.**

Marsalek, R. (2014). Particle size and zeta potential of ZnO. *APCBEE Procedia*, *9*, 13–17.

Micochova, P., Chadha, A., Hesseloj, T., Fraternali, F., Ramsden, J. J., & Gupta, R. K. (2021, September 9). Rapid inactivation of SARS-CoV-2 by titanium dioxide surface coating. *Wellcome Open Research*, *6*, 56.

Moshikur, R., Ali, M. K., Moniruzzaman, M., & Goto, M. (2021). Recent advances in surface-active ionic liquid-assisted self-assembly systems for drug delivery. *Current Opinion in Colloid & Interface Science*, *56*, Article 101515.

Pan, M., Yang, J., Liu, K., Yin, Z., Ma, T., Liu, S., Xu, L., & Wang, S. (2020). Noble metal nanostructured materials for chemical and biosensing systems. *Nanomaterials*, *10*, 209.

Ratner, B. D. (2019). Biomaterials: Been there, done that, and evolving into the future. *Annual Review of Biomedical Engineering*, 171–191.

Roco, M. C. (2003). Nanotechnology: Convergence with modern biology and medicine. *Current Opinion in Biotechnology*, *14*(3), 337–346.

Shao, J., Zhang, J., Jiang, C., Lin, J., & Huang, P. (2020). Biodegradable titanium nitride MXene quantum dots for cancer phototheranostics in NIR-I/II biowindows. *Chemical Engineering Journal*, *400*, 126009. ISSN 1385–8947.

Shao, J., Zhang, R., Li, X., Wang, Y., & Chen, Z. (2023). Titanium nitride quantum dots for NIR-I/II photoacoustic imaging-guided photothermal therapy. *Advanced Materials*, *35*(12), 2300123.

Shiflett, M. (2020). *Commercial applications of ionic liquids*. Cham, Switzerland: Springer, p. 288.

Singh, V. (2024). *Theranostics: Integrated diagnostics and therapy using nanomedicine*. https://doi.org/10.1007/978-3-031-72467-1_17

Tang, B., Chen, H., Peng, H., Wang, Z., & Huang, W. (2018). Graphene modified TiO_2 composite photocatalysts: Mechanism, progress and perspective. *Nanomaterials*, *8*, 105.

Tao, W., Zhu, X., Yu, X., Zeng, X., Xiao, Q., Zhang, X., Ji, X., Wang, X., Shi, J., Zhang, H., Mei, L., & Liu, N. (2020). Black phosphorus nanosheets as a robust delivery platform for cancer theranostics. *Journal of Controlled Release*, *321*, 209–226.

Thangadurai, D., Islam, S., Sangeetha, J., & Cruz-Martins, N. (Eds.). (2022). *Biogenic nanomaterials: Structural properties and functional applications*. Boca Raton, FL: CRC Press.

Tsai, H., Shrestha, S., Vilá, R. A., Huang, W., Liu, C., Hou, C. H., Huang, H. H., Wen, X., Li, M., Wiederrecht, G., & Cui, Y. (2021). Bright and stable light-emitting diodes made with perovskite nanocrystals stabilized in metal-organic frameworks. *Nature Photonics*, *15*, 843–849.

Vaishampayan, V., Kapoor, A., & Gumfekar, S. P. (2023). Enhancement in the limit of detection of lab-on-chip microfluidic devices using functional nanomaterials. *The Canadian Journal of Chemical Engineering*, *101*, 5208.

Wang, L., Feng, W., Su, M., Guo, T., Jiang, B., & Deng, Y. (2024). Ionic liquid-functionalized nanohybrids for efficient removal of heavy metals from wastewater. *Chemical Engineering Journal*, *481*, 148532.

Wang, S., McGuirk, C. M., Ross, M. B., Wang, S., Chen, P., Xing, H., Liu, Y., & Mirkin, C. A. (2017). General and direct method for preparing oligonucleotide-functionalized metal-organic framework nanoparticles. *The Journal of the American Chemical Society, 139*(29), 9827–9830.

Wu, M.-X., & Yang, Y.-W. (2017). Metal-organic framework (MOF)-based drug/cargo delivery and cancer therapy. *Advanced Materials*, *29*(23), 1606134.

Yan, J., Wang, Q., Yang, J., Rutter, P., Xing, M., & Li, B. (2023). Chemical synthesis of innovative silver nanohybrids with synergistically improved antimicrobial properties. *International Journal of Nanomedicine*, *18*, 2295–2305.

Zhang, X., Li, Y., & Wang, J. (2023). Mesoporous TiO_2 nanoparticles coated with polydopamine for NIR/UV light-responsive drug delivery. *Journal of Materials Chemistry B*, *11*, 4567–4578.

Zhang, Y., Li, H., Wang, J., & Liu, X. (2024). Magnetotactic bacteria-enabled biosynthesis of Fe_3O_4/ZnO heterostructures for magnetically recyclable photocatalysis. *Advanced Functional Materials*, *34*(8), 2305678.

Zhang, Y., Wang, Q., Xu, J., & Ma, S. (2012). Synthesis of Pd/ZnO nanocomposites with high photocatalytic performance by a solvothermal method. *Applied Surface Science, 258*, 10104–10109.

10 Challenges and Future Direction of Nanotechnology in Biomedical Applications

Surya Prakash DV, Sandeep Sirohi, Parnika Vashist, and Anand Kumar Nelapati

10.1 INTRODUCTION

Nanotechnology has been embraced with increasing frequency in medicine. This is known as nanomedicine, a completely novel, autonomous branch of the science of biology. The use of nanomaterials for the creation of biological devices and nanosystems, as well as nano-electronic biosensors and other biological machineries, are the primary applications of nanomedicines in the medical profession (Liu et al., 2017). Nanotechnology has effectively appeared as a very promising cancer intervention method employing medication delivery systems based on nanoparticles. In addition, this nanotechnology has garnered significant attention in recent years due to its enormous potential for illness monitoring, diagnosis, and therapy. Scientists from educational institutions and companies worldwide have concentrated more on this prominent field. There are numerous new routes that nanomedicine is taking. First, it has been discovered in tissue engineering that advanced biomaterials' nanostructure plays a critical role in how the materials interact with biological systems (Kashyap et al., 2023). Another example is chip systems with micro and nano-level structures created for highly accurate diagnostic techniques, including the identification of disorder markers in blood. The field is expanding at an unimaginable rate, and it is certain that many new technologies will be introduced in the years to come that will further advance disease screening and therapy for the benefit of both patients and society. Nevertheless, there are certain fundamental difficulties the field faces (Kaushik et al., 2018). A lack of knowledge of the intricate relationship among the synthetic materials are creating and the biological field in which they interact is possibly commonality throughout all technological advancements in the field. This ignorance is at the protein, cellular, and entire organism levels. It is evident that factors such as surface chemistry, material softness, and nanoscale to macroscale morphology all influence the biological behavior of the technologies we are attempting to create, but, over the coming decades, we must progressively enhance our capacity to comprehend and record these effects. A discussion of the

DOI: 10.1201/9781003563723-10

state of knowledge on intravenous drug delivery systems based on nanoparticles and their medical applications serves as an example of this issue. Nonetheless, there are a number of discussions, disagreements, and brainstorming sessions among academics, medical professionals, and industry scientists on the definition of nanomedicines. A number of regulatory bodies worldwide have expressed their opinions and provided different definitions for nanotechnology and nanomedicines (Kothamasu et al., 2012). The U.S. Food and Drug Administration (FDA) defines nanotechnology as a field of technology that enables researchers to develop, investigate, and work with materials that are measured in nanometers (billionths of a meter), which may vary in their intrinsic physical, chemical, and biological characteristics. National Institutes of Health (NIH) described nanomedicines as highly specific molecular-level medical interventions for the treatment of disease or the restoration of damaged bone, muscle, other tissues, or nerves. Additionally, the European Science Foundation's Forward Look Nanomedicine program has defined nanomedicine as a field of medicine that uses nanoscale instruments, typically smaller than 1000 nm, to comprehend the complexities of a disease's pathophysiology and then diagnose, prevent, and treat it (Mora-Huertas et al., 2010). Nanomedicines have emerged as the most intriguing, promising, and extensively researched method in the field of innovative medication delivery and diagnostics throughout the past few decades. This is evident from the emergence of several promising nanomedicine candidates, including enhanced drug delivery, imaging, and diagnostics, and/or regenerative treatments, which have been approved by various regulatory bodies worldwide. Health agencies have confirmed the important role that technologies play in disease monitoring, treatment, and progression management. Biomedical nanotechnology focuses on exploring nanoscience to enhance health and well-being, ultimately aiming for personalized health management. It is also clear that the use of nanotechnology-assisted methods improves the sensitivity, affordability, and accessibility of targeted illness diagnosis and therapy (Yuchong et al., 2016). Nanosystems' adjustable performance, which is being studied in biomedical research, is beneficial for the creation of treatments that take patient profiles into account, and individualized health management. The advent of numerical approaches, such as artificial intelligence, combining deep and machine learning, and bioinformatics, has helped to analyze predictions and trends, in addition to the noteworthy aspects of nano-assisted approaches (Acharya and Sahoo, 2011). Such data is helpful for risk assessment, therapeutic optimization, and understanding epidemic variations. At the same time, fast and efficient analysis depends on proper bioinformatics administration. The internet of medical things (IoMT) is a medical nanotechnology technique for analysis, storage, and data sharing, and is now being promoted with great effort. IoMT results are helpful when transferring biomedical technology from the lab to the field. Efforts are underway to convert electronic health into intelligent health with these results in mind.

10.2 BIOMEDICAL APPLICATIONS

The incorporation of biological, chemical and physical sciences to develop treatments, improve patient outcomes, and enhance their general state of health is referred to as biomedical applications (Park, 2016). This interdisciplinary discipline uses engineering concepts to develop therapeutic approaches, diagnostic instruments, and medical equipment. For instance, biomedical engineering has made it possible to create sophisticated prosthetics that are more comfortable and functional than ever before, as well as medical imaging technologies like ultrasounds, CT scans, and MRIs that are crucial for the diagnosis and ongoing monitoring of a variety of medical disorders (Xie et al., 2021). Additionally, biocompatible materials have been created to replace or repair tissues that are damaged, as in the case of pacemakers, implants, and artificial joints, assisting in the restoration of physiological functions along with improving the quality of life for patients. Personalized medicine, in which medications and treatments are customized to each patient's specific genetic composition, has been made possible in recent years by advances in molecular biology and biotechnology (Couvreur and Vauthier, 2006). This individualized strategy has enormous promise for treating complicated illnesses like cancer, as focused treatments can target particular mutations to produce better results with fewer adverse effects. Gene therapy is another area of biomedical applications, where genetic information is inserted or changed within an individual's cells to treat or prevent disease, providing hope for conditions like genetic disorders and some forms of blindness that were previously incurable. Developments in tissue engineering are also helping to create organs that can be created in a lab, which could reduce the need for organ donors and solve the transplant shortage. In addition, utilizing biomaterials in drug delivery systems enables the development of more effective and regulated release mechanisms for pharmaceuticals, guaranteeing that they reach the intended location in the body and boosting their effectiveness (Almeida et al., 2011). In general, biomedical applications keep transforming healthcare by encouraging innovation in illness prevention, diagnosis, and treatment, ultimately enhancing the quality of life for patients everywhere. By utilizing the concepts of nanotechnology, nanopharmaceuticals have transformed modern medicine's medication delivery methods and therapeutic approaches. These cutting-edge formulations address significant shortcomings of traditional medicines by employing nanoparticles (NPs) and nanocarriers (NCs) to provide improved targeting capabilities, increased bioavailability, and decreased toxicity. The numerous nanopharmaceuticals' clinical achievements highlight their revolutionary influence on healthcare.

10.2.1 Nanomicelles

Nanomicelles are 5–100 nm structures that may absorb hydrophilic and hydrophobic substances. When amphiphilic molecules come together at the concentration at which micelles form (CMC), they are created. The particles can form in both aqueous and non-aqueous solutions, with the polar region forming the micelle's exterior phase and the nonpolar region forming its interior. Micelles often have a spherical shape, depending on the solutions' pH, surfactant content, and ionic strength. However, occasionally, they can also have an ellipsoid or cylindrical shape (Wolinsky and Grinstaff, 2008). The micelle formation is influenced by the quantity of surfactants, the ability of micelles to form depends on the concentration of the solution and the chain length of the surfactant molecules. Micelles tend to form at lower concentrations when the molecule's chain is longer. A reduced critical micelle concentration is also required if the solution contains dissolved ions. Alcohols have an impact on the CMC as the temperature rises, the CMC value increases from methanol to butanol (Chou, 2004). The CMC also rises with temperature. Micelles are often formed by surfactant molecules, which can be cationic, ionic, or nonionic detergents (Deng et al., 2020). A combination of lipids and detergents may be present in certain nano-micelles. The amounts of lipids in the micelles determine the CMC and the average quantity of detergent molecules. Hydrophobic medications are soluble in polymeric micelles that are created when amphiphilic block copolymers self-assemble in an aqueous medium (Anwarul et al., 2018). It is the most effective way to improve the medication's solubility and bioavailability. The micelle structures' ineffective drug-loading capacities, inadequate cellular interactions with neutral micelles, and poor physical in vivo stability are their drawbacks. Various applications of nanomicelles are displayed in Table 10.1.

10.2.2 Metal and Metal Oxide Nanoparticles

MNPs and MONPs are the most widely employed nanomaterials because of their tiny size and huge surface area, which provide innovative approaches to illness diagnosis and treatment. Because of their special qualities, metal-based nanocomposites are also frequently used in a variety of applications. Widely used in various fields due to their unique physical, chemical, and biological properties, metals like gold, silver, and platinum exhibit excellent conductivity, antimicrobial activity, and stability, making them valuable in medicine, electronics, and catalysis. Silver nanoparticles, for example, are widely used in antibacterial coatings, while gold nanoparticles are explored for drug delivery and cancer therapy. The designs of magneto plasmonic nanohybrids, which make use of collaborative features, are given considerable attention. The design of magneto plasmonic nanohybrids (Chen et al., 2019), which take use of synergistic features for biomedical applications, is given considerable attention.

TABLE 10.1
Nanomicelles Applications for Supporting Human Health

S.No	Active Principle Loaded in Nanomicelles	Applications	References
1	Curcumin nanomicelles	Asthenoterat ozoospermia therapy	Erenler et al., 2023
2	Polyplex nanomicelles	Muscle-Targeted mRNA Delivery	Cheng et al., 2013
3	Casein nanomicelles	pharmaceutics, Nutraceutics, and cosmetics	Li et al., 2023
4	Celastrol-loaded nanomicelles	Corneal neovascularization therapeutics	Kim, 2007
5	Cholesteryl succinyl silane with gold nanoshells	Cancer therapy	Ariga and Fakhrullin, 2021

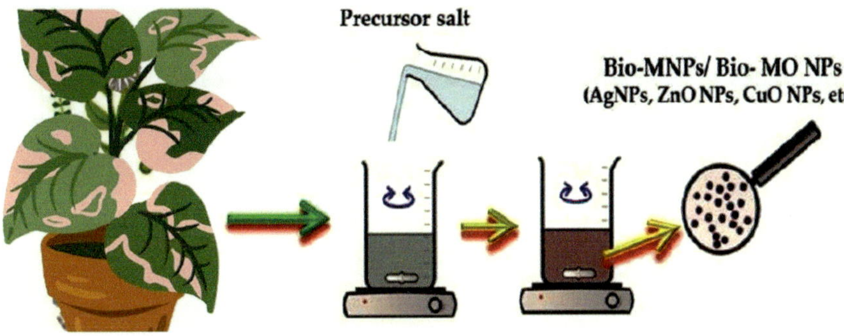

FIGURE 10.1 Schematic representation of "green" synthesis of MNPs/MONPs. The "green" produced nanoparticles have a variety of effects, such as antifungal, antibacterial, and anticancer qualities. Due to these broad operations, nanoparticles are now known for their wide range of biological and electronic applications, along with their use in wastewater treatment and the textile industry. Therefore, CuO NPs, ZnO NPs, MgO NPs, Fe_2O_3NPs, Fe_3O_4NPs, AgNPs, and AuNPs – all phytosynthesized nanoparticles – exhibited exceptional effectiveness of light-induced degradation for organic dyes in wastewater (Shi et al., 2017).

Physical and chemical techniques, as well as electrochemical or photochemical techniques, can be used to create MNPs and MONPs. Research has increasingly focused on the synthesis of particles through biological methods, which are cost effective and biocompatible, and non-toxic (Nair et al., 2016), because physical methods involve costly synthesis and low yield, while chemical methods are dangerous because they involve dangerous chemicals bound to the surface of these particles. This process is referred to as "green or biosynthesis." Various microorganisms have been found to biosynthesize MNPs/MONPs. The "green" synthesis of MNPs/MONPs is shown in Figure 10.1.

Phytoplants are the most commonly used bio-nano-factories for the "green" synthesis of MNPs/MONPs due to their abundance, safety, renewability, and the presence of various biological compounds that surround the nanoparticles and confer biological activity (Farokhzad and Langer, 2009). They also have stability, biocompatibility, and little to no toxicity. There are three different ways to create nanoparticles with plants: the first is by creating them inside living plants or through intracellular pathways; the second is by creating them with plant extracts; and the third is by creating them with phytochemicals. The extracellular pathway for nano synthesis is used in the final two techniques. Proteins, flavonoids, terpenoids (Vashist et al., 2016), organic acids, alkaloids, and other primary and secondary metabolites are present in the plant. These substances function as manufacturing and bioreducing agents to produce nanoparticles. Table 10.2 lists a few instances of MNPs/MONPs and their biotherapeutic applications. These are a rapidly evolving field of study, valued for their distinctive properties and wide-ranging applications. However, challenges like scalability, toxicity, and stability still need to be addressed before these nanoparticles can be more broadly adopted. With ongoing research, it is anticipated that the use of metal and metal oxide nanoparticles will increase in everyday technologies, fostering

TABLE 10.2
Various Types of MNPs/MONPs and Their Biotherapeutics

S.No	MNPs/MO NPs	Applications	References
1	PtNPs	Anti-colitis agent Cancer therapy	Riehemann et al., 2009
2	AuNPs	Antimicrobial agent	Jokerst et al., 2011
3	TiO_2NPs	Drug delivery Antibacterial agent	Gu et al., 2023
4	Fe_2O_3NPs	Antioxidant agent Antimicrobial agent	Kaushik et al., 2016
5	ZnO NPs	Anticancer agent Antimicrobial agent	Madhuri, 2023

innovation across various sectors, including clean energy and healthcare. These nanoparticles continue to revolutionize multiple industries, but ongoing research is needed to address potential toxicity and environmental impact concerns.

10.2.3 Prebiotics, Probiotics, and Postbiotics in Nanopharmaceuticals

The intestinal microbiome is a highly complex ecological community. Understanding how its composition influences both physical and mental health highlights the importance of familiarizing oneself with its key components: probiotics, prebiotics, and postbiotics. Probiotic supplements can help to partially restore and influence a changed microbiome (Bobo et al., 2016). Probiotics show great promise in the treatment and prevention of a variety of illnesses, including cancer, cardiovascular disease, inflammatory disorders, and neurological diseases. Nevertheless, because probiotics are living microbes, their clinical uses present difficulties. Their effectiveness is restricted by biopharmaceutical limitations, such as vulnerability to severe stomach disorders and bile salts. Probiotic viability during in vivo transit is hampered by digestive tract conditions. One viable way to deal with this problem is through encapsulation technology (Xu et al., 2022). Information about the probiotic's antibacterial and antioxidant properties after encapsulation is lacking. The drawbacks of conventional encapsulation techniques are their vulnerability to high temperatures, their greater capsule sizes, and their inability to regulate particle sizes. Probiotic biopharmaceutical barriers can be enhanced by the transition from conventional methods to novel strategies, such as encapsulation utilizing nanoparticles, nanobio films, biofibers and nanocoatings for probiotics (Ferrari, 2005). Moreover, probiotic-derived outer membrane vesicles (OMVs) incorporating MnO_2nanozymes have been developed to further improve the therapeutic effect of nano probiotics. These OMVs can attach to inflamed colonic epithelium and efficiently remove excess reactive oxygen species from the digestive system. This therapy showed negligible systemic toxicity. Probiotics, such as *Bifidobacterium* probiotics modified with artificial enzymes, are essential for improving the directing and maintaining biocompatible synthetic enzymes allowing for efficient and sustainable scavenging of elevated ROS levels, thereby reducing inflammatory factors. Prebiotics, in contrast to probiotics, are food for probiotics rather than live things. These are ballast materials, such galactooligosaccharides or inulin that enter the big intestine as nutrition for beneficial bacteria since they cannot be broken down in the small intestine (Zhu et al., 2019). As a result, prebiotics can be utilized to supplement probiotics. Complex carbohydrates and fiber, which are present in a wide variety of plant foods, are the primary components of prebiotics. Because humans lack the enzyme necessary to break down fiber, the majority of the fiber included in plant-based foods passes through the intestine largely undamaged. However, fiber can be metabolized by colonic microorganisms and converted into other substances. Because of their innate ability to protect the encapsulated compounds while they are passing through the upper gastrointestinal (GI) tract, prebiotics are the best components for oral drug administration and nano-encapsulation. Rather, postbiotics are produced during digestion following the breakdown of microbial fibers (Berrouiguet et al., 2018). One type of bacteria may produce compounds that serve as the prebiotic or food source for another type of bacteria. Short-chain fatty acids (SCFAs) are a class of postbiotic chemicals that are very beneficial to health. Butyrate is among the most thoroughly researched SCFAs. This substance serves as a fuel source for the cells lining the colon, promoting gut health. Butyrate also modulates the immune system and helps reduce inflammation. It has an impact on brain function and can increase the synthesis of the hormone glucagon-like peptide 1 (GLP-1), which reduces hunger (Torchilin, 2014). Extracellular NPs generated by beneficial bacteria are essential for providing unique health-promoting capabilities, as numerous in vivo and in vitro studies have repeatedly shown. These effects go beyond the digestive area to include systemic effects, which is how the new idea of postbiotics was born. A schematic depiction of the symbiotic relationship within the microbiome is shown in Figure 10.2.

10.3 CHALLENGES

It is anticipated that nanomedicine will lead to new discoveries in the treatment of a number of incurable diseases; nevertheless, this will require a sincere worldwide endeavor to successfully translate laboratory innovations into clinical counterparts for the benefit of humanity (Tomitaka et al., 2017). These critical elements of treatment, such as diagnostics, improved targeted therapies, less side effects, and improved therapeutic monitoring, could be accomplished by nanomedicines such as nanotherapeutics and nanopharmaceuticals. These benefits will undoubtedly raise people's quality of life and help make healthcare more cost effective. The field of nanomedicine is still in its infancy, despite its prospective benefits, which include the ability to efficiently transport hydrophobic active substances, bypass biological barriers, and selectively target infection areas. Due to many difficulties and roadblocks at various stages of development, the majority of nanomedicine research and innovations is currently limited to the laboratory stage, with only a few nanoparticle-based medications approved for clinical use. Doxil, the first FDA-approved nanodrug formulation in 1995, is one such example that can extend the duration of drug circulation and prevent the RES because it uses the PEGylation technology. This

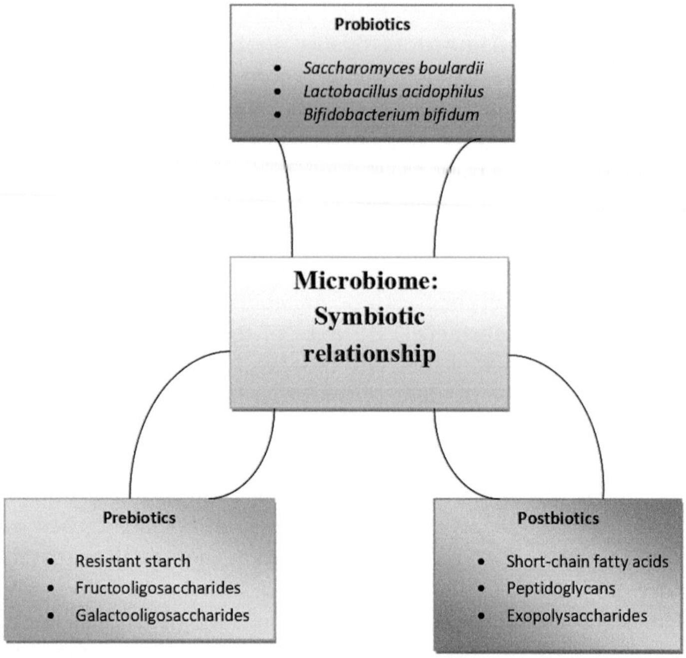

FIGURE 10.2 Schematic representation of symbiotic relationship in microbiome. Probiotics, prebiotics, and postbiotics all have crucial functions in the microbiome's symbiotic connection that supports gut health. Live helpful bacteria known as probiotics help maintain the gut microbiota's equilibrium. Conversely, prebiotics are indigestible fibers that serve as nourishment for these advantageous microorganisms, promoting their growth. When probiotics are active, they produce metabolic byproducts called postbiotics, like short-chain fatty acids, which can improve gut health. All three of these components work in concert to produce a balanced environment, which encourages a diverse, ranging healthy microbiome and enhances one's overall health.

nano-formulation's durability and precise release of the medication, doxorubicin, at the tumor site are its primary characteristics (Hillaireau and Couvreur, 2009). Between 1995 and 2017, around 50 nanopharmaceuticals were approved by the FDA and made available for clinical use. The distinct features of three-dimensional assembly with several nanoscale components are what make nanomedicine so alluring. Although nanomedicine is so complex, to ensure a consistent product with stable characteristics of physicochemical and biological properties, rigorous characterization of physicochemical properties, careful design and engineering, and a validated manufacturing process are essential for reproducible scale-up (Tiwari et al., 2019). Compared to traditional medications, nanomedicine's safety and regulatory concerns require more thought. Therefore, reviewing and summarizing the difficulties and constraints encountered during the creation and subsequent commercialization of nanomedicine products is crucial, as is talking about possible solutions to hasten the expansion of this significant subject. It is still difficult to successfully transition nanomedicine advances from pre-clinical feasibility demonstration to clinical evidence of therapeutic efficacy; however, numerous barriers have been identified as key scientific challenges in delivering nano-engineered products to healthcare recipients.

10.3.1 Biological Barriers and Drug Targeting

Drugs with a nano-based formulation are able to successfully penetrate a number of biological barriers and enter the microenvironment of illness locations. For instance, oral administration nanoparticles must be highly stable in the gastrointestinal tract, able to traverse the intestinal epithelium while preserving high systemic bioavailability of medications after overcoming multiple challenges (De Jong and Born, 2008). Intravenous injection (IV) is the sole effective method for delivering large therapeutic molecules, such as proteins, peptides, and polynucleotides, in contrast to the majority of small molecules administered orally. Drugs in circulation still need to get past a number of biological obstacles to reach their micro targets after systemic administration. A key hurdle to treating illnesses of the central nervous system is the blood-brain barrier (BBB), which prevents about 99% of big, hydrophilic molecules from entering the central nervous system, including the brain and its surrounding cerebrospinal fluid. As a result, brain targeted delivery is hampered. There are numerous potential routes via which solute molecules or drug-loaded nanoparticles can penetrate the BBB. Delivering nanomedicine carrying therapeutic compounds into solid tumors is another significant challenge faced by formulators. Extensive areas of tumors with a high concentration of cancer cells and dense stromal tissue remain poorly perfused, further hindering the distribution of medication within the tumor, despite the fact that in the tumor the distribution of vasculature varies significantly, with certain areas being more permeable than others (Jiang et al., 2010). Disrupted lymphatic drainage in tumors leads to an increase in IFP (interstitial fluid pressure), presenting an additional significant barrier to effective drug delivery. This is believed to be a key factor contributing to reduced drug extravasation and transvascular transport, even in the presence of a leaky cancer microvasculature, thereby hindering the movement of molecules into the tumor's interstitial space. The ability of various nanoparticle-based delivery methods, such as liposomes, polymer micelles, and peptide or protein nanoparticles, to deliver medications is being carefully examined (Habib and Singh, 2021). The tumor vasculature is extremely permeable and leaky, and because lymphatic drainage is inadequate, the enhanced permeability and retention (EPR) effect causes passive nanoparticle buildup. As a result of the macromolecules' continued accumulation in the tumor microenvironment, tumor medication delivery via EPR was significantly enhanced. Pegylated liposomal formulations, such as those containing paclitaxel and doxorubicin, were among the first nanomedicines to be commercially available. Managing the pharmacokinetics and biodistribution of nanoparticles by adjusting their physicochemical characteristics is the main concern of this passively targeted nanomedicine (Subramanian et al., 2024). Active transport can lower systemic drug exposure by using active biological transporters, even though passive absorption has certain benefits. The medications have been more effective since. They are precisely targeted to the place of action. The structured architecture of the active targeting nanoparticles makes it easier to incorporate different targeting active moieties, such as oligonucleotides, proteins, peptides, receptors, and tiny molecule ligands (Langer and Tirrell, 2004). By efficiently transporting medications to the intended locations and so promoting cellular uptake of encapsulated therapeutic substances, it can lessen off-target toxicity to organs. Ligands improve cancer treatment by binding drugs to receptors that are present in large numbers on their surfaces. Furthermore, big, biologically active, compound nanoparticles incorporating protein transduction domains and cell-penetrating peptides can facilitate uniform delivery of the agents; otherwise, they cannot efficiently reach cancer cells. Furthermore, tumor endothelial cells are another potential target of nanomedicine. $\alpha 2\beta 3$, $\alpha vb3$, and $\alpha 5\beta 1$ integrins are bound by the cyclic and linear variants of oligopeptides RGD, giving liposomes and other nanoparticles their ability to penetrate tumors (Leach et al., 2019). Nanoparticles that have undergone RGD alteration provide cytotoxic agents to tumor tissue and provide notable antitumor effects. The effectiveness and affinity of a target and its particular ligand determine active targeting. Additionally, in order to achieve both high targeting efficiency and optimal internalization, it is crucial to adjust the density of targeting ligands per nanocarrier.

10.3.2 Analysis and Characterization of Nano-Formulations

When compared to traditional pharmaceutical formulations, nanomedicine is a complicated alternative made up of several components that instead fulfill a specific purpose. Therefore, it is crucial to detect and characterize such excipients in addition to the active ingredient. To do this, more advanced and suitable analytical testing techniques are needed to characterize and quantify each formulation component (Sumer and Gao, 2008). Additionally, it is necessary to look into how these elements interact with the active agent or ingredients, taking into account both their physicochemical characteristics and biological behaviors. As a result, formulators currently face difficulties in developing nanomedicine from both a technical and a regulatory standpoint. The key physicochemical properties of nanomedicine typically include size, size distribution, structure, surface characteristics, surface charge, porosity, and overall stability. However, due to their variable nature, these characteristics are challenging to describe in the produced nanomedicine products. For example, polydispersity (PD) is an important measure of particle heterogeneity in terms of structural size (Gao et al., 2013). Thus, even if formulations of nanomedicine have the same structural size, differences in polydispersity (PD) can conduct to noticeable variations in their behavior, such as drug release rate, stability, targeting properties, and toxicity in vivo. Characterizing the stability of nanomedicine is another issue the formulator frequently faces. Due to their excellent physicochemical properties polymers have been utilized in the products of nanomedicine for development. However, these materials' biodegradable qualities will also be affected by processing variable parameters, which also affect the characteristics of products when they are stored in solutions or even as lyophilized powder. Therefore, it's critical to enhance the quality evaluation of those biodegradable materials using established and repeatable standards. Another common problem with nanocarriers over time is in vivo biodistribution (Zafar et al., 2020). Once administered in vivo, nanomedicines may interact with biomolecules and biofluids to change their physicochemical characteristics, including structural size, conglomeration, and release profile, as well as change how the nanomedicine functions in biological systems. To establish in vivo-in vitro correlation, it is crucial to thoroughly characterize the nanomedicine products using both in vitro and in vivo models under clinically relevant conditions (Greene et al., 2014). Even though the fluorescence or radiolabeling methods can now be used to obtain pictorial biodistribution of nanoparticles and their accumulation in bio-models, evaluating mass-balance information remains challenging, yet it is essential for tracking the entire administered dose, ensuring safety, and, as a result, assessing toxicity. Additionally, one of the nanoparticle formulation components is chemically linked to radiolabeling and fluorescence emitters, which are easily degraded, and the internal environment does not always stay stable. Therefore, tracking the degraded fluorescence or radiolabeling component, rather than the medication or the nanoparticle as a whole, becomes a challenge, it may produce inconsistent and incorrect data. Furthermore, compared to the same nanoparticles without radio labeled or fluorescence alteration, it is possible that the dispersion pattern of these chemically changed nanoparticles will differ. Finally, individual tracking may be required for nanomedicines with multiple components and function of delivering and distributing various therapeutic and imaging compounds (Jain, 2005). To make sure that the created formulations include all key properties needed for the desired therapeutic impact and steady effectiveness with minimal side effects, a range of characterization techniques is essential. These include quantifying both active and inactive ingredients along with impurities, measuring particle size and distribution using light scattering, determining surface charge, imaging nanoparticles via microscopy, and employing technical methods designed to describe the in vivo behavior of nanoparticles.

10.3.3 Scale-Up and Manufacturing

Controlling important parameters, batch-to-batch stability, and applicability are the most difficult issues in pharmaceutical development. With well-characterized nanoparticles, small-scale nanomedicine processes may be reproducible, and the outcomes of their preclinical and clinical research may be satisfactory. However, regulating the physicochemical processes of nanomaterials during large-scale production is challenging, leading to batch-to-batch variability and potential failures in various clinical trials (Hu et al., 2020). Most nano-formulations, such as nanoparticles, are intricate three-dimensional products composed of multiple distinct components. These multicomponent systems and their unique configuration make it extremely difficult to regulate the manufacturing process. These considerations make it challenging to manufacture and scaleup nanomedicine. Doxil, one of the first FDA approved nanomedicines, faced manufacturing and sterility problems and was discontinued in November 2011 (Vashist et al., 2016). The Doxil shortage lasted until 2014, when different manufacturing processes were used, which raised the cost of the drug. To ensure reproducibility during large-scale manufacturing, it is essential to accurately identify the elements and comprehend their interactions in the early phases of development. Generally, there are various approaches for preparing nanoparticles. Top-down methods involve creating nano-entities by breaking down macroparticles through techniques such as milling, while bottom-up methods involve assembling micro components into functional structures, such as through monomer polymerization. For the production of nano medicinal formulations, several techniques are commonly employed, including centrifugation, sonication, milling, filtration, emulsification, lyophilization, and high-speed or high-pressure homogenization (Kontham et al., 2022). When scaling up the production of nanomedicines, it is crucial to select the appropriate methods and processing parameters. These parameters include the active compounds, organic solvent type, emulsifiers/cross-linkers/stabilizers, pressure, temperature, and pH. Using inappropriate conditions could lead to unintended impurities and alterations in the chemical structure of the therapeutic agents. In particular, macromolecules like proteins and peptides are highly susceptible to changes in their chemical structure and conformation due to processes like coagulation (Ross et al., 2004), denaturation, degradation, and cross-linking. As a result, producing nanomedicine is not that easy; instead, it requires carefully planned, accurate, and tested production processes with stringent quality-controlling parameters. The manufacture and scaling up of nanomedicine are hampered by the comparatively high cost of raw materials, the requirement for complex machinery, and the multistep production process, which drives up the cost of producing nanotherapeutics. Therefore, the clinical efficacy of nanomedicine medications is more sought after than that of conventionally available treatments in pattern to offset the development and fabrication expenses of products. Pharmaceutical businesses may be discouraged from producing nano-formulations on a wide scale due to these factors. Scaling up and producing nanomedicine comes with distinct challenges due to the high level of precision required at the nanoscale. Unlike traditional drug manufacturing, nanomedicine demands meticulous control over particle size, stability, and reproducibility to ensure consistent therapeutic performance. Various advanced methods, including high-pressure homogenization, nanoprecipitation, and microfluidics, are employed to enable large-scale production while preserving quality. Regulatory requirements are also a key factor, as nanomedicines must adhere to strict safety and efficacy guidelines. With ongoing advancements, innovations in automation and process optimization are helping to transition nanomedicine from research labs to large-scale commercial production, making it more widely available for clinical applications.

10.3.4 Pharmacology and Safety Challenges

The pharmacological advantages and safety profiles of nanomedicine are significantly influenced by its physical and chemical properties. Even minor adjustment composition and minor modifications to the finished products could have a major impact on the pharmacology and toxicity of nanomedicine (Das et al., 2017). Designing the formulation's pharmacokinetic parameter is the fundamental prerequisite for achieving the intended pharmacological profile of a successful medication, including nanomedicine. Furthermore, the majority of researchers and pharmaceutical corporations evaluate nanomedicine using the usual criteria of pharmacological molecules. This is because small-molecule active substances typically diffuse across biological barriers more easily, maintaining the medication concentration in the blood at equilibrium to reach the levels desired by the target tissue. Furthermore, one crucial factor in determining PK and, consequently, the outcome of any pharmaceutical formulation is the assessment of the drug concentration in plasma (De Carvalho and Conte-Junior, 2021). Nevertheless, this methodology cannot be assumed to be correct and may have inherent flaws if it is used in nanomedicine. Therefore, distinct nanomedicines require different PK methods with varied indications. For instance, evaluating the characteristics of pharmacology at the exact target site may be more relevant for assessing the pharmacological effect and reproducibility of nanomedicine products than the traditional method of quantifying drug behavior in plasma. Additionally, the bioequivalence of pharmaceutical products based on nanotechnology could be utilized to assess their efficacy and resolve concerns about toxicity to human health. Nanomedicine products' nanoscale size can mimic intracellular macromolecules such as proteins, polysaccharides, and enzymes involved in cell signaling, which could result in undesirable biological interactions. Nowadays, nanotoxicology is a separate area of study, and there is a wealth of information about the toxicity of various nanoparticles. However, since traditional drug toxicity assays may not be adequate for assessing these nanomedicines, evaluating the toxicity of nanomaterials remains challenging, especially in terms of long-term toxicity. As a result, the need for sophisticated complementary tests in addition to the accepted standard for assessing the toxicity of nanomedicine products arises and some of the characteristics that influence how well nanomedicine drugs and nanoproducts work at the nano-bio interface (Yang et al., 2023). Therefore, any product including nanomedicine may have unique problems and so need unique assessments. In the pharmaceutical industry, "toxicity" typically refers to both acute and chronic toxicity. Studies on chronic toxicity take a lot time, and evaluating the data is more difficult. Sometimes immuno toxicity from in vitro tests cannot easily transfer to humans due to the lack of an appropriate animal model. However, free radicals stress, erythrocyte destruction, immune activation are typically included in acute toxicity. Both the nanoparticles and the biologics they contain, such fragments of antibodies, and nucleic acids, can act as antigen sources and stimulate an immune response. The physicochemical parameters of nanoparticles, including their size, charge, solubility, surface features, and hydrophobicity, can also influence their immunogenicity.

10.3.5 Regulatory Challenges

Though several nanomedicine products for cancer treatment have been licensed by the US FDA and European Medicines Agency (EMA), the FDA, EMA, and other regulatory agencies have not yet established precise standards for medication products incorporating these types of materials. Only individual benefit and risk assessment can be used to make regulatory judgments when there is insufficient information available for the evaluation of nanomedicine goods or therapies (Blanco et al., 2015). Because of this, the regulatory process takes a long time and calls for a highly qualified specialist cutting-edge technologies, which could cause delays. Alongside clinical trials and the approval process, regulatory considerations are crucial for the development of innovative technologies that quantify, characterize, and monitor the quality of nanomedicine products. Therefore, comprehensive regulatory criteria for characterization, quality control, and assessing the safety of nanomedicine products are urgently needed. Nonetheless, definitions, policies, and collaboration in this field are being developed and enhanced over time (Peer et al., 2007). In June 2014, the FDA published industry guidelines for nano-formulations and FDA-Regulated Products. According to these guidelines, nanomaterials are designed materials with dimensions ranging from 1 nm to 100 nm. To advance regulatory procedures for characterizing nanomedicine products, the FDA and the European Technology Platform on Nanomedicine intend to collaborate with the European Nano-Characterization Laboratory and Nanotechnology Characterization Laboratory. Enhancing and standardizing the criteria for approving safe products of nanomedicine is a crucial priority for regulatory authorities in the field of nanomedicine therapies (Rao et al., 2022). In addition to the aforementioned controls and reviews, more sophisticated and multipurpose instruments must be created to describe the complexity in order to enhance the nanomedicine approval procedure. Regulating nanomedicine is complex because it doesn't fit neatly into traditional drug approval systems. Since nanoparticles interact differently with the body compared to regular medicines, their safety isn't always predictable, raising concerns about toxicity and long-term effects. Another challenge is the lack of standardized testing, as different countries and agencies have their own guidelines, making global approval a slow and complicated process. Manufacturing is also tricky small variations in production can change how the nanomedicine works, making consistency difficult to maintain. Additionally, there's confusion about how to classify nanomedicines, as they sometimes blur the line between drugs, devices, and biological treatments. With limited long-term data, regulators must be extra cautious, balancing the need for innovation with ensuring public safety. Developing clear, universal guidelines is crucial for the future of nanomedicine.

10.4 CONCLUSION

Current concerns regarding the use of nanotechnology in the biomedical and pharmaceutical industries are presented in this article. To create an effective nanosystem that can safely transport therapeutic drug concentrations, properties of nanocarriers must be thoroughly investigated. Current developments in nanopharmaceutical design were highlighted. Bio nano-formulations, in particular, can offer appealing qualities. For instance, biomimetic and bio-inspired techniques such as covering NPs with synthetic or natural cell membranes camouflage that increases the appeal of nanopharmaceuticals in bioapplications can guarantee biocompatibility and stealth qualities. In personalized medicine, nanomedicine has enormous potential to transform medication administration and treatment. The creation of multifunctional nanoparticles, targeted drug carriers, and theranostic agents that can deliver drugs and perform diagnostic imaging at the same time are examples of future directions in nanomedicine. Utilizing the special qualities of nanoparticles, such as surface functionalization, drug release control and pharmacokinetics based on particle size, scientists can create patient-specific formulations that have lower systemic toxicity and increased therapeutic efficacy. Wearable technology, smartphone apps, and remote monitoring systems are just a few examples of the digital health innovations that have the potential to revolutionize customized medicine. These technologies facilitate early disease identification, treatment optimization, and patient involvement by enabling real-time data collection, individualized feedback, and ongoing monitoring of patient health parameters. Predictive analytics, personalized decision support tools, and artificial intelligence algorithms are some of the future directions in digital health that will enable patients and healthcare professionals to make well-informed treatment decisions. Regulations and policy frameworks will be essential as customized medicine develops to guarantee patient safety, effectiveness, and access to cutting-edge treatments. The creation of adaptive routes, accelerated review procedures, and value-based reimbursement models that are adapted to the particular customized treatments are some examples of future regulatory directions. To create clear rules, expedite regulatory routes, and promote innovation while protecting public health, regulatory authorities must work with industry partners, patient advocacy organizations, and healthcare stakeholders. Utilizing natural materials (raw) and valuing bio-wastes should be the focus of scientific research when selecting precursor materials for development of nano-drugs because they are inexpensive, abundant, and offer intriguing qualities. Because they are abundant in nature and utilized in the drug industry, plants are a useful source of biological chemicals that can be utilized to create nano-biopharmaceuticals. Additionally, plants serve as bio nanofactories for the environmentally friendly synthesis of nanoparticles with potential uses in the biomedical industry.

REFERENCES

Acharya, S., and Sahoo, S.K., 2011. PLGA nanoparticles containing various anticancer agents and tumour delivery by EPR effect. *Adv. Drug Deliv. Rev.* 63, 170–183.

Almeida, J.P.M., Chen, A.L., Foster, A., and Drezek, R.J.N., 2011. In vivo biodistribution of nanoparticles. *Int. J. Nanomed.* 6, 815–835.

Anwarul, H., Mahboob, M., Adnan, M., et al., 2018. Nanoparticles in tissue engineering: Applications, challenges and prospects. *Int. J. Nanomedicine.* 13, 5637–5655.

Ariga, K., and Fakhrullin, R., 2021. Nanoarchitectonics on living cells. *RSC Adv.* 11, 18898–18914.

Berrouiguet, S., Perez-Rodriguez, M.M., Larsen, M., Baca-García, E., Courtet, P., and Oquendo, M., 2018. From eHealth to iHealth: Transition to participatory and personalized medicine in mental health. *J. Med. Intern. Res.* 20(1), 1–9.

Blanco, E., Shen, H., and Ferrari, M., 2015. Principles of nanoparticle design for overcoming biological barriers to drug delivery. *Nat. Biotechnol.* 33, 941–951.

Bobo, D., Robinson, K.J., Islam, J., Thurecht, K.J., and Corrie, S.R., 2016. Nanoparticle-based medicines: A review of FDA-approved materials and clinical trials to date. *Pharm. Res.* 33, 2373–2387.

Chen, J., Liu, J., Yaping Hu, Y., Tian, Z., and Zhu, Y., 2019. Metal-organic framework-coated magnetite nanoparticles for synergistic magnetic hyperthermia and chemotherapy with pH-triggered drug release. *Sci. Technol. Adv. Mater.* 20, 1043–1054.

Cheng, R., Meng, F., Deng, C., Klok, H.A., and Zhong, Z., 2013. Dual and multi-stimuli responsive polymeric nanoparticles for programmed site-specific drug delivery. *Biomaterials.* 34, 3647–3657.

Chou, K.C., 2004. Structural bioinformatics and its impact on biomedical science. *Curr. Med. Chem.* 11, 2105–2134.

Couvreur, P., and Vauthier, C., 2006. Nanotechnology: Intelligent design to treat complex disease. *Pharm. Res.* 23, 1417–1450.

Das, D., Maity, N., and Anuradha, H.V., 2017. Nanotechnology: A revolution targeted drug delivery. *Int. J. Basic Clin. Pharmacol.* 6, 2766–2773.

De Carvalho, A.P.A., and Conte-Junior, C.A., 2021. Food-derived biopolymer kefiran composites, nanocomposites and nanofibers: Emerging alternatives to food packaging and potentials in nanomedicine. *Trends Food Sci. Technol.* 116, 370–386.

De Jong, W.H., and Born, P.J., 2008. Drug delivery and nanoparticles: Applications and hazards. *Int. J. Nanomed.* 3, 133–149.

Deng, S., Gigliobianco, M.R., Censi, R., and Di Martino, P., 2020. Polymeric nanocapsules as nanotechnological alternative for drug delivery system: Current status, challenges and opportunities. *Nanomaterials.* 10, 847.

Erenler, R., Gecer, E.N., Hosaflioglu, I., and Behcet, L., 2023. Green synthesis of silver nanoparticles using Stachys spectabilis: Identification, catalytic degradation, and antioxidant activity. *Biochem. Biophys. Res. Commun.* 659, 91–95.

Farokhzad, O.C., and Langer, R., 2009. Impact of nanotechnology on drug delivery. *ACS Nano.* 3, 16–20.

Ferrari, M., 2005. Cancer nanotechnology: Opportunities and challenges. *Nat. Rev. Cancer.* 5, 161–171.

Gao, W., Hu, C.M.J., Fang, R.H., Luk, B.T., Su, J., and Zhang, L., 2013. Surface functionalization of gold nanoparticles with red blood cell membranes. *Adv. Mater.* 25, 3549–3553.

Greene, C.S., Tan, J., Ung, M., Moore, J.H., and Cheng, C., 2014. Big data bioinformatics. *J. Cell. Physiol.* 229, 1896–1900.

Gu, Z., Meng, S., Wang, Y., Lyu, B., Li, P., and Shang, N., 2023. A novel bioactive postbiotics: From microbiota-derived extracellular nanoparticles to health promoting. *Crit. Rev. Food Sci. Nutr.* 63, 6885–6899.

Habib, S., and Singh, M., 2021. Recent advances in lipid-based nanosystems for gemcitabine and gemcitabine–combination therapy. *Nanomaterials.* 11, 597.

Hillaireau, H., and Couvreur, P., 2009. Nanocarriers' entry into the cell: Relevance to drug delivery. *Cell. Mol. Life Sci.* 66, 2873–2896.

Hu, J., Wu, X., Wu, F., et al., 2020. TiO_2 nanoparticle exposure on lettuce (*Lactuca Sativa L.*): Dose-dependent deterioration of nutritional quality. *Environ. Sci. Nano.* 7(2), 501–513.

Jain, K.K., 2005. Nanotechnology-based drug delivery for cancer. *Technol. Cancer Res. Treat.* 4, 407–416.

Jiang, X., Rocker, C., Hafner, M., Brandholt, S., Dorlich, R.M., and Nienhaus, G.U., 2010. Endo-and exocytosis of zwitterionic quantum dot nanoparticles by live HeLa cells. *ACS Nano.* 4, 6787–6797.

Jokerst, J.V., Gambhir, S.S., and Liu, A., 2011. Molecular imaging with theranostic nanoparticles. *Acc. Chem. Res.* 44, 1050–1060.

Langer, R., and Tirrell, D.A., 2004. Designing materials for biology and medicine. *Nature.* 428, 487–492.

Leach, D.G., Young, S., and Hartgerink, J.D., 2019. Advances in immunotherapy delivery from implantable and injectable biomaterials. *Acta Biomater.* 88, 15–31.

Li, J., Sun, M., Liu, L., et al., 2023. Nano probiotics for remodeling the pro-inflammatory microenvironment and microbiome in the treatment of colitis. *Nano Lett.* 23, 8593–8601.

Liu, D., Yang, F., Xiong, F., and Gu, N., 2017. The smart drug delivery system and its clinical potential. *Theranostics.* 7, 1306–1323.

Kashyap, B.K., Singh, V.V., Solanki, M.K., Kumar, A., Ruokolainen, J., Kesari, K.K., 2023. Smart nanomaterials in cancer theranostics: Challenges and opportunities. *ACS Omega.* 8, 14290–14320.

Kaushik, A., Jayant, R.D., Bhardwaj, V., and Nair, M., 2018. Personalized nanomedicine for CNS diseases. *Drug Discov. Today.* 23, 1007–1015.

Kaushik, A., Tiwari, S., Jayant, R.D., Marty, A., and Nair, M., 2016.Towardsdetection and diagnosis of Ebola virus disease at point-of-care. *Biosens. Bioelectron.* 75, 254–272.

Kim, K.Y., 2007. Nanotechnology platforms and physiological challenges for cancer therapeutics. *Int. J. Nanomed.* 3, 103–110.

Kontham, S., Mandava, K., Dosa, S., Mohd, F.U., Mohammed, O.A., and Mohammad, A.U., 2022. Review on facile synthesis of cerium oxide nanoparticles and their biomedical applications. *Inorg. Nano-Met. Chem.* 52, 1183–1195.

Kothamasu, P., Kanumur, H., Ravur, N., Maddu, C., Parasuramrajam, R., and Thangavel, S., 2012. Nanocapsules: The weapons for novel drug delivery systems. *Bioimpacts BI.* 2, 71–81.

Madhuri, K., 2023. A review on the functions, preparation and future aspects of nanocapsules. *Int. J. Sci. Res. Arch.* 8, 421–426.

Mora-Huertas, C.E., Fessi, H., and Elaissari, A., 2010. Polymer-based drug-delivery nanocapsules. *Int. J. Pharm.* 385, 113–142.

Nair, M., Jayant, R.D., Kaushik, A., and Sagar, V., 2016.Getting in to the brain: Potential of nanotechnology in the management of neuro AIDS. *Adv. Drug Deliv. Rev.* 103, 202–217.

Park, K., 2016. Facing the truth about nanotechnology in drug delivery. *ACS Nano.* 10, 8453–8456.

Peer, D., Karp, J.M., Hong, S., and Farokhzad, O.C., 2007. Nanocarriers as an emerging platform for cancer therapy. *Nat. Nanotechnol.* 2, 751–760.

Rao, C., Liao, D., Pan, Y., Zhong, Y., Zhang, W., Ouyang, Q., Alireza, N.E., and Liu, J., 2022. Novel formulations of metal-organic frameworks for controlled drug delivery. *Expert Opin. Drug Deliv.* 19, 1183–1202.

Riehemann, K., Schneider, S.W., Luger, T.A., Godin, B., Ferrari, M., and Fuchs, H., 2009. Nanomedicine – Challenge and perspectives. *Angew. Chem. Int. Ed.* 48, 872–897.

Ross, J.S., Schenkein, D.P., Pietrusko, R., et al., 2004. Targeted therapies for cancer. *Am. J. Clin. Pathol.* 122, 598–609.

Shi, J., Kantoff, P.W., Wooster, R., and Farokhzad, O.C., 2017. Cancer nanomedicine: Progress, challenges and opportunities. *Nat. Rev. Cancer.* 17, 20–37.

Subramanian, R., Ponnanikajamideen, M., Samuel Rajendran, R., Alshehri, M.A., Alasmari, A., Panneerselvam, C., and Periyasamy, S., 2024. TiO2 nanoparticles: Green synthesis, characterization, and investigation of antimicrobial properties, and developmental toxicity in zebrafish (Danio rerio) embryos. *Drug Chem. Toxicol.* 47, 90–100.

Sumer, B., and Gao, J., 2008. Theranostic nanomedicine for cancer. *Int. J. Nanomed.* 3, 137–140.

Tiwari, S., Sharma, V., Mujawar, M., Mishra, Y.K., Kaushik, A., and Ghosal, A., 2019. Biosensors for epilepsy management: State-of-art and future aspects. *Sensors.* 19, 1525.

Tomitaka, A., Arami, H., Raymond, A., et al., 2017. Development of magneto-plasmonic nanoparticles for multimodal image-guided therapy to the brain. *Nanoscale.* 9, 764–773.

Torchilin, V.P., 2014. Multifunctional, stimuli-sensitive nanoparticulate systems for drug delivery. *Nat. Rev. Drug Discov.* 13, 813–827.

Vashist, A., Kaushik, A., Vashist, A., et al., 2016. Recent trends on hydrogel based drug delivery systems for infectious diseases. *Biomater. Sci.* 4, 1535–1553.

Wolinsky, J.B., and Grinstaff, M.W., 2008. Therapeutic and diagnostic applications of dendrimers for cancer treatment. *Adv. Drug Deliv. Rev.* 60, 1037–1055.

Xie, W., Zhang, S., Pan, F., Chen, S., Zhong, L., Wang, J., and Pei, X., 2021. Nanomaterial-based ROS-mediated strategies for combating bacteria and biofilms. *J. Mater. Res.* 36, 822–845.

Xu, C., Ban, Q., Wang, W., Hou, J., and Jiang, Z., 2022. Novel nano-encapsulated probiotic agents: Encapsulate materials, delivery, and encapsulation systems. *J. Control. Release.* 349, 184–205.

Yang, H., Liao, D., Cai, Z., Zhang, Y., Nezamzadeh-Ejhieh, A., Zheng, M., Liu, J., Bai, Z., and Song, H., 2023. Current status of Fe-based MOFs in biomedical applications. *RSC Med. Chem.* 14, 2473–2495.

Yuehong, Y.I.N., Zeng, Y., Chen, X., and Fan, Y., 2016. The internet of things in healthcare: An overview. *J. Indus. Inform. Integr.* 1, 3–13.

Zafar, F., Jahan, N., Rahman, K.U., Asi, M.R., and Zafar, W.U.I., 2020. Nanosuspension enhances dissolution rate and oral bioavailability of *Terminalia arjuna* bark extract in vivo and in vitro. *Asian Pac. J. Trop. Biomed.* 10, 164–171.

Zhu, S., Zeng, M., Feng, G., and Wu, H., 2019. Platinum nano particles as a therapeutic agent against dextran sodium sulfate-induced colitis in mice. *Int. J. Nanomed.* 14, 8361–8378.

Index

Note: Page numbers in *italics* indicate a figure and page numbers in **bold** indicate a table on the corresponding page.

C

D

O

P

T

W

X

For Product Safety Concerns and Information please contact our
EU representative GPSR@taylorandfrancis.com Taylor & Francis
Verlag GmbH, Kaufingerstraße 24, 80331 München, Germany